Stanfield's
Essential Medical Terminology

FIFTH EDITION

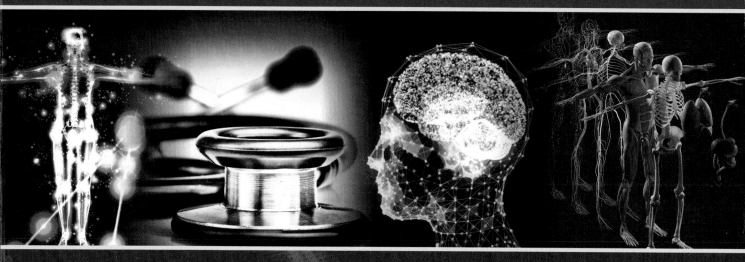

Nanna Cross, PhD
Chicago, Illinois

Dana McWay, JD, RHIA, FAHIMA
Saint Louis University
Saint Louis, Missouri

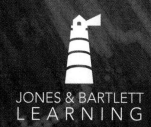

JONES & BARTLETT
LEARNING

World Headquarters
Jones & Bartlett Learning
5 Wall Street
Burlington, MA 01803
978-443-5000
info@jblearning.com
www.jblearning.com

Jones & Bartlett Learning books and products are available through most bookstores and online booksellers. To contact Jones & Bartlett Learning directly, call 800-832-0034, fax 978-443-8000, or visit our website, www.jblearning.com.

16026-0

Production Credits

VP, Product Management: David D. Cella
Director of Product Management: Cathy L. Esperti
Product Assistant: Allyson Larcom
Vendor Manager: Nora Menzi
Senior Production Editor, Navigate: Leah Corrigan
Director of Marketing: Andrea DeFronzo
Marketing Manager: Michael Sullivan
VP, Manufacturing and Inventory Control: Therese Connell
Composition and Project Management: Exela Technologies

Cover Design: Kristin E. Parker
Text Design: Kristin E. Parker
Rights & Media Specialist: Robert Boder
Media Development Editor: Troy Liston
Cover Image (Title Page, Part Opener, Chapter Opener): © teekid/iStock/Getty Images, © Anatomy Insider/Shutterstock, © Adrian Grosu/Shutterstock, © Hubis/Shutterstock, © Kamira/Shutterstock
Printing and Binding: LSC Communications
Cover Printing: LSC Communications

Library of Congress Cataloging-in-Publication Data

Names: Cross, Nanna, author. | McWay, Dana C., author. | Preceded by (work): Stanfield, Peggy. Essential medical terminology.
Title: Stanfield's essential medical terminology / Nanna Cross and Dana McWay.
Other titles: Essential medical terminology
Description: Burlington, MA : Jones & Bartlett Learning, [2020]. | Preceded by Essential medical terminology / Peggy Stanfield, Y.H. Hui, Nanna Cross. Fourth edition. 2013. | Includes bibliographical references and index.
Identifiers: LCCN 2018003928 | ISBN 9781284142211 (pbk. : alk. paper)
Subjects: | MESH: Terminology as Topic | Problems and Exercises
Classification: LCC R123 | NLM W 15 | DDC 610.1/4—dc23 LC record available at https://lccn.loc.gov/2018003928

6048

Printed in the United States of America
22 21 20 19 18   10 9 8 7 6 5 4 3 2 1

Dedication

The Fifth Edition of *Stanfield's Essential Medical Terminology* is dedicated to the authors of previous editions—Y. H. Hui and Peggy S. Stanfield—and to all students and practitioners in the health professions.

—Nanna Cross

To my husband Patrick, my sons Conor, William, and Ryan, and daughter-in-law Michelle, whose support and love I treasure, and to my granddaughter Catalina for the pleasure she provides to my life.

—Dana McWay

Brief Contents

Contents

Preface

The Fifth Edition of *Stanfield's Essential Medical Terminology* is a brief, user-friendly text designed to aid students in mastering the medical vocabulary and terms they will encounter in allied health, nursing, and medical careers. The terms have been selected on the basis of their utility, practical value, and application to the real world of the healthcare work environment.

The intended audience includes students in nursing, nursing assistants/aides, vocational/practical nurses, medical secretaries, medical technologists, medical librarians, medical assistants, physician's assistants, and other persons in the allied health and paramedical fields. This text is designed for use in one-semester or two-semester courses, as it provides students with the basic principles of medical terminology and teaches vocabulary by applying terms in practical examples.

It also offers a great deal of flexibility to instructors as well as students. Our recommendation is to progress through the table of contents as written. In any learning process, studying the information progressively provides sequence of thought and ensures that one does not overlook critical information.

The student, especially one studying independently of a formal class lecture, should read each chapter thoroughly and complete all exercises.

ORGANIZATION

Our intention was to create a text that would serve the needs of both instructors and students. We strove to create a text that is concise and thorough, thematically unified, easy to read, beautifully illustrated, and fully supplemented with supporting material to assure mastery of the material. We hope that both instructors and students will find *Stanfield's Essential Medical Terminology* a satisfactory and rewarding experience in teaching and learning medical terminology.

The text is organized into five units:

- Unit I: Word Parts and Medical Terminology (Chapters 1–2)
- Unit II: Root Words, Medical Terminology, and Patient Care (Chapters 3–6)
- Unit III: Abbreviations (Chapters 7–8)
- Unit IV: Review (Chapter 9)
- Unit V: Medical Terminology and Body Systems (Chapters 10–20)

Every chapter is organized into two components:

- Materials to Be Learned
- Progress Check

Basically, we provide didactic content in digestible pieces via Materials to Be Learned and then provide students the opportunity to stop and test their comprehension with Progress Check. This creates a building-block approach to learning the content.

We also continue to include full color illustrations of the human anatomy detailing the major body systems, special senses, and skin. These figures provide an anatomic reference for all the medical terms in the text as well as reinforce anatomy and physiology knowledge.

GENERAL GUIDELINES

So, we offer the following guidelines to both instructors and students:

1. Read the table of contents to determine the syllabus or match up the contents to a prepared syllabus.
2. After studying the basis of pronunciation, students may start with any of the remaining chapters in Units I–IV. Chapters 10–20 (Unit V), which discuss body systems, can be taught in any order.
3. For each chapter, the study procedure is simple. Read the Materials to Be Learned a few times and proceed with the Progress Check. Students may want to repeat or review chapter materials before taking a test.
4. Once a chapter is started, finish it before proceeding to the next one.
5. Complete each chapter from beginning to end. Do not begin randomly within a chapter.
6. When students begin Unit V, they will find that each chapter contains an overview of a body system. Each body system can be studied in more depth with an anatomy and physiology text.
7. We encourage students to develop their own methods of memorizing unfamiliar words. The interactive audio glossary is a helpful tool in learning the correct pronunciation. Word associations are useful. Flashcards are a useful adjunct to study. Studying in pairs also is helpful for most students.
8. Students should review completed materials as often as possible to refresh their memories.
9. Answers to all Progress Check exercises from all chapters are provided in Appendix A. Most instructors prefer that students do not look at the answers until they have completed the assigned exercise.

KEY BOX FEATURES

Clinical Notes: Designed to assist the student in applying chapter lessons to real-world examples by showing how medical terms and abbreviations are used in patient health records.

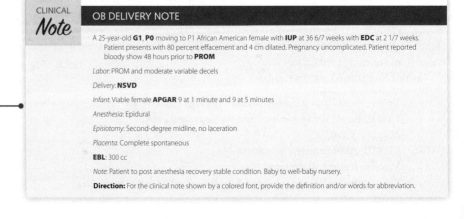

CLINICAL *Note*

OB DELIVERY NOTE

A 25-year-old **G1**, **P0** moving to P1 African American female with **IUP** at 36 6/7 weeks with **EDC** at 2 1/7 weeks. Patient presents with 80 percent effacement and 4 cm dilated. Pregnancy uncomplicated. Patient reported bloody show 48 hours prior to **PROM**

Labor: PROM and moderate variable decels

Delivery: **NSVD**

Infant: Viable female **APGAR** 9 at 1 minute and 9 at 5 minutes

Anesthesia: Epidural

Episiotomy: Second-degree midline, no laceration

Placenta: Complete spontaneous

EBL: 300 cc

Note: Patient to post anesthesia recovery stable condition. Baby to well-baby nursery.

Direction: For the clinical note shown by a colored font, provide the definition and/or words for abbreviation.

Confusing Medical Terminology: Identify and differentiate between confusing medical terms. Many medical terms derive from Latin and Greek, among other European languages. Sometimes, two terms with different medical meaning may differ only in one letter in their spellings. Sometimes, two terms with different medical meanings may sound alike, though their spellings are completely different. Sometimes, two terms with the same medical meanings may be spelled entirely differently. Obviously, it is not possible to explain or list all such variations in a book of this size. Samples are provided in a special box, starting in Chapter 1.

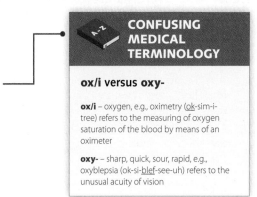

CONFUSING MEDICAL TERMINOLOGY

ox/i versus oxy-

ox/i – oxygen, e.g., oximetry (<u>ok</u>-sim-i-tree) refers to the measuring of oxygen saturation of the blood by means of an oximeter

oxy- – sharp, quick, sour, rapid, e.g., oxyblepsia (ok-si-<u>blef</u>-see-uh) refers to the unusual acuity of vision

Pharmacology and Medical Terminology: Address the connection between drugs and medical terms. Most of us are familiar with terms such as ulcer, chemotherapy, and antibiotic treatments. This text does not have a chapter on pharmacology and medical terms. Instead, we have provided boxes in Chapters 11–20, which relate medical terminology to drugs and their targeted medical treatments. Although they are examples, they provide you with some perspectives about prescription and over-the-counter drugs. The ultimate objective is for you to learn some medical terms in pharmacology.

PHARMACOLOGY AND MEDICAL TERMINOLOGY

Drug Classification	antiemetic (an-ti-e-<u>met</u>-ic)	antineoplastic (an-tih-nee-oh-<u>plass</u>-tik)	immunosuppressant (im-moo-noh-suh-<u>press</u>-ant)
Function	prevents nausea and vomiting associated with chemotherapy and radiation therapy	prevents the development, growth, or reproduction of cancerous cells	suppresses the body's natural immune response to an antigen, as in treatment for transplant patients
Word Parts	**anti** = against; **emesis** = vomiting; **tic** = pertaining to	**anti-** = against; **ne/o** = new; **plas/o** = formation; **-tic** = pertaining to	**immun/o** = immunity, **suppressant** = pertaining to lower, to control
Active Ingredients (examples)	chlorpromazine (Thorazine); dexamethasone (Baycadron)	fluorouracil (Adrucil); methotrexate (Rheumatrex Dose Pack)	cyclosporine (Sandimmune); azathioprine (Imuran)

Allied Health Professions: Explain types of professions available in the allied health field.

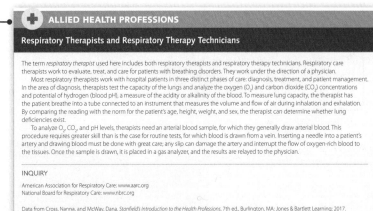

ALLIED HEALTH PROFESSIONS

Respiratory Therapists and Respiratory Therapy Technicians

The term *respiratory therapist* used here includes both respiratory therapists and respiratory therapy technicians. Respiratory care therapists work to evaluate, treat, and care for patients with breathing disorders. They work under the direction of a physician.

Most respiratory therapists work with hospital patients in three distinct phases of care: diagnosis, treatment, and patient management. In the area of diagnosis, therapists test the capacity of the lungs and analyze the oxygen (O_2) and carbon dioxide (CO_2) concentrations and potential of hydrogen (blood pH), a measure of the acidity or alkalinity of the blood. To measure lung capacity, the therapist has the patient breathe into a tube connected to an instrument that measures the volume and flow of air during inhalation and exhalation. By comparing the reading with the norm for the patient's age, height, weight, and sex, the therapist can determine whether lung deficiencies exist.

To analyze O_2, CO_2, and pH levels, therapists need an arterial blood sample, for which they generally draw arterial blood. This procedure requires greater skill than is the case for routine tests, for which blood is drawn from a vein. Inserting a needle into a patient's artery and drawing blood must be done with great care; any slip can damage the artery and interrupt the flow of oxygen-rich blood to the tissues. Once the sample is drawn, it is placed in a gas analyzer, and the results are relayed to the physician.

INQUIRY

American Association for Respiratory Care: www.aarc.org
National Board for Respiratory Care: www.nbrc.org

Data from Cross, Nanna, and McWay, Dana. *Stanfield's Introduction to the Health Professions*, 7th ed., Burlington, MA: Jones & Bartlett Learning; 2017.

NEW! Box features describing medical conditions or treatments in infants, children, or teens to illustrate examples across the life span.

> **Box 18-1 What are Cochlear Implants and when are they Used?**
>
> Imagine hearing sound for the first time! Activation of a cochlear implant after surgical placement is a joyful occasion for the patient, family, and the entire healthcare team.
>
> A cochlear implant is an electronic device that restores partial hearing to those with severe to profound hearing loss. Unlike a hearing aid, the implant does not make sound louder or clearer. Instead, the device bypasses damaged parts of the auditory system and directly stimulates the nerve of hearing, allowing those who are profoundly deaf to receive sound. An implant does not restore normal hearing. Instead, it can give a deaf person a representation of sounds in the environment and the means to understand speech.
>
> Most often, surgery can successfully treat problems with the outer and middle ear, including the eardrum. However, when there is nerve deafness from damaged hair cells, hearing aids are not beneficial and a cochlear implant is appropriate. Candidates for a cochlear implant are children or adults with profound deafness because of damage to the inner ear. For children who were deaf at birth, the goal is to place the cochlear implant by 18 months of age to allow for the development of language skills comparable to the child's peers. An artificial cochlear placed in a child or adult who became deaf after a hearing loss will require less speech therapy after a cochlear implant than a child who has been deaf from birth. An entire team of health professionals—the physician, audiologist, nurse, social worker and speech and language pathologist—supports the patient and family after cochlear implant surgery.
>
> *Source:* National Institutes of Deafness and Other Communication Disorders. National Institutes of Health. *Cochlear Implants.* https://www.nidcd.nih.gov/health/cochlear-implants

Full Color Illustrations and Photographs for Clinical Disorders: There is an old adage "A picture is worth a thousand words." We believe it is true, so we have included in this edition new full color illustrations and photographs showing common clinical disorders and their assorted medical terms to enhance your understanding and identification of diseases and how they may be treated.

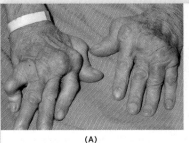 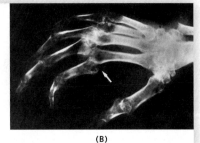

(A)   (B)

FIGURE 17-13 (A) Advanced joint deformities caused by rheumatoid arthritis. **(B)** Radiograph illustrating destruction of articular surfaces and anterior dislocation of the base of index finger as a result of joint instability.

Courtesy of Leonard V. Crowley, MD, Century College.

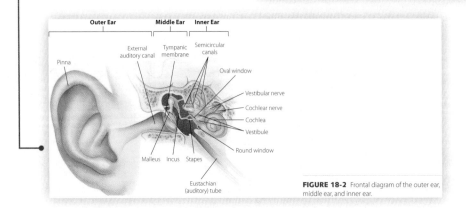

FIGURE 18-2 Frontal diagram of the outer ear, middle ear, and inner ear.

What Is New and Improved in the Fifth Edition?

As we move forward in the advancing fields of medicine and health practices, we find an increasing need to make changes and add new material. We received many valuable suggestions and comments from reviewers and have included constructive input where appropriate. We hope that the resulting changes will continue to improve the contents of *Stanfield's Essential Medical Terminology, Fifth Edition,* and facilitate learning medical terminology.

NEW! Clinical Notes added! These notes support understanding of what health records look like and what content is contained within them. Clinical Notes can be found in each chapter, immediately before the Progress Check section.

REVISED! Addresses Roles of Medical and Health Professions! Explanations of the roles of various medical and health professions are provided throughout the text. A listing of Allied Health Professionals can be found in Chapter 1, with further explanation of the definitions and pronunciations of these professions in Chapter 6. A separate enclosure highlighting an Allied Health Profession is featured at the beginning of Chapters 10–20. This highlighted feature describes in detail the work performed by the Allied Health Professional selected as the focus of the chapter. These explanations support the concept of core competencies for interprofessional education as identified by the Interprofessional Educational Collaborative (IPEC) in its 2016 Update to Core Competencies for Interprofessional Collaborative Practice.[1]

REVISED! Attention to Latin and Greek Origins! Attention is given to the Latin and Greek backgrounds of the medical terms students are to learn. Chapter 1 provides an explanation why so many terms derive from the Latin and Greek languages. Chapters 11–20 include tables that explain the Latin or Greek origin of medical terms used in diagnosing and treating diseases or disorders of a specific medical system.

REVISED! Chapter 1 is substantially revised to address the reasons to learn medical terminology, why correct pronunciation of medical terms is important, and the need to understand eponyms, homonyms, and synonyms.

---

[1] Interprofessional Education Collaborative (2016). Core competencies for interprofessional collaborative practice: 2016 Update. Washington DC: Interprofessional Educational Collaborative.

The Learning and Teaching Package

We have compiled a strong package to support both the instructor and the student.

THE TEACHING PACKAGE FOR THE INSTRUCTOR

Instructor's Manual: The instructor's manual provides a spectrum of information—clinical case histories, practice tests, and student activities. It serves two important purposes—providing a wide selection of teaching materials and a reduction in class preparation time. For example, by using clinical case histories to supplement a complex topic in the classroom, the instructor can usually elicit enthusiastic participation and enliven classroom presentations.

Video Links: This document provides informative and instructive YouTube video links either to be shown in the classroom, or for students to view as self-study to drive home key concepts or interesting information.

Answer Keys for Case Studies and Clinical Notes.

Slides in PowerPoint™ format for each chapter.

Test Bank for each chapter.

THE LEARNING PACKAGE FOR THE STUDENT

Case Studies: A set of 19 interactive, printable PDFs in which to apply the concepts learned in the book to real-world scenarios.

Interactive eBook for access anytime anywhere.

Progress Checks: Printable and interactive PDFs to help drive home the core concepts and information found in each chapter.

Printable Study Sheets: Use these printable study sheets to enhance retention.

Audio Glossary: Search for key words and terms and hear their correct pronunciations.

Flash Cards: Use these helpful flashcards to review key terms.

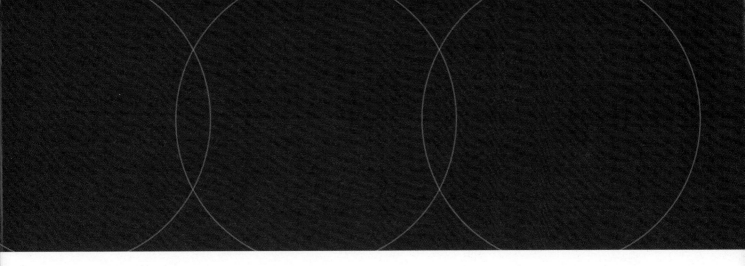

Acknowledgments

We acknowledge the invaluable assistance and advice provided by the staff and Health Science team at Jones & Bartlett Learning, who have helped move this edition from manuscript to publication: Cathy Esperti, Allyson Larcom, Nora Menzi, Robert Boder, Troy Liston, Andrea DeFronzo, Rachael Souza, and Therese Connell. Thanks also to the production staff whose dedicated work and professionalism are evident in the quality of their work. You are the best judge.

We also extend our appreciation to the many students and their instructors for their continued use of *Stanfield's Essentials of Medical Terminology* through its first four editions. We have tried to provide you with the updates and new information that you have asked for. We hope our mutual relationships continue with this Fifth Edition and beyond.

In addition, we would like to extend a special thank you to our Ancillary Author Amy Veit, RHIA. She is an Instructor for Health Information Management at the Center for Nursing and Allied Health Sciences, Saint Charles Community College, in Dardenne Prairie, Missouri.

Reviewers

We sincerely thank our reviewers who offered many valuable suggestions. Your comments were very helpful, and we incorporated as many of them into this edition as allocated page space would permit.

Colleen L. Croxall, PhD
Director, School of Health Sciences, Eastern Michigan University

James W. Ledrick, BS, MD
Adjunct Professor, Grand Valley State University

Mirella G. Pardee, MSN, MA, RN
Associate Professor, University of Toledo

Linda Treitler, RN, MSN
Assistant Professor, Midwestern State University

J. Ryan Walther, MHA, RT(R), ARRT
El Centro College School of Allied Health and Nursing

Linda Wenn, BA
Business Technology Instructor, Central Community College

David J. White, PhD, MA
Senior Lecturer, Baylor University

About the Authors

NANNA CROSS

Nanna Cross, PhD, has worked as a faculty member in dietetic and physician education programs teaching clinical nutrition courses and supervising dietetic interns in clinical practicums, and has also taught courses online. Dr. Cross worked as a clinical dietitian at the University of Missouri Hospitals and Clinics and as a consulting dietitian for Home Care, Hospice, Head Start, and Long-Term Care facilities. She is the coauthor of *Stanfield's Introduction to Health Professions* and a contributing author for several food science texts.

DANA McWAY

Dana McWay, JD, RHIA, FAHIMA, is both a lawyer and a health information management professional. She works as an adjunct faculty member at Saint Louis University in programs focusing on health informatics and information management, pre-law studies, and alternative dispute resolution. She is licensed to practice law in Missouri and Illinois. She is a Fellow of the American Health Information Management Association and an award-winning author. She serves as a voting member of the Institutional Review Board at Washington University School of Medicine, from 1992 to present. She has written and published extensively on matters related to the intersection of law, ethics, and health informatics. She is the co-author of *Stanfield's Introduction to Health Professions*.

UNIT 1

Medical Terminology

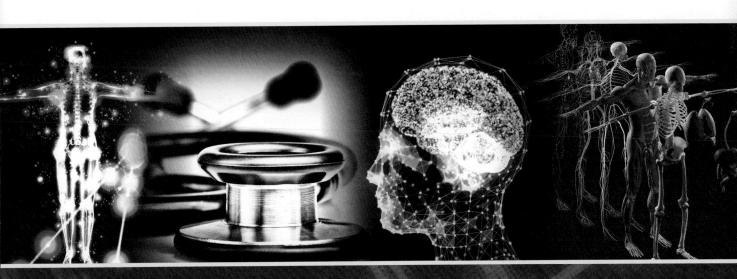

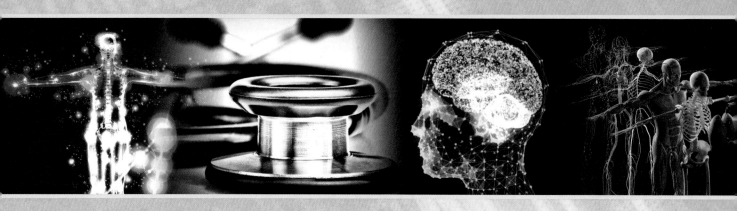

CHAPTER 1

Word Pronunciations

OBJECTIVES

After completing this chapter and the exercises, the student should be able to:

1. Identify how learning medical terminology is valuable to healthcare professionals.
2. Recall the reasons why many medical terminologies derive from the Latin and Greek languages.
3. Summarize the value of learning correct pronunciation of medical terms.
4. Provide examples of specific rules for pronunciation of medical terms.

LESSON ONE	Materials to Be Learned

PART 1: INTRODUCTION

A time once existed when the doctor, nurse, and an aide or two was all that were involved in caring for a patient. Not much interaction occurred beyond this grouping unless the physician called for a conference with selected individuals. Healthcare facilities today are run by teams of medical personnel, including doctors, nurses, aides, pharmacists, laboratory personnel, health information managers, technicians, dietary personnel, and social service workers. All have important roles to play in patient care and recovery. For the team approach to function properly, these teams need to speak a common language: medical terminology.

Medical terminology is the language of the healthcare industry, including those involved in the delivery of direct patient care and those who support the healthcare industry but do not provide direct patient care. Becoming fluent in this language serves as the basic foundation for practicing any health care-related career. Medical terminology offers those who learn it a standard of correctness or acceptability of words used across the full range of healthcare professions.

This concept of a standard approach makes possible a shared understanding of the same words. This shared understanding offers other benefits as well, including:

1. Improved communication between and among healthcare professionals.
2. Improved interaction between humans and the technology used in health care such as electronic health records.
3. Ease in performing clinical proceedings.
4. Improved efficiency in the delivery of clinical care.
5. Faster and more accurate documentation of healthcare conditions and treatments.
6. Improved comprehension of reports and medical literature.
7. A uniform language that can be used across countries to describe the same idea, condition, or instrument.
8. Increased trust among healthcare professionals due to the use of fundamental medical terms with a shared understanding.

While medical terminology has been influenced by many languages, the majority of terms used are derived from Greek and Latin. Examples of medical terms and the languages from which they derive are seen in **Table 1-1**. Most of the terms commonly used to describe the clinical observation and treatment of patients derive from Greek, while those terms used to describe anatomy derive most often from Latin. The reasons for these derivations are historical. Ancient Greece produced medical scientists whose names are not only known today (Hippocrates and Galen), but also whose theories formulated much of the knowledge of medicine until the middle of the 18th century. When Greek influence declined across the ancient world, many Greeks migrated to Rome where the Latin language predominated. As part of this migration, they brought with them the language they used to describe medicine. For most of the following centuries, many medical textbooks were written in Latin but included Greek words that described medical terms. One such textbook, authored by Andreas Vesalius in 1543, described human anatomy and was used for centuries until the middle of the 18th century. Combined together, these influences informed past individuals of their knowledge of medical science. As new ideas, conditions, or instruments were developed, those individuals built upon these terms to form many of the compound words that we know in medical terminology today.

TABLE **1-1** Examples of Medical Terms and Their Language of Origin	
Language of Origin	**Medical Terms**
French	Massage Passage Plaque Pipette
Greek	Cardiology Gastritis Nephropathia
Italian	Belladonna Influenza Varicella
Latin	Cor Ren Ventriculus

Because of the way medical terminology developed over time, some terms have more than one word root. For example, one word root for the term kidney is *nephr* from the Greek language, while a second word root for kidney is *ren* from the Latin language. Similarly, the term ped sometimes means child as in pediatrician, while other times it means foot as in pedestrian. This is because the term *pediatr* refers to child and arose from Greek sources, while the term *pedestri* means foot in Latin. More information about word roots can be found in Chapter 2, Word Parts and Word Building Rules.

Sometimes, medical terms can be confusing. For example, two terms with different medical meaning may differ only in one letter of their spellings. Sometimes, two terms with different medical meanings may sound alike even though their spellings are completely different. Sometimes, two terms with the <u>same</u> medical meaning may be spelled entirely differently. While it is not possible to explain or list all such variations in a textbook of this size, some examples are provided in all the chapters in special boxes.

This confusion is often the result of using eponyms, homonyms, and synonyms. *Eponyms* are proper names given to a body part, disease, instrument, procedure, or technique based on the name of the person who discovered or perfected it. Some healthcare professionals find it easier to say the eponym rather than say the body part, disease, instrument, procedure, or technique. The problem with eponyms is that the word or phrase by itself does not clearly describe or otherwise provide useful information about the body part, disease, instrument, procedure, or technique that is the subject of discussion. The current trend is to move away from eponyms to terms that more fully describe what is being discussed. Until such time eponyms are eliminated, it will remain important for healthcare professionals to know about them. Some examples are included in **Table 1-2**.

Homonyms are words with the same or nearly the same sound but different meanings. As mentioned earlier, homonyms pose the danger of creating misunderstandings, causing potential risks in delivering patient care. Some examples are included in **Table 1-3**.

Synonyms are words that have the same or nearly the same meaning as another word but are spelled differently. They are considered alternate words with the same meaning. Some examples are included in **Table 1-4**.

The best way to learn medical terminology is to become familiar with the structure and the most commonly used components. This science-based vocabulary follows a

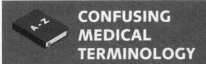

CONFUSING MEDICAL TERMINOLOGY

ileum versus ilium

ileum – last portion of small intestine, from jejunum to cecum, e.g., a part of the small intestine is the ileum (il-e-um)

ilium – one of the bones of each half of the pelvis, e.g., the ilium (il-i-um) is part of the pelvic arch

TABLE **1-2** Medical Eponyms

Eponyms	Meaning
Adam's apple	laryngeal prominence in the neck
Bell's palsy	form of facial paralysis
Down's syndrome	a genetic birth defect causing mental retardation, a characteristic facial appearance, and multiple malformations
Grave's disease	goiter of the thyroid
Hansen's disease	leprosy
Heimlich maneuver	abdominal thrust to clear an airway obstructed by a foreign object
Parkinson's disease	degenerative disorder of the motor system
Tommy John surgery	reconstruction of the ulnar collateral ligament

TABLE **1-3** Medical Homonyms

Homonym with Meaning	Homonym with Meaning
Anuresis – lack of urine; inability to urinate	Enuresis – bed-wetting
Aural – pertaining to hearing	Oral – pertaining to the mouth
Ensure – to make certain of	Insure – to provide protection, often in a monetary sense
Galactorrhea – abnormal flow of breast milk	Galacturia – milk-like appearance to the urine
Malleolus – rounded lateral projections of bone at the ankle	Malleus – outermost of the three small bones of the ear
Osteal – pertaining to a bone	Ostial – pertaining to an opening
Pancreas – a body part	Pancrease – a naturally occurring enzyme
Prostate – a body gland	Prostrate – laying prone

TABLE **1-4** Medical Synonyms

Synonyms	Meaning
Hypodermic, subcutaneous	under the skin
Morto, necro, thanto	death
Myocardial infarction, cardiac infarction, coronary thrombosis	heart attack
Thoracentesis, thoracocentesis, pleurocentesis	surgical puncture and drainage of the thoracic cavity

systematic methodology, with each term containing two or three components that can be broken down into parts. This systematic methodology forms the basis for the remaining chapters of this textbook and is used in the everyday world of healthcare professionals, including the ones listed at the end of this chapter.

PART 2: PRONUNCIATION

Among the most essential points in learning medical terminology is to determine the correct pronunciation of a given word. Knowing how to articulate the sound of the word, what syllable to stress, and the melody or pitch to use makes pronunciation not only easier for those who say the words but also for those with whom the speaker interacts. Misspelled or mispronounced words may signal a wrong meaning to the listener, making it extremely important that rules for spelling and pronunciation are followed. Correctly pronouncing medical terms supports the common understanding among healthcare professionals, described earlier in this chapter.

The pronunciation of each medical term is governed by specific rules. Pronunciation is indicated by a simple phonetic respelling of the term and the use of *diacritical markings*, which are marks added to a letter that help signal how the letter should be pronounced. The following rules illustrate the simple phonetic respelling and the dia-critical markings of terms:

1. The primary accent is indicated by an underlining, e.g., cerebellum (ser-e-<u>bel</u>-um).
2. The secondary accent is indicated by (´), e.g., ser´-<u>e</u>-bel-um.
3. When an unmarked vowel ends a syllable, it is long, e.g., immune (i-mun´).
4. When a syllable ends with a consonant, its unmarked vowel is short, e.g., cranial (<u>kra</u>-ne-al).

For ease of interpretation, the phonetic spellings used in this text have no other diacritical markings. However, the following basic rules apply to all pronunciation and are listed here for ease of interpretation of medical terms.

An unmarked vowel ending a syllable is *long*: It is indicated by a macron (¯):

a urease (<u>u</u>-re-ās); abate (ah-bāt)
e electroscope (e-lek-tro-scōp); lead (lēd)
i askaracide (as-<u>kar</u>-i-sīd); bile (bīl)
o ohms (ōmz); ionophere (i-on-o-phēr); hormone (hor-mōn)
u union (ūn-ion); ampule (am-pūl)
oo oophoron (oo-fōr-on)

A short vowel that *is* the syllable or that *ends* the syllable is indicated by a breve (˘):

a apophysis (ă-<u>pof</u>-i-sis)
e edema (ĕ-<u>dēm</u>-ah); effusion (ĕ-<u>fūs</u>-ion)
i immunity (ĭ-<u>mūn</u>-ĭ-te´); oxidation (oks´-sĭ-<u>da</u>-shun)
o otic (ŏ-tic); official (ŏ-<u>fish</u>-al)
u avoirdupois (av-er-dŭ-poiz)
oo book (book)

➕ ALLIED HEALTH PROFESSIONS

- *Communication impairment professionals*:   Speech-language pathologists, audiologists
- *Dentistry*:   Dentists, dental hygienists, dental assistants, dental laboratory technicians
- *Dietetics*:   Dietitians, nutritionists, dietetic technicians, dietetic assistants
- *Emergency medical services*:   Emergency medical technicians and paramedics
- *Health Information Personnel*:   Health information administrators, health information technicians, medical transcriptionists, medical librarians
- *Imaging modalities*:   Radiologic technologists and technicians, radiation therapists
- *Managers and counselors*:   Health services managers, genetic counselors
- *Medicine*:   Cardiovascular technologists and technicians, nuclear medicine technologists, surgical technologists, medical assistants
- *Mental health professionals*:   Psychologists, substance abuse and behavioral disorder counselors
- *Nursing*:   Registered nurses, advanced practice registered nurses, licensed practical nurses, licensed vocational nurses
- *Occupational therapy*:   Occupational therapists, occupational therapy assistants and aides
- *Optometry*:   Dispensing opticians, ophthalmic laboratory technicians
- *Pharmacy*:   Pharmacists, pharmacy technicians, pharmacy aides
- *Physical therapy*:   Physical therapists, physical therapist assistants and aides
- *Respiratory care practitioners*:   Respiratory therapists, respiratory therapy technicians
- *Veterinary medicine*:   Veterinary technologists and technicians, animal care and service workers
- *Miscellaneous technologists and technicians*:   Clinical laboratory (medical) technologists and technicians; medical, dental, and ophthalmic laboratory technicians; nursing, ophthalmic, personal care, psychiatric, and home health aides, medical assistants

Data from Cross N, McWay D. *Standfield's Introduction to the Health Professions*, 7th ed. Burlington, MA: Jones & Bartlett; 2017.

CLINICAL *Note* | Introduction: Physician Progress Note

S: Forty-seven-year-old Caucasian female with complaint of numbness on the right side of face. No other right-sided weakness. Symptoms began 48 hours previous to this visit for assessment. Patient has no other complaints at this time

O: Upon physical examination; **HEENT**: negative except for slight facial droop on the right side; NEURO: **WNL** other than facial droop; NECK: supple without masses or **adenopathy**; CHEST: negative; CARDIO: negative; BP: 100/70; ABDOMINAL: negative; PELVIC: deferred

A: Probable **Bell's Palsy R/O TIA/CVA**

P: **CT** with contrast to rule out TIA/CVA

Direction: For the portions of the clinical note shown by a colored font, provide the definition and/or words for abbreviation.

LESSON TWO	Progress Check

FILL IN

Fill in the blanks to make a complete, accurate sentence:

1. Most medical terms are derived from the _____ and _____ languages.

2. A _____ refers to two or more words that have the same or nearly the same meaning as another word but are spelled differently.

3. A _____ refers to words with the same or nearly the same sound but different meanings.

4. A _____ refers to proper names given to a body part, disease, instrument, procedure, or technique based on the name of the person who discovered or perfected it.

5. A _____ signals how a word should be pronounced.

6. Knowing what _____ to stress aids in pronouncing words correctly.

TRUE OR FALSE

Check T for statements that are true and F for statements that are false.

T ❑ F ❑ 1. Medical terminology serves as a common basis among healthcare careers.

T ❑ F ❑ 2. Healthcare professionals work independently and not as part of a team.

T ❑ F ❑ 3. One cannot learn medical terminology by breaking a word into component parts.

T ❑ F ❑ 4. Learning the correct pronunciation of a word is not critical to the study of medical terminology.

T ❑ F ❑ 5. Correctly pronouncing medical terms supports a common understanding among healthcare professionals.

CHAPTER 2

Word Parts and Word Building Rules

OBJECTIVES

After completing this chapter and the exercises, the student should be able to:

1. List the basic parts of a medical term.
2. Define the terms *word root, combining vowel, combining form, prefix,* and *suffix*.
3. State the rules for building medical terms.
4. Divide medical words into their component parts.
5. Build medical words using combining forms, prefixes, and suffixes.
6. Use multiple word roots in a compound word.

LESSON ONE	Materials to Be Learned

PARTS OF A MEDICAL TERM

Words have power. The words we speak and the words we write provide the opportunity to do much good in the world. If we do not understand these words fully, we risk creating misinterpretations or even causing harm to a patient. For these reasons, it is important to learn how medical terms are comprised. Doing so allows one to learn how these terms are used in science and patient care. An illustration of the many terms used in health care is seen in **Figure 2-1**.

Often, medical terms will describe an underlying disease or disorder. A *disease* involves an external influence such as a bacterium, virus, or mutation that overpowers the body's defenses. A *disorder* is a disruption within a body system. While sometimes used interchangeably, there is a difference between the two terms. Other times, medical terms will describe a sign or a symptom. A *sign* is an objective indication of an illness, for example,

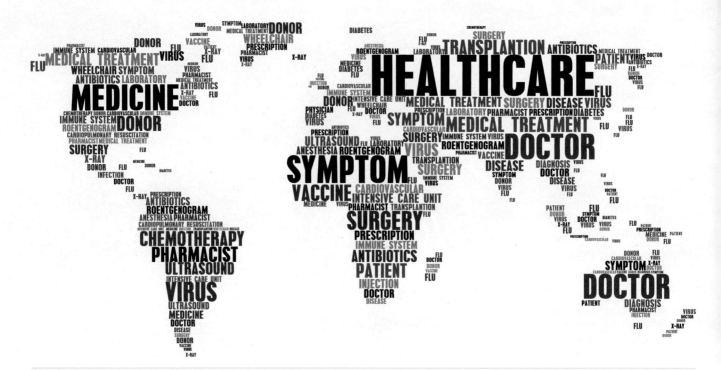

FIGURE 2-1 Sample of words used in health care.
Vector Tradition/Shutterstock

something that can be observed or detected by a patient or medical professional. By contrast, a *symptom* is a subjective indication of an illness, for example, something a patient may feel.

Words, including medical terms, are composed of three basic parts: word roots, prefixes, and suffixes. How the parts are combined determine their meaning. Changing any part of a word changes its meaning. Spelling and pronunciation also are very important because some medical terms sound similar and some sound exactly alike but are spelled differently, and therefore have different meanings. For example, *phagia* (fay-jee-ah) means eating or swallowing and *phasia* (fay-zee-ah) means with speech.

Examples of words that are pronounced exactly alike but spelled differently are the terms *ileum* (ill-ee-um) and *ilium* (ill-ee-um). Ileum is part of the small intestine and ilium is part of the hipbone.

1. **Prefix**: The word or element attached to the *beginning* of a word root to modify its meaning. Not all medical words have a prefix. A prefix keeps its same meaning in every term in which it is used. *When defining a medical term that has both a prefix and a suffix, define the suffix first, the prefix next, and the word root last.*

    Note in the following example how the meaning of the word changes: **peri–** = prefix for around, **cardi** = root word for heart, and **–itis** = suffix for inflammation.

    Term: <u>pericarditis</u>
    Definition: <u>inflammation around the heart (muscle)</u>

2. **Word root**: The *meaning* or *core* part of the word. Medical terms have one or more roots. By adding prefixes and suffixes to a word root, the meaning of a word is changed. Most medical words have at least one word root and some have several. Word roots are joined by a combining vowel. A word root will have the

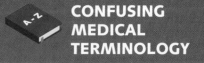

CONFUSING MEDICAL TERMINOLOGY

aphasia versus **apraxia**

aphasia – a language disorder characterized by either an inability to talk but able to understand or an inability to understand but with the ability to talk

apraxia – inability to perform a skilled and learned motor activity, despite no impairment in motor or sensory functions and coordination

same meaning in every word that contains it. When a word root is joined to a suffix or to other root words to make a compound word, it requires the use of a combining vowel.

3. *Combining vowel*: Usually an "o" and occasionally an "i" used between compound word roots or between a word root and a suffix. Combining vowels make word pronunciation easier. When a vowel is added to a root word, it is called a *combining form*. It is usually marked with a diagonal, e.g., **arthr/o**. Combining vowels are kept between compound words even if the second word root does begin with a vowel, e.g., **gastr/oentero/logy**. Compound words are two or more root words joined with a combining vowel. Compound words also may have a suffix, which is joined to the word by a combining vowel. When the suffix begins with a vowel (usually an "i"), the combining vowel on the root word is dropped. When the suffix begins with a consonant, the combining vowel is kept. Examples are:

- **mening/o** = root word and combining vowel and **-itis** = suffix. The word is spelled *meningitis*, dropping the "o." The term means inflammation of the meninges.
- **hem/o** = root word and combining vowel and **-rrhage** = suffix. The word is spelled *hemorrhage*, keeping the "o." The term means escape of blood from the vessels. If the suffix and the combining vowel are the same vowel, the duplicate vowel is also dropped, e.g., **cardi/o** = root word for heart and **-itis** = suffix. The word is spelled *carditis* (only one "i" is used). It means inflammation of the heart (muscle).

4. *Suffix*: The word part or element attached to the end of a root word to modify its meaning. Not all root words have a suffix and some words have two suffixes, e.g., **psych/o/log/ic/al**. When a medical term has two suffixes (as *psychological* does), they are joined and considered as one suffix, that is, **-ic/al** = **-ical**. Some suffixes are attached to a prefix only, e.g., **dia-** = prefix and **-rrhea** = suffix or *diarrhea*. When they form a complete word, as in this example (*diarrhea*), the resulting word may be considered a root word, depending on its use.

The literal meaning of a word may be shortened through usage, by common consent, or when understood without being expressed. Please note the following two premises when studying:

1. Many columns carry the heading "word root." This is taken to mean that items under this column can be the word root itself or a word root with /o, that is, a combining form. This practice is to avoid excess repetition of the term "combining form" throughout the book.

2. About 3–5% of the medical terms in this book, which have not been presented in the lessons, are included in the practice exercises. This is designed to:
- Encourage students to use the dictionary because the practice exercises are all open book.
- Provide students an opportunity to practice dividing those words into their respective components according to the rules in the book.
- Give the instructor a choice whether to include these additional words.
- Some textbooks on medical terminology use the same technique; others do not. Feedback from students and instructors will be noted. Word parts combine in various ways, as can be seen in **Table 2-1**.

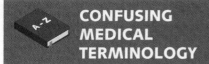

CONFUSING MEDICAL TERMINOLOGY

-stasis versus -stalsis

-stasis – control, stop, e.g., hemostasis (he-mo-<u>sta</u>-sis) refers to the interruption of blood flow or arrest of bleeding by the physiological properties of vasoconstriction and coagulation or by surgical means

-stalsis – contraction, e.g., peristalsis (per-uh-<u>stawl</u>-sis) refers to successive waves of involuntary contraction passing along the walls of a hollow muscular structure (as the esophagus or intestine) and forcing the contents onward

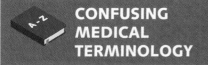

CONFUSING MEDICAL TERMINOLOGY

ante- versus anti-

ante- – before, forward, e.g., antepartum (an-te-<u>par</u>-tum) refers to occurring before childbirth

anti- – against, counter, e.g., anticoagulant (an-te-ko-<u>ag</u>-u-lant) is an agent that slows down the clotting process

TABLE 2-1 Parts of a Medical Term

Word Parts	Examples	Medical Terms
prefix + word root	**anti-** (prefix meaning against) + **thyroid** (root word for thyroid gland)	*antithyroid* • literal definition: against the thyroid • actual usage: (agent) suppressing thyroid activity
word root + suffix	**gastr** (word root for stomach) + **-ic** (suffix meaning pertaining to)	*gastric* • definition: pertaining to the stomach
combining form (word root + combining vowel) + suffix	**cardi** (root word for heart) + **/o** (a combining vowel) + **-logy** (suffix meaning study of)	*cardiology* • definition: study of the heart
prefix + suffix	**an-** (prefix meaning no, without) + **-emia** (suffix meaning blood)	*anemia* • literal definition: without (or no) blood • actual usage: decreased number of red blood cells or decreased hemoglobin in the cells
prefix + root word + suffix	**epi-** (prefix meaning above, over) + **gastr** (root word for stomach) + **-algia** (suffix meaning pain)	*epigastralgia* • literal definition: pain above the stomach • actual usage: pain in the upper region of the abdomen
compound word* + suffix	**ot/o** (root word for ear) + **rhin/o** (root word for nose) + **laryng/o** (root word for throat or larynx) + **-logy** (suffix meaning study of)	*otorhinolaryngology* • definition: the branch of medicine dealing with diseases of the ear, nose, and throat

* Two or more root words connected with a combining vowel.

LISTING OF WORD PARTS

You may or may not know most of the words presented in the table. Do not be concerned if you do not. There will be plenty of opportunities to learn more about them. In the next section, you are provided with listings of word parts. Eventually, you will have to be familiar with all of them. Here are some steps that will help you to learn:

1. Go through the lists of word parts once or twice.
2. Check your knowledge by covering all but the first column and see if you can provide meanings for some of the words.

PREFIXES, WORD ROOTS WITH COMBINING FORMS, AND SUFFIXES

Many of the prefixes, combining forms, word roots, and suffixes are indicated in the four tables appearing in this section (**Tables 2-2** through **2-5**).

TABLE 2-2 Prefixes Commonly Used in Medicine

Prefix	Definition	Word Example	Pronunciation	Definition
a-, an-	no, not, without, lack of, apart	**an**oxia	an-okʹ-se-ah	lack of sufficient oxygen in the blood
ad-	toward, near, to	**ad**hesion	ad-heʹ-zhun	union of two surfaces that are normally separate

Prefix	Definition	Word Example	Pronunciation	Definition
bi-	two, double	**bi**cuspid	bi-kus´-pid	having two cusps
de-	down, away from	**de**generate	de-jen´-er-ate	to change from a higher to a lower form
di-	two, double	**di**plopia	di-plo-pe-ah	double vision
dia-	through, between	**dia**lysis	di-al´-i-sis	diffusion of solute molecules through a semipermeable membrane
dif-, dis-	apart, free from, separate	**dif**fusion	di-fu´-zhun	state or process of being widely spread
dys-	bad, difficult, painful	**dys**functional	dis-fungk´-zhun-al	disturbance, impairment, or abnormality of an organ
ec-, ecto-	out, outside, outer	**ecto**derm	ek-to-derm	outermost of the three primitive germ layers of the embryo
end-, endo-	within, inner	**endo**metrium	en-do-me´-tre-um	mucous membrane lining the uterus
ep-, epi-	upon, over, above	**epi**dural	ep-i-du-ral	situated upon or outside the dura mater
eu-	good, normal	**eu**phoria	u-fo´-re-ah	an exaggerated feeling of mental and physical well-being
ex-, exo-	out, away from	**ex**crete	ek-skreet´	to throw off or eliminate, as waste matter, by normal discharge
extra-	outside, beyond	**extra**uterine	ek-strah-u´-ter-in	situated or occurring outside the uterus
hyper-	above, beyond, excessive	**hyper**tension	hi-per-ten´-shun	persistently high blood pressure
hypo-	below, under, deficient	**hypo**dermic	hi-po-der´-mik	Beneath the skin
in-	in, into, not	**in**fusion	in-fu´-zhun	steeping a substance in water to obtain its soluble principles
mega-	large, great	**mega**lgia	meg-al-je-ah	a severe pain
meta-	beyond, over, between, change	**meta**stasis	me-tas´-tah-sis	transfer of a disease from one organ to another not directly connected to it
para-	beside, alongside, abnormal	**para**colitis	par´-ah-ko-li´-tis	inflammation of the outer coat of the colon
poly-	many, much, excessive	**poly**cystic	pol´-e-sis´-tik	containing many cysts
post-	after, behind	**post**natal	post-na´-tal	occurring after birth, with reference to the newborn
pre-	before, in front of	**pre**menstrual	pre-men´-stroo-al	preceding menstruation
pro-	before, in front of	**pro**otic	pro-ot´-ik	in front of the ear
super-	above, beyond	**super**nutrition	soo-per-nu-trish´-un	excessive nutrition
supra-	above, beyond	**supra**costal	soo-prah-kos´-tal	above or outside the ribs

TABLE 2-3 Word Roots and Combining Forms for Body Parts

Word Part	Definition	Word Example	Pronunciation	Definition
abdomin/o	abdomen	**abdomin**ocystic	ab-dom´-i-no-<u>sis</u>-tic	pertaining to the abdomen and gallbladder
aden/o	gland	**aden**itis	ad´-e-<u>ni</u>-tis	inflammation of a gland
an/o	anus	**an**oplasty	an´-oh-<u>plas</u>-te	plastic repair of the anus
andr/o	men	**andr**oid	<u>an</u>-droid	resembling a man
angi/o	vessel	**angi**ectomy	an´-je´-<u>ek</u>-to-me	excision of part of a blood vessel or lymph vessel
appendage	attached to or outgrowth	**append**ectomy	<u>ah</u>-pen-dek´-to-me	excision of the vermiform appendix
appendic/o	appendix	**appendic**olysis	ah-<u>pen</u>-di-kol´-i-sis	surgical separation of adhesions binding the appendix
arteri/o	artery	**arteri**ogram	ar-<u>te</u>-re-o-gram´	an x-ray picture of an artery
arthr/o	joint	**arthr**ocele	<u>ar</u>-thro-sel	a joint swelling
cardi/o	heart	**cardi**ology	<u>kar</u>-de-ol´-ogy	study of the heart
cephal/o	head	**cephal**ic	se´-phăl-ic	pertaining to the head
cerebr/o	cerebrum (part of the brain)	**cerebr**al	ser´-e-<u>bral</u>	pertaining to the brain
cyst/o	bladder	**cyst**ocele	<u>sis</u>-toh-seel	hernia of the bladder into the vagina
cyt/o	cell	**cyt**ology	si´-toh-lōgy	study of the body cells
encephal/o	brain	**encephal**oma	en-sef´-ah-<u>lo</u>-mah	a swelling or tumor of the brain
enter/o	intestines	**enter**itis	en-<u>ter</u>-i´-tis	inflammation of the intestine (usually small intestine)
esophag/o	esophagus	**esophag**ism	e-<u>sof</u>-ah-jism	spasm of the esophagus
gastro/o	stomach	**gastro**pathy	gas-<u>trop</u>-ah-the	any disease of the stomach
gloss/o	tongue	**gloss**odynia	glos´-o-<u>din</u>-e-ah	pain in the tongue
gyne	woman	**gyne**phobia	jin´-e-<u>fo</u>-be-ah	morbid aversion to women
hem/o	blood	**hem**atoma	he-<u>ma</u>-toh´-mah	blood clot in an organ or under the skin
hepat/o	liver	**hepat**ocele	<u>hep</u>-ah-to-sel	hernia of the liver
hyster/o	uterus	**hyster**olith	<u>his</u>-ter-o-lith´	a uterine calculus (stone)
ile/o	ileum (small intestine)	**ile**us	<u>il</u>-e-us	intestinal obstruction
irid/o	iris (eye)	**irid**omalacia	ir´-i-do-mah-<u>la</u>-she-ah	softening of the iris

Word Part	Definition	Word Example	Pronunciation	Definition
kerat/o	cornea of eye; horny substance	**kerat**orrhexis	ker´-ah-to-<u>rek</u>-sis	rupture of the cornea
lamina, lamin/o	thin, flat part of vertebra	**lamin**otomy	lam´-i-<u>not</u>-o-me	transection of a vertebral lamina
lapar/o	abdominal wall	**lapar**orrhaphy	lap´-ah-<u>ror</u>-ah-fe	suture of the abdominal wall
lingua	tongue	nigra**lingua**	ni-gra-<u>ling</u>-gwah	black tongue
lob/o	lobe, as of lung or brain	**lob**otomy	lo-<u>bot</u>-o-me	cutting of nerve fibers connecting a lobe of the brain with the thalamus
mamm/o	breast	**mamm**ogram	<u>mam</u>-o-gram	x-ray recording of breast tissue
mast/o	breast	**mast**itis	mas-<u>ti</u>-tis	inflammation of the breast
my/o	muscle	**my**ocarditis	mi´-o-kar-<u>di</u>-tis	inflammation of the heart muscle
myel/o	bone marrow; spinal cord	**myel**ocyte	<u>mi</u>-e-lo-sit´	immature cell of bone marrow
myring/o	eardrum	**myring**oplasty	mi-<u>ring</u>-o-plas´-te	surgical reconstruction of the eardrum
nephr/o	kidney	**nephr**itis	ne-<u>fri</u>-tis	inflammation of the kidney
neur/o	nerve	**neur**algia	nu-<u>ral</u>-je-ah	pain in a nerve
oophor/o	ovary	**oophor**ocystosis	o-of´-o-ro-sis-<u>to</u>-sis	formation of an ovarian cyst
ophthalm/o	eye	**ophthalm**orrhagia	of-thal´-mo-<u>ra</u>-je-ah	hemorrhage from the eye
orchi/o	testicle	**orchi**opathy	or´-ke-<u>op</u>-ah-the	any disease of the testes
orchid/o	testicle	**orchid**orrhaphy	or´-ki-<u>dor</u>-ah-fe	surgical fixation of an undescended testis into the scrotum by suturing
oste/o	bone	**oste**oporosis	os´-te-o-po-<u>ro</u>-sis	abnormal thinning of the skeleton
ot/o	ear	**ot**itis	o-<u>ti</u>-tis	inflammation of the ear
pancreat/o	pancreas	**pancreat**ogenous	pan´-kre-ah-<u>toj</u>-e-nus	arising in the pancreas
pharyng/o	pharynx	**pharyng**ismus	far´-in-<u>jis</u>-mus	muscular spasm of the pharynx
phleb/o	vein	**phleb**otomy	fle-<u>bot</u>-o-me	incision of a vein
pneum/o	lungs (air or gas)	**Pneum**onectomy	nu´-mo-<u>nek</u>-to-me	excision of lung tissue
proct/o	rectum	**proct**odynia	prok´-to-<u>din</u>-e-ah	pain in the rectum
prostat/o	prostate gland	**prostat**itis	pros´-tah-<u>ti</u>-tis	inflammation of the prostate
pyel/o	pelvis of kidney	**pyel**ectasis	pi´-e-<u>lek</u>-tah-sis	dilation of the renal pelvis

(continues)

TABLE **2-3** (*continued*)

Word Part	Definition	Word Example	Pronunciation	Definition
rect/o	rectum and/or anus	**rect**ocele	<u>rek</u>-to-sel	hernial protrusion of part of the rectum into the vagina
ren/i	renal (kidney)	**ren**iform	<u>ren</u>-i-form	kidney-shaped
rhin/o	nose	**rhin**itis	ri-<u>ni</u>-tis	inflammation of the mucous membrane of the nose
sacr/o	sacrum	**sacr**olumbar	sa´-kro-<u>lum</u>-bar	pertaining to the sacrum and loins
salping/o	fallopian tube	**salping**ocyesis	sal-ping´-go-ci-<u>e</u>-sis	development of an embryo in the uterine tube; a tubal pregnancy
splen/o	spleen	**splen**optosis	sple-nop-<u>to</u>-sis	downward displacement of the spleen
spondyl/o	vertebra	**spondyl**odymus	spon´-di-<u>lod</u>-i-mus	twin fetuses united by the vertebrae
steth/o	chest	**steth**ospasm	<u>steth</u>-o-spasm	spasm of the chest muscles
stomat/o	mouth	**stomat**omalacia	sto-mah-to-ma-<u>la</u>-she-ah	softening of the structures of the mouth
ten/o	tendon	**ten**dolysis	ten-<u>dol</u>-i-sis	the freeing of tendon adhesions
thorac/a	thorax (chest)	**thorac**entesis	tho´-rah-sen-<u>te</u>-sis	surgical puncture and drainage of the thoracic cavity
thyr/o	thyroid gland	**thyr**oxine	thi-<u>rok</u>-sin	a hormone of the thyroid gland that contains iodine
trache/o	trachea	**trache**oscopy	tra´-ke-<u>os</u>-ko-pe	inspection of the interior of the trachea
tympan/o	eardrum	**tympan**um	<u>tim</u>-pah-num	part of the cavity of the middle ear, in the temporal bone
ureter/o	ureter	**ureter**opathy	u-re´-ter-<u>op</u>-ah-the	any disease of the ureter
vas/o	vessel	**vas**cular	<u>vas</u>-ku-lar	pertaining to blood vessels
ven/i	vein	**ven**ipuncture	<u>ven</u>´-i-punk-chur	surgical puncture of a vein

TABLE **2-4** Suffixes Used in Surgery

Suffix	Definition	Word Example	Pronunciation	Definition
-age	related to	tri/**age** (three)	tre-<u>ahzh</u>	sorting out and classification of casualties to determine priority of treatment
-centesis	surgical puncture	arthro/**centesis** (joint)	ar´-thro-sen-<u>te</u>-sis	puncture of a joint cavity for aspiration of fluid

Suffix	Definition	Word Example	Pronunciation	Definition
-cid	kill	germi/**cid**al (germ)	jer-mi-si-dal	destructive to pathogenic microorganisms
-cis	cut, kill, excise	circum/**cis**ion (around)	ser-kum-sizh´-un	surgical removal of the foreskin of the penis
-clasis	to break down, refracture	oste/o**clasis** (bone)	os´-te-ok-lah-sis	surgical fracture or refracture of bones
-desis	binding, stabilization	arthr/o**desis** (joint)	ar´-thro-de-sis	surgical fusion of a joint
-ectomy	excision, removal	append/**ectomy**	ap´-en-dek-to-me	excision of the vermiform appendix
-iatry	healing (by a physician)	psych/**iatry** (mind)	si´-ki-ah-tre	healing of the mind
-ion	process	excerebrat**ion** (brain)	ek-ser-e-bra´-shun	process of removal of the brain
-lysis	loosen, free from adhesions, destruction	enter/o**lysis** (intestine)	en´-ter-ol-i-sis	surgical separation of intestinal adhesions
-osis	condition of	necr/**osis** (death)	ne-kro-sis	death of cells or tissues
-os/tomy	mouth, forming an opening	col/**ostomy** (colon)	ko-los-to-me	the surgical creation of an opening between the colon and the body surface
-pexy	fixation, suspension	gastro/**pexy** (stomach)	gas-tro-pek´-se	surgical fixation of the stomach
-plasty	formation, plastic repair	rhino/**plasty** (nose)	ri-no-plas´-te	plastic surgery of the nose
-stasis	stop/control	hemo/**stasis** (blood)	he-mo-sta´-sis	stopping the escape of blood by either natural or artificial means
-therapy	treatment	chemo/**therapy** (drug)	ke-mo-ther´-ah-pe	treatment of illness by medication
-tomy	incision, to cut into	phlebo/**tomy** (vein)	fle-bot-o-me	incision of a vein
-tripsy	to crush	litho/**tripsy** (stone)	lith-o-trip´-se	the crushing of a stone in the bladder

TABLE 2-5 Suffixes for Diagnoses and Symptoms

Suffix	Definition	Word Example	Pronunciation	Definition
-algia	pain	cephal/**algia** (head)	sef´-a-lal-je-ah	headache
-cele	hernia, swelling	hepat/o**cele** (liver)	hep-ah-to-sel	hernia of the liver
-dynia	pain	cephal/o**dynia** (head)	sef´-ah-lo-din-e-ah	pain in the head
-ectasis	dilation, expansion	bronchi/**ectasis** (bronchus)	brong´-ke-ek-tah-sis	chronic dilation of one or more bronchi
-emia	blood	poly/cyth/**emia** (many)	pol-e-si-the´-me-ah	increase in total red cell mass of the blood

(continues)

TABLE 2-5 (*continued*)

Suffix	Definition	Word Example	Pronunciation	Definition
-gen	producing, beginning	carcin/o/**gen** (cancer)	car-<u>sin</u>-o-jen	any substance that causes cancer
-gram	record, picture	encephal/o/**gram** (brain)	en-<u>sef</u>-ah-lo-gram	the x-ray film obtained by encephalography
-graph	instrument for recording	cardi/o/**graph** (heart)	<u>kar</u>-de-o-graf´	an instrument used for recording electrical activity of the heartbeat
-graphy	process of recording	roentgen/o/**graphy**	rent´-gen-<u>og</u>-rah-fe	x-ray films (roentgenograms) of internal structures of the body
-iasis	abnormal condition, formation of, presence of	chole/lith/**iasis** (gallstone)	ko´-le-li-<u>thi</u>-ah-sis	the presence or formation of gallstones
-itis	inflammation	gastr/**itis** (stomach)	gas-<u>tri</u>-tis	inflammation of the stomach
-logy	study of	bio/**logy** (life)	bi-<u>ol</u>-o-je	scientific study of living organisms
-malacia	softening	oste/o/**malacia** (bone)	os´-te-o-mah-<u>la</u>-she-ah	softening of the bones resulting from vitamin D deficiency
-megaly	enlargement	hepat/o/**megaly** (liver)	hep´-aht-o-<u>meg</u>-ah-le	enlargement of the liver
-meter	instrument for measuring	crani/o/**meter** (cranium)	kra´-ne-<u>om</u>-e-ter	an instrument for measuring skulls
-metry	process of measuring	pelvi/**metry** (pelvis)	pel-<u>vim</u>-e-tre	measurement of the capacity and diameter of the pelvis
-oid	resemble	lip/**oid** (fat)	<u>lip</u>-oid	fatlike; lipid (resembling a fat)
-oma	tumor	aden/**oma** (gland)	ad´-e-<u>no</u>-mah	a benign skin tumor in which the cells are derived from glandular epithelium
-osis	abnormal condition	dermat/**osis** (skin)	der´-mah-<u>to</u>-sis	any skin disease, especially one not characterized by inflammation
-pathy	disease	nephr/o/**pathy** (kidney)	ne-<u>frop</u>-ah-the	disease of the kidneys
-penia	decrease, deficiency	leuk/o/cyto**penia** (white cell)	loo-ko-sit-o-<u>pe</u>-ne-ah	reduction of the number of leukocytes (white blood cells), the count being 5,000/mm³ or less
-phagia	eating, swallowing	dys/**phagia** (difficult)	dis-<u>fa</u>-je-ah	difficulty in swallowing or eating
-phasia	speech	a/**phasia** (without)	ah-<u>fa</u>-zhe-ah	defect or loss of the power of expression by speech, writing, or signs, or of comprehending spoken or written words
-phobia	fear	acr/o/**phobia** (extremities or top)	ak´-ro-<u>fo</u>-be-ah	morbid fear of heights

Suffix	Definition	Word Example	Pronunciation	Definition
-plegia	paralysis	hemi/**plegia** (half)	hem´-e-<u>ple</u>-je-ah	paralysis of one side of the body
-ptosis	prolapse, falling, dropping	hyster/o/**ptosis** (uterus)	his´-ter-op-<u>to</u>-sis	metroptosis; downward displacement or prolapse of the uterus
-rrhage	burst forth	hem/o/**rrhage** (blood)	<u>hem</u>-o-rij	the escape of blood from the vessels; excessive bleeding
-rrhea	discharge, flow	men/o/**rrhea** (menses)	men´-o-<u>re</u>-ah	normal menstruation
-rrhexis	rupture	angi/o/**rrhexis** (blood vessel)	an´-je-or-<u>ek</u>-sis	rupture of a vessel, especially a blood vessel
-sclerosis	hardening	arteri/o/**sclerosis** (artery)	ar-te´-re-o-skle-<u>ro</u>-sis	a group of diseases characterized by thickening and loss of elasticity of the arterial walls
-scopy	examination, view	oto/**scopy** (ear)	o-<u>tos</u>-ko-pe	examination of the ear by means of the otoscope
-spasm	involuntary contraction, twitching of a muscle	blephar/o/**spasm** (eyelid)	<u>blef</u>-ah-ro-spazm	spasm of the eyelids

In summary, the important elements of a medical term are:

1. *Root*: The foundation of the term
2. *Prefix*: The word beginning
3. *Suffix*: The word ending
4. *Combining vowel*: A vowel that links the root word to the suffix or to other root words
5. *Combining form*: A combination of the root word(s) and the combining vowel

The rules for building medical words from these elements are:

1. A prefix is always placed at the beginning of the word.
2. A suffix is always placed at the end of the word.
3. When more than one root word is used, it is a compound word and requires the use of a combining vowel to separate the words, even if the root word begins with a vowel.
4. When defining medical terms, begin with the suffix and read backward.
5. If the word also contains a prefix, define the suffix first, prefix second, and root word(s) last.
6. When using compound words that relate to parts of the body, anatomic position determines which root word comes first.

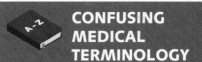

CONFUSING MEDICAL TERMINOLOGY

an/o versus ana- versus an-

an/o – anal origin or anus, e.g., anorectal (a-no-<u>rek</u>-tal) refers to the anal opening of the rectum

ana- – back, again, up, e.g., anaplasia (an-uh-<u>pley</u>-zhuh) refers to a reversion (back, again) of differentiation in cells and is characteristic of malignant tumors

an- – no, not, or without, e.g., anacusis (an-ah-<u>ku</u>-sis) refers to without hearing

CLINICAL
Note

Physician Office Visit Note

Maria Brown, a 64-year-old Hispanic female, presents at the office today for follow up of her **gastralgia** and **aphasia** (residual of previous stroke). Patient continues physical therapy and occupational therapy for aphasia with good progress.

Patient appears well nourished in no apparent distress. Patient is one week status post **EGD** prior to this visit. EGD showed active bleeding from a gastric ulcer. **Cautery** was used to achieve **hemostasis** without complication. Gastralgia has ceased and peristalsis is evident in all **abdominal quadrants**.

Will follow up in 6 weeks.

Direction: For the portions of the clinical note shown by a colored font, provide the definition and/or words for abbreviation.

LESSON TWO   Progress Check Part A

FILL IN

Fill in the blanks to make a complete, accurate sentence:

1. A _____ is an indication of illness that can be observed by someone objectively.

2. A disruption to the body's system is referred to as a _____.

3. A subjective indication of an illness is called a _____.

4. A _____ refers to an external influence that overpowers the body's defenses.

5. The three basic parts of a medical term are _____, _____, and _____.

MATCHING

Match the following word elements with their meaning:

Word Element	Meaning
1. aden/o	**a.** brain
2. bronch/o	**b.** uterus
3. encephal/o	**c.** abdominal wall
4. gloss/o	**d.** bronchus
5. hyster/o	**e.** bone
6. irid/o	**f.** gland
7. lapar/o	**g.** tongue
8. oste/o	**h.** iris

SPELLING AND DEFINITION

Circle the letter of the correct spelling and then define the combining form:

1. **(a)** oophor/o   **(b)** ophoor/o   **(c)** oorphor/o
Definition: _____

2. **(a)** prosct/o   **(b)** proct/o   **(c)** prost/o
Definition: _____

3. **(a)** neuphr/o   **(b)** neprect/o   **(c)** nephr/o
    Definition: _____

4. **(a)** rhinit/o   **(b)** rhin/o   **(c)** rhen/o
    Definition: _____

5. **(a)** orchi/o   **(b)** oorch/o   **(c)** orche/o
    Definition: _____

6. **(a)** salcr/o   **(b)** salp/o   **(c)** sacr/o
    Definition: _____

7. **(a)** salpr/o   **(b)** salping/o   **(c)** salpen/o
    Definition: _____

8. **(a)** myring/o   **(b)** mirang/o   **(c)** myleng/o
    Definition: _____

9. **(a)** pharang/o   **(b)** pharyng/o   **(c)** pragyn/o
    Definition: _____

10. **(a)** spongyl/o   **(b)** sphondyl/o   **(c)** spondyl/o
    Definition: _____

11. **(a)** urotor/o   **(b)** uroter/o   **(c)** ureter/o
    Definition: _____

12. **(a)** chondr/o   **(b)** cholondr/o   **(c)** chodol/o
    Definition: _____

13. **(a)** chost/o   **(b)** cost/o   **(c)** costol/o
    Definition: _____

14. **(a)** vast/o   **(b)** vas/o   **(c)** vein/o
    Definition: _____

15. **(a)** ven/o   **(b)** vin/o   **(c)** vein/o
    Definition: _____

16. **(a)** erythr/o   **(b)** eythry/o   **(c)** erythrey/o
    Definition: _____

DEFINING MEDICAL WORD ELEMENTS

Provide the medical root word for the following terms:

1. man _____

2. woman _____

3. heart _____

4. head _____

5. chest _____

6. bone _____

7. brain _____

8. stomach _____

9. liver _____

10. gallbladder _____

11. mouth _____

12. tongue _____

13. breast _____

14. muscle _____

15. nerve _____

BUILDING MEDICAL WORDS

Using all word elements necessary, build medical words that mean:

1. Inflammation of a tendon _____

2. Removal of the thyroid gland _____

3. Incision into the trachea _____

4. Any disease of the intestine _____

5. Pain in the nerves _____

6. Inflammation in the urinary bladder _____

7. Inflammation in a joint _____

8. Removal of the spleen _____

9. An eye specialist _____

10. An X-ray picture of a blood vessel _____

11. Stones in the gallbladder _____

12. An obstructed artery _____

13. Removal of a lung _____

14. An X-ray picture of the spinal cord _____

15. Instrument for examining the ear _____

16. Incision into a vein _____

17. Removal of the prostate gland _____

18. Rupture of a vessel in the cerebrum _____

19. Inflammation of the esophagus _____

20. Incision into the thorax _____

21. Excessive sugar in the blood _____

LESSON TWO   Progress Check Part B

MATCHING

Match the following word elements with their meaning:

Word Element	Meaning
1. -ectomy	**a.** tumor
2. -ostomy	**b.** abnormal condition
3. -otomy	**c.** rupture
4. -rrhaphy	**d.** resembling
5. -rrhage	**e.** discharge
6. -rrhea	**f.** burst forth
7. -rrhexis	**g.** cut into
8. -oid	**h.** suture
9. -oma	**i.** surgical removal
10. -osis	**j.** mouth, surgical creation

SPELLING AND DEFINITION

Circle the correct spelling and then define the word element:

1. **(a)** -centesis   **(b)** -centisis   **(c)** -senticis   **(d)** -cinteses
    Definition: _____

2. **(a)** -clysis   **(b)** -clasis   **(c)** -claxis   **(d)** -clasy
    Definition: _____

3. **(a)** -ectasy   **(b)** -ectosis   **(c)** -ectasis   **(d)** -eclasis
    Definition: _____

4. **(a)** -malachi   **(b)** -melacia   **(c)** -malazia   **(d)** -malacia
    Definition: _____

5. **(a)** -plegia   **(b)** -plagia   **(c)** -phlagia   **(d)** -pelagia
    Definition: _____

6. **(a)** -tosis   **(b)** -ptosis   **(c)** -protosis   **(d)** -tsosis
    Definition: _____

7. **(a)** -slerosis   **(b)** -schlerosis   **(c)** -sclerosis   **(d)** -shlerosis
    Definition: _____

8. **(a)** -magaly   **(b)** -mejally   **(c)** -magely   **(d)** -megaly
    Definition: _____

9. **(a)** -cele   **(b)** -cely   **(c)** -cili   **(d)** -ceal
    Definition: _____

10. **(a)** -isis   **(b)** -iasis   **(c)** -iatis   **(d)** -iesis
    Definition: _____

BUILDING MEDICAL WORDS

Using all word elements necessary, build medical words that mean:

1. A headache _____

2. Taking X-ray films of internal body structures _____

3. Inflammation of the stomach _____

4. Formation of gallstones _____

5. Increase in red cell mass _____

6. Softening of the bones _____

7. Surgical puncture of a joint _____

8. Removal of blood from a vein _____

9. Repair of a broken nose _____

10. Scientific study of living organisms _____

11. Enlargement of the liver _____

12. Any skin disease _____

13. Excision of the appendix _____

14. Healing of the mind _____

15. Incision into the brain _____

16. Treatment of illness by medication _____

17. Stopping the flow of blood _____

18. A substance that causes cancer _____

19. Disease of the kidneys _____

20. Loss of the power of speech _____

DEFINING MEDICAL TERMS

Define the following medical terms:

1. Osteoclasis _____

2. Enterolysis _____

3. Lithotripsy _____

4. Necrosis _____

5. Circumcision _____

6. Adenoma _____

7. Dysphagia _____

8. Leukopenia _____

9. Hemiplegia _____

10. Acrophobia _____

UNIT II

Root Words, Medical Terminology, and Patient Care

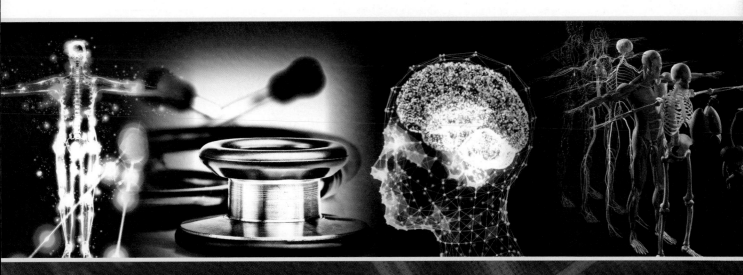

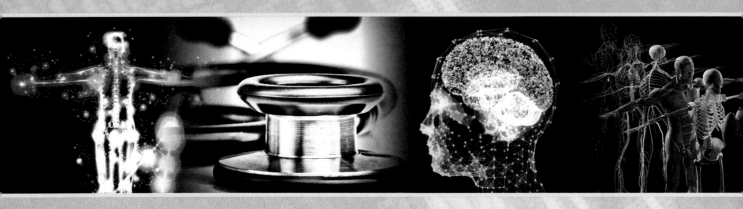

CHAPTER

3

© teekid/iStock/Getty Images

Bacteria, Color, and Some Medical Terms

OBJECTIVES

After completing this chapter and the exercises, the student should be able to:

1. Define the term bacteria and describe how bacteria can be both a beneficial and destructive force.
2. List and define the five major types of bacteria.
3. List and define prefixes that deal with color.
4. Change the meaning of a given word root by adding appropriate prefixes. Define, spell, and pronounce the new word.
5. Define, spell, and pronounce medical words used in this chapter.

LESSON ONE	Materials to Be Learned

ROOT WORDS FOR BACTERIA

Bacteria are minute organisms visible under a microscope that are composed of single cells and exist either on their own (independent or free living) or dependent upon another organism for life (parasite). Bacteria fall within the definition of *microbe*: a minute organism typically visible under a microscope that may be bacteria, fungi, or a protozoan parasite.

Bacteria can exist in multiple shapes and sizes. The most common way to classify them is by their shape and appearance; DNA sequencing can also be used to classify bacteria types. Bacteria are located everywhere and can live in many types of environments, including soil, the ocean, and the human body.

Not all bacteria cause disease and some are considered beneficial to maintaining health. For example, bacteria play a role in curdling milk into yogurt or in aiding digestion. Alternatively, they can be a destructive force, causing meningitis, tuberculosis, cholera, or pneumonia. Examples of bacteria are seen in **Figure 3-1**.

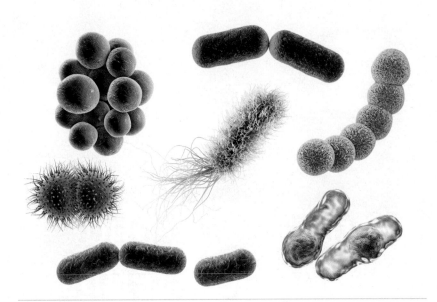

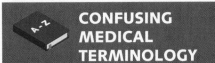

CONFUSING MEDICAL TERMINOLOGY

fasci/o versus faci/o

fasci/o – fascia, fibrous band, e.g., fasciculation (fuh-sik-yuh-<u>ley</u>-shuh) refers to a brief spontaneous contraction affecting a small number of muscle fibers

faci/o – the face, form, e.g., facioplegia (fa-shi-o-<u>ple</u>-jia) refers to facial paralysis

FIGURE 3-1 Bacteria: Staphylococci, Streptococci, Neisseria, Clostridium, Rod Shaped, *Escherichia coli*, Klebsiella.

© Kateryna Kon/Shutterstock

Scientists study bacteria not only to find cures for life-threatening diseases like malaria and typhoid fever, but also to create building blocks and tools for future research and treatment. For example, the study of bacteria has led to development of the field of *genomic medicine*, the study of genes and heredity. New tools have been created from studying bacteria that help to understand genes, how they work, and what happens when something goes wrong with a gene. These tools help not only treating physicians, but also epidemiologists, archeologists, researchers, forensic scientists, and historians. An entirely new multibillion dollar industry called *biotechnology* has emerged as a result. It involves any technological application that uses biological systems, living organisms, or derivatives thereof, to make or modify products or processes for specific use. The tables included in this chapter identify root words for bacteria (**Table 3-1**), prefixes for color, and commonly used prefixes.

TABLE 3-1 Root Words for Bacteria

Root Word	Definition	Word Example	Pronunciation	Definition
bacillus*	bacteria that are rod-shaped (plural is bacilli)	strepto**bacillus**	strep´-to-bah-<u>sil</u>-lis	rod-shaped bacteria that grow in twisted chains
coccus*	bacteria that are round in shape (plural is cocci, pronounced "coc´-seye")	strepto**coccus**	strep´-to-<u>kok</u>-us	round bacteria that grow in twisted chains
dipl/o	pairs; bacteria that grow in pairs	**dipl**ococcus	dip´-lo-<u>kok</u>-us	round bacteria that grow in pairs
staphyl/o	bunches, like grapes; bacteria that grow in clusters	**staphyl**ococcus	staf´-i-lo-<u>kok</u>-us	round bacteria that grow in clusters
strept/o	twisted; bacteria that grow in twisted chains	**strepto**coccus	strep-to-<u>kok</u>-us	round bacteria that grow in twisted chains

* Both "bacillus" and "coccus" are Latin and considered regular scientific words. They are neither word roots nor combining forms. Although some consider them suffixes when written as "-bacillus" and "-coccus," others disagree. We place them under the heading "root word" because we do not want to start another column or invent another heading.

PREFIXES FOR COLOR

The prefixes used to denote color are very useful. The color of the cells, body fluids and reactions, skin, growths, and rashes are important indications used in diagnosing and treating conditions and diseases. **Table 3-2** contains definitions and examples of some of the more commonly used prefixes for color.

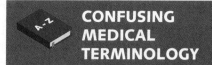

CONFUSING MEDICAL TERMINOLOGY

-cele versus celi/o

-cele – cyst, hernia, herniation, e.g., pharyngocele (fah-rin-jo-sel) refers to herniation of the throat

celi/o – abdomen, e.g., celioma (se-le-o-mah) an abdominal tumor

TABLE 3-2 Prefixes for Color

Prefix	Definition	Word Example	Pronunciation	Definition
alb-	white	**alb**ino	al-bi-no	a person with white hair, very pale skin, and nonpigmented irises
chlor/o-	green	**chlor**ophyll	klo-ro-fil	any of a group of green pigments that are involved in oxygen-producing photosynthesis
chrom/o-	color	**chrom**ocyte	kro-mo-sit	any colored cell or pigmented corpuscle
cirrh/o-	orange-yellow	**cirrh**osis	si-ro-sis	interstitial inflammation of an organ, particularly the liver (cirrhosis of the liver), showing orange-yellow discoloration in organ pigments
cyan/o-	blue	**cyan**osis	si´-ah-no-sis	a bluish discoloration of skin and mucous membranes
erythr/o-	red	**erythr**ocyte	e-rith-ro-sit	a red blood cell or corpuscle containing hemoglobin and transporting oxygen
leuk/o-	white	**leuk**ocyte	loo-ko-sit	white cell; a colorless blood corpuscle whose chief function is to protect the body against microorganisms causing disease
lutein/o-	saffron yellow	**lutein**	loo-te-in	a lipochrome from the corpus luteum, fat cells, and egg yolk
melan/o-	black	**melan**oma	mel´-ah-no-mah	malignant melanoma—"black tumor"
poli/o-	gray	**poli**omyelitis	po´-le-o-mi´-e-li-tis	an acute viral disease marked clinically by fever, sore throat, headache, vomiting, and often stiffness of the neck and back. It may attack the gray matter of the central nervous system (CNS) and brain, hence the common name "polio"
purpur/o	purple	**purpur**a	per-pyr-a	any of several hemorrhagic states characterized by spots and patches of purplish discoloration resulting from leaking of blood into the skin and mucous membranes
rhod/o-	red	**rhod**opsin	ro-dop-sin	visual purple; a photosensitive purple-red chromoprotein in the retinal rods
rubi/o-	reddish, redness	**rub**ella	roo-bel-ah	German measles; a mild viral infection marked by a pink macular rash, fever, and lymph node enlargement
xanth/o-	yellowish	**xanth**ochromia	zan´-tho-kro-me-ah	yellowish discoloration, as of the skin or spinal fluid

COMMONLY USED MEDICAL PREFIXES

The prefixes in **Table 3-3** are commonly used in medical terminology. Many have been defined previously. They also appear throughout the text, especially as they relate to body systems. They are included in this chapter for easy reference.

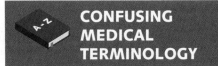

CONFUSING MEDICAL TERMINOLOGY

-rrhage versus -rrhea

-rrhage – bursting forth, e.g., hemorrhage (<u>hem</u>-er-ij) refers to a profuse discharge of blood, as from a ruptured blood vessel; bleeding

-rrhea – flow, discharge, e.g., prostatorrhea (pros-tat-or-<u>re</u>-ah) refers to discharge from the prostate

TABLE 3-3 Commonly Used Prefixes

Prefix	Definition	Word Example	Pronunciation	Definition
a-, an-	without, not	**a**febrile	a-<u>feb</u>-ril	without fever
		anoxia	an-<u>ok</u>-se-ah	absence of oxygen supply to tissues despite adequate perfusion of the tissue by blood; often used interchangeably with hypoxia to indicate reduced oxygen supply
acro-	extremities; top or extreme point	**acro**dermatitis	ak-ro-der´-mah-<u>ti</u>-tis	inflammation of the skin of the hands or feet
aero-	air	**aero**bic	ar-<u>o</u>-bik	produced in the presence of oxygen
		an**aero**bic	an-ar-<u>o</u>-bik	produced without oxygen
aniso-	unequal	**aniso**cytosis	an-i´-so-si-to-sis	presence in the blood of erythrocytes showing excessive variations in size
brady-	slow	**brady**cardia	brad´-e-<u>kar</u>-de-ah	slowness of the heartbeat, as evidenced by slowing of the pulse rate to < 60
de-	take away, remove	**de**hydrate	de-<u>hi</u>-drat	remove water from, to dry; to lose water, become dry
dia-	through (as in running through)	**dia**rrhea	di´-ah-<u>re</u>-ah	abnormally frequent evacuation of watery stools
dif-, dis-	apart, free from, separate	**dif**fusion	di-fu´-zhun	state or process of being widely spread
dys-	bad, painful, difficult	**dys**tocia	dis-<u>to</u>-se-ah	abnormal labor or childbirth
		dysmenorrhea	dis´-men-or-re-ah	painful menstruation
ec-, ecto-	out, outside, outer	**ecto**derm	ek´-to-derm	outermost of the three primitive germ layers of the embryo

Prefix	Definition	Word Example	Pronunciation	Definition
end-, endo-	within, inner	**endo**metrium	<u>en</u>-do-me´-tre-um	mucous membrane lining the uterus
eu-	good, easy	**eu**phoria	u-<u>fo</u>-re-ah	bodily comfort; well-being; absence of pain or distress
		euthanasia	u´-thah-<u>na</u>-zhe-ah	easy or painless death; mercy killing; deliberate ending of life of a person suffering from an incurable disease
extra-	outside, beyond	**extra**uterine	ek-strah-u´-ter-in	situated or occurring outside the uterus
hemi-	one side, half	**hemi**plegia	hem´-e-<u>ple</u>-je-ah	paralysis of one side of the body
hemo-	blood	**hemo**lysis	he-<u>mol</u>-i-sis	separation of the hemoglobin from the red cells and its appearance in the plasma
hetero-	different	**hetero**sexual	het´-er-o-<u>seks</u>-u-al	one who is sexually attracted to persons of the opposite sex
homo-	same	**homo**sexual	ho´-mo-<u>seks</u>-u-al	one who is sexually attracted to persons of the same sex
	resembling each other	**homo**geneous	ho´-mo-<u>je</u>-ne-us	of uniform quality, composition, or structure throughout
hydro-	water	**hydro**therapy	hi´-dro-<u>ther</u>-a-pe	the treatment of disease by the internal or external use of water
		hydrocephalus	hi´-dro-<u>sef</u>-ah-lus	a congenital or acquired condition marked by dilation of the cerebral ventricles and an accumulation of cerebrospinal fluid within the skull
hyper-	above normal, excessive, beyond	**hyper**tension	hi-per-<u>ten</u>-shun	persistently high arterial blood pressure; it may have no known cause or be associated with other diseases
hypo-	under, below normal	**hypo**glycemia	hi´-po-gli-<u>se</u>-me-ah	deficiency of glucose concentration in the blood, which may lead to nervousness, hypothermia, headache, confusion, and sometimes convulsions and coma
in-	in, into, not	**in**fusion	<u>in</u>-fu´-zhun	steeping a substance in water to obtain its soluble principles
iso-	equal, same	**iso**tonic	i´-so-<u>ton</u>-ik	of equal tension
		isothermal	i´-so-<u>ther</u>-mal	having the same temperature
lip-	fat	**lip**idemia	lip´-i-<u>de</u>-me-ah	hyperlipidemia: a general term for elevated concentrations of any or all of the lipids in the plasma
mal-	bad, poor	**mal**aise	mal-<u>az</u>	a vague feeling of bodily discomfort
		malocclusion	mal´-o-<u>kloo</u>-zhun	absence of proper relations of opposing teeth when the jaws are in contact

(continues)

TABLE **3-3** (continued)

Prefix	Definition	Word Example	Pronunciation	Definition
mega-	large, great	**mega**lgia	meg-al´-je-ah	a severe pain
		megavitamin	meg´-ah-<u>vi</u>-tah-min	a dose of vitamin(s) vastly exceeding the amount recommended for nutritional balance
megalo-	large (enlarged)	acro**megal**y	ak´-ro-<u>meg</u>-ah-le	abnormal enlargement of the extremities of the skeleton—nose, jaws, fingers, and toes
meno-	menses (menstruation)	**meno**pause	<u>men</u>-o-pawz	cessation of menstruation
noct-	night	**noct**uria	nok-<u>tu</u>-re-ah	excessive urination at night
nyct-	night	**nyct**uria	nik-<u>tu</u>-re-ah	excessive urination at night
pan-	all, every	**pan**demic	pan-<u>dem</u>-ik	a widespread epidemic disease
para-	beside, beyond, accessory to	**para**cystic	par´-ah-<u>sis</u>-tik	situated near the bladder
per-	through	**per**forate	<u>pur</u>-fo-rat	to make a hole or holes through, as by punching or boring; to pierce, penetrate
peri-	around	**peri**toneum	per´-i-to-<u>ne</u>-um	the serous membrane lining the walls of the abdominal and pelvic cavities
poly-	many, much	**poly**uria	pol´-e-<u>u</u>-re-ah	excessive secretion of urine
post-	following, after	**post**partum	post-<u>par</u>-tum	occurring after childbirth, with reference to the mother
		postoperative	post-<u>op</u>-ra-tiv	following surgery
pre-	before	**pre**natal	pre-<u>na</u>-tal	preceding birth
pro-	preceding, coming before	**pro**gnosis	prog-<u>no</u>-sis	a forecast of the probable course and outcome of a disorder
pyo-	pus	**pyo**genic	pi´-o-<u>jen</u>-ik	producing pus
		pyorrhea	pi-o-<u>re</u>-ah	a copious discharge of pus
re-	put back	**re**hydrate	re-<u>hi</u>-drat	to restore water or fluid content to the body
super-	above, beyond	**super**nutrition	soo-per-nu-trish´-un	excessive nutrition
supra-	above, beyond	**supra**costal	soo-prah-kos´-tal	above or outside the ribs
syn-	going together, united	**syn**thesis	<u>sin</u>-the-sis	creation of a compound by union of elements composing it, done artificially or as a result of natural processes
		syndrome	<u>sin</u>-drome	a set of symptoms occurring together
tachy-	fast	**tachy**cardia	tak´-e-<u>kar</u>-de-ah	abnormally rapid heart rate

CLINICAL *Note*

History and Physical

Gary Smith is a 35-year-old white male with a complaint of fatigue, sore throat, muscle pain, and itching of the skin.

Physical exam:

Height/Weight: 6'0" 215 lbs

HEENT: Head is **normocephalic**. Eyes appear **jaundiced**. Ears are normal; no fluid or pain. Throat is red with **pustules** on both sides. Patient is post-tonsillectomy at age 10.

Cardio pulmonary: Normal breath sounds, no wheezing or rales. No cardiac arrhythmias

BP: 130/75

T: 99.8 (37.6)

Neuro: Within normal limits

Skin: Jaundiced in appearance

Gastrointestinal: Tender with enlarged liver. Some enlargement of the spleen. Bowel sounds normal.

Urinary: No tenderness, no difficulty with urination.

Genital exam: Deferred

Impression: An ill-appearing gentleman with obvious jaundice and tenderness near the liver and spleen. Suspect early **cirrhosis**. Possible Hepatitis. Possible Strep Infection.

Plan: Bloodwork to include **CBC**, Chem panel, Liver Function: **SGOT**, **SGPT**, Bilirubin, Albumin, Total Protein, Hep A, Hep B, Hep C. **Rapid strep** with Throat culture for sensitivity.

Direction: For the portions of the clinical note shown by a colored font, provide the definition and/or words for abbreviation.

LESSON TWO   Progress Check

FILL IN

Fill in the blanks to make a complete, accurate sentence:

1. A _____ is a minute organism that may be bacteria, fungi, or a protozoan parasite.

2. _____ is the study of genes and heredity.

3. _____ are minute organisms visible under a microscope that are composed of single cells.

4. The industry that applies technology to biological systems and living organisms is called _____.

MULTIPLE CHOICE

Circle only one answer unless directed otherwise:

1. A bacterium that grows in a twisted chain is called
   a. coccus
   b. diplo
   c. strepto
   d. staphylo

2. Bacteria that are rod-shaped are called
   a. coccus
   b. diplo
   c. bacillus
   d. staphylo

3. Round bacteria that grow in clusters are called
    a. streptococcus
    b. staphylococcus
    c. streptobacillus
    d. diplococcus

4. Round bacteria that grow in twisted chains are called
    a. streptobacillus
    b. diplococcus
    c. staphylococcus
    d. streptococcus

5. Round bacteria that grow in pairs are called
    a. streptobacillus
    b. diplococcus
    c. staphylococcus
    d. streptococcus

6. Rod-shaped bacteria that grow in twisted chains are called
    a. streptobacillus
    b. diplococcus
    c. staphylococcus
    d. streptococcus

MATCHING

Match the terms on the left to their correct color on the right:

Prefix	Color
1. erythr/o	a. white
2. lutein	b. green
3. chrom/o	c. orange-yellow
4. poli/o	d. yellowish
5. melan/o	e. saffron yellow
6. cyan/o	f. black
7. albus	g. blue
8. rhod/o	h. red
9. cirrh/o	i. gray
10. xanth/o	j. purple
11. rubor	k. any color
12. chlor/o	
13. leuk/o	
14. purpur/o	

WRITE IN THE PREFIX

Write in the correct prefix for each term given:

1. Extremities _____

2. Unequal _____

3. Different _____

4. Painful _____

5. Same _____

6. Equal _____

7. Poor _____

8. Large _____

9. Every _____

10. Following _____

11. Blood _____

DEFINE THE PREFIX

State the meaning of the following prefixes:

1. mal _____
2. dys _____
3. megalo _____
4. hyper _____
5. tachy _____
6. hypo _____
7. brady _____
8. de _____
9. re _____
10. hydro _____
11. para _____
12. peri _____
13. poly _____
14. pre _____
15. pro _____
16. per _____
17. syn _____
18. noct _____
19. nyct _____
20. dia _____
21. peri _____
22. pyo _____

© teekid/iStock/Getty Images

Body Openings and Plural Endings

OBJECTIVES

After completing this chapter and the exercises, the student should be able to:

1. Provide definitions for and use each term for the openings or orifices in the human body.
2. Identify singular and plural endings and provide word examples with pronunciations.

LESSON ONE	Materials to Be Learned

BODY OPENINGS

Body openings, sometimes referred to as orifices, are cavities or passages in the body. The term orifice derives from two Latin word roots: *os* meaning mouth and *facere* meaning to make. Terms for openings in the human body are listed in **Table 4-1** and examples of openings typically found in the human body are listed in **Table 4-2**. Visual examples of body openings are seen in **Figures 4-1** and **4-2**.

TABLE 4-1 Body Openings Terms

Term	Pronunciation	Definition or Usage
aperture	ap-er-chur	an opening or orifice
canal (alimentary)	kah-nal	the musculomembranous digestive tube extending from the mouth to the anus
canal (vaginal)	kah-nal	the canal in the female from the vulva to the cervix uteri that receives the penis in copulation
cavity	kav-i-te	a hollow place or space, or a potential space, within the body or one of its organs
constriction	kon-strik-shun	making something narrow; to contract; to close (an opening)
dilatation, dilation	dil´-ah-ta-shun, di-la-shun	stretched beyond normal dimensions; the widening of something; expansion, opening
foramen	for-ra-men	a natural opening or passage, especially one into or through a bone
hiatus	hi-a-tus	a gap, cleft, or opening
introitus	in-tro-itus	opening or entrance to a canal or cavity such as the vagina
lumen	loo-men	opening within a hollow tube or organ
meatus	me-a-tus	urinary passage or opening
orifice	or-i-fis	any orifice such as the anal orifice
os	os	mouth opening; os uteri: mouth of the uterus or cervix
patent	pa-tent	adjective, meaning open or not plugged, as in "the tube is patent"
perforation	per-fo-ra-shun	a hole in something, e.g., perforation of the stomach wall by a gastric ulcer
stoma	sto-mah	artificial opening established by colostomy, ileostomy, or tracheostomy
ventricle	ven-tri-kul	a small cavity or chamber, as in the brain or heart

TABLE 4-2 Examples of Human Body Openings

Term	Pronunciation	Definition or Usage
anus	ey-nuh-s	defecation
ear canal	kah-nal	sense of hearing
mouth	mouth	eating; breathing; vocalization
nasolacrimal duct	ney-zoh-lak-ruh-muh-l duhkt	carries tears from the lacrimal sac into the nasal cavity
nipple	nip-uh-l	to carry breastmilk
nares (nostril)	nair-eez	breathing; sense of smell

Term	Pronunciation	Definition or Usage
urinary meatus	yoor-uh-ner-ee mee-ey-tuhs	childbirth; menstruation; sexual intercourse
vagina	vuh-jahy-nuh	ejaculation; urination

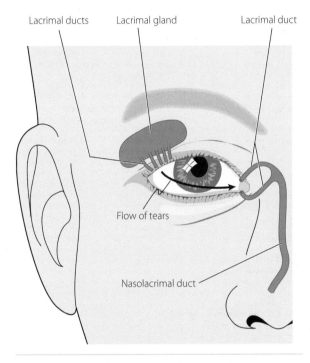

FIGURE 4-1 The lacrimal gland, the lacrimal sac, and the nasolacrimal duct.

© Blamb/Shutterstock.

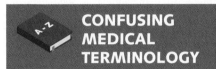

strata versus striae

strata – plural of stratum, layers, e.g., strata (strey-tuh) of tissues refer to layers of tissues

striae – striae (strahy-ee) refers to a slight or narrow furrow, ridge, stripe, or streak, especially one of a number in parallel arrangement, e.g., striae of muscle fiber, as in stretch marks

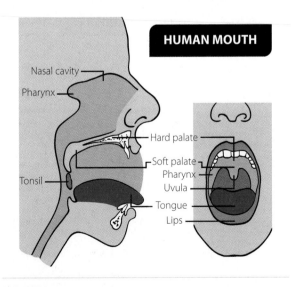

FIGURE 4-2 The human mouth.

© Udaix/Shutterstock.

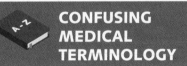

hidr/o versus hydr/o

hidr/o – sweat, e.g., hidropoiesis (hid-roh-poi-ee-sis) refers to the production of sweat

hydr/o – water, relating to water, e.g., hydrencephalomeningocele (hi-dren-cefal-o-men-in-jo-sel) refers to herniation of brain substance and meninges caused by a defect, with accumulation of cerebrospinal fluid along with brain substance in the sac

PLURAL ENDINGS

Many medical terms have special plural forms. They are based on the ending of the word. Some of them are made plural in the same way you learned in English class. For example:

1. Adding an "s" to a singular noun, e.g., singular, abrasion; plural, abrasions.
2. Singular nouns that end in "s" or "ch" form plurals by adding "es," e.g., singular, abscess; plural, abscesses.
3. Singular nouns that end in "y" preceded by a consonant form plurals by changing the "y" to "i" and adding "es," e.g., singular, artery; plural, arteries.

The following rules are commonly used for forming plurals for medical terms. If the word:

1. Ends in "a," retain the "a," and add "e," e.g., singular, bursa, vertebra; plural, bursae, vertebrae.
2. Ends in "is," drop the "is," and add "es," e.g., singular, crisis, diagnosis; plural, crises, diagnoses.
3. Ends in "ix" or "ex," drop the "ix" or "ex," and add "ices," e.g., singular, index, appendix; plural, indices, appendices.
4. Ends in "on," drop the "on," and add "a," e.g., singular, ganglion; plural, ganglia.
5. Ends in "um," drop the "um," and add "a," e.g., singular, ovum; plural, ova.
6. Ends in "us," drop the "us," and add "i," e.g., singular, nucleus, fungus; plural, nuclei, fungi.
7. Ends in "oma," drop the "oma," and add "omata," e.g., singular, carcinoma, fibroma; plural, carcinomata, fibromata.

There are exceptions to the rules. Some terms have more than one acceptable plural. If in doubt, consult your medical dictionary. **Table 4-3** lists the plural endings to medical terms.

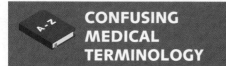

CONFUSING MEDICAL TERMINOLOGY

sarc/o versus sacr/o

sarc/o – flesh (connective tissue), cancer of connective tissue, e.g., sarcocele (sar´-kosel) refers to a fleshy tumor or sarcoma of the testis

sacr/o – sacrum, e.g., sacrum (sak-ruhm) refers to a bone resulting from the fusion of two or more vertebrae between the lumbar and the coccygeal regions in humans being composed usually of five fused vertebrae and forming the posterior wall of the pelvis; it means the area of the tailbone

TABLE 4-3 Plural Endings

Singular	Word Example	Pronunciation	Plural	Word Example	Pronunciation
a	bursa	ber-sah	ae	bursae	bur-sae
	vertebra	vur-ta-bra		vertebrae	vur-te-bre
ax	thorax	thor-aks	aces	thoraces	thor-a-sez
en	lumen	loo-men	ina	lumina	lu-mina
	foramen	for-ra-men	ina	foramina	for-ra-mina
is	crisis	kri-sis	es	crises	kri-ses
	diagnosis	di´-ag-no-sis		diagnoses	di´-ag-no-sez
	femoris	fe´-mo-ris	a	femora	fe´-mo-ra

Singular	Word Example	Pronunciation	Plural	Word Example	Pronunciation
ix	appendix	ah-pen-diks	ices	appendices	ah-pen-dises
inx	meninx	me-ninks	inges	meninges	me-nin-ges
nx	phalanx	fa-lanks	ges	phalanges	fa-lan-ges
oma	carcinoma	kahr-si-no-mah	omata	carcinomata	kahr-si-no-ma-ta
	fibroma	fi-bro-mah	Omata	fibromata	Fi-bro-ma-ta
on	spermatozoon	sper´-ma-to-zo-on	a	spermatozoa	sper´-ma-to-zo-a
um	diverticulum	di´-ver-tik-u-lum	a	diverticula	di´-ver-tik-u-la
	ovum	o-vum		ova	o-va
us	nucleus	nu-kli-us	i	nuclei	nu-clei
	thrombus	throm-bus		thrombi	throm-bi
ur	femur	fe-mur	ora	femora	fem-ora
y	artery	ar-ter-e	ies	arteries	ar-ter-es
	ovary	o-var-e		ovaries	o-var-es

CLINICAL Note

ED Discharge Note

HPI: 18-month-old healthy male presented with **epistaxis** and pain in the nasal **cavity**

Allergies: **NKDA**

Medication: None

Physical examination: HEENT: Normal other than some bleeding from the left **nare**. **BP**/Temp: WNL

ED course: Patient placed in a **supine** lying position and an **otorhinolaryngology examination** performed. Visualization of the nasal cavity showed a foreign object lodged just **anterior** to the middle turbinate of the left nare. The foreign body was removed with direct instrumentation.

Discharge summary: Mother stated that the child was playing with food while having lunch in his high chair and began crying. Upon checking, mother noticed child's nose was bleeding. Mother attempted to stop bleeding by tilting the head back and pinching nares. Mother thought she felt a lump within the soft portion of the left nare. Upon examination in the ED, it was noted that a foreign object was lodged within the left nare. Child was gently restrained by mother as forceps were used to withdraw a portion of what turned out to be a French fry. Epistaxis was controlled and child discharged to mother's care with instructions to return if bleeding reoccurred.

Direction: For the portion of the clinical note shown by a colored font, provide the definition and/or words for abbreviation.

LESSON TWO	Progress Check

SPELLING AND DEFINITION

Circle the letter of the correctly spelled word and define it:

1. **(a)** apurchur   **(b)** aperchur   **(c)** aperture   **(d)** apurchure
Definition: _____

2. **(a)** constriction   **(b)** constrictuve   **(c)** conscriture   **(d)** consctrition
Definition: _____

3. **(a)** foramine   **(b)** foramen   **(c)** formanen   **(d)** formaine
Definition: _____

4. **(a)** hitias   **(b)** hiateus   **(c)** hitrois   **(d)** hiatus
Definition: _____

5. **(a)** orifice   **(b)** orafus   **(c)** orafice   **(d)** orifux
Definition: _____

6. **(a)** introtoitus   **(b)** introitus   **(c)** introtois   **(d)** introices
Definition: _____

7. **(a)** ventracle   **(b)** vintricle   **(c)** ventricle   **(d)** veintricle
Definition: _____

8. **(a)** loomen   **(b)** lumen   **(c)** louman   **(d)** lumine
Definition: _____

WORD CONSTRUCTION

The following questions pertain to *plural endings*. For each singular ending listed, write the correct change to make it *plural*:

1. a _____

2. ax _____

3. en _____

4. is _____

5. ix _____

6. inx _____ or ex _____

7. nx _____

8. om _____

9. on _____

10. um _____

11. us _____

12. ur _____

13. y _____

The following medical words have *plural* endings. Write in the *singular* for each term listed:

14. vertebrae _____

15. thoraces _____

16. lumina _____

17. crises _____

18. ovaries _____

19. arteries _____

20. diverticula _____

21. nuclei _____

22. meninges _____

23. diagnoses _____

24. spermatozoa _____

25. femora _____

26. appendices _____

27. ova _____

28. thrombi _____

BUILDING MEDICAL TERMS

Using all word elements necessary, build medical words that mean:

1. A hollow space within the body _____

2. Stretched open beyond normal dimensions _____

3. A natural opening through a bone _____

4. The opening within an artery _____

5. Opening from the colon to the outside of the body made by surgery _____

6. A small chamber in the brain _____

7. An unplugged tube _____

8. The hollow space that extends from vulva to cervix _____

9. The tube extending from mouth to anus _____

10. A gap or cleft that allows a part of the alimentary canal to protrude through the diaphragm _____

11. Paralysis affecting all four limbs _____

DEFINITIONS

Define these body parts used in this chapter:

1. Femur _____

2. Meninx _____

3. Thorax _____

4. Bursa _____

5. Phalanx _____

6. Artery _____

7. Foramen _____

8. Ovary _____

9. Appendix _____

10. Spermatozoon _____

11. Erythrocyte _____

12. Diverticuli _____

13. Os _____

14. Introitus _____

15. Ventricle _____

CHAPTER

5

Numbers, Positions, and Directions

© teekid/iStock/Getty Images

OBJECTIVES

After completing this chapter and the exercises, the student should be able to:

1. Identify the location of any given body part.
2. Use appropriate prefixes to describe the direction of any movement and part of the body.
3. Give the meaning of prefixes that denote number and define given examples.
4. Identify commonly used prefixes that describe locations.
5. Describe body positions that indicate placement of a patient for a procedure or treatment.
6. Define the three major systems of weight and measurement used most often in medicine.
7. Convert Celsius to Fahrenheit or Fahrenheit to Celsius as needed.
8. Recognize commonly used symbols and abbreviations.
9. Define given word elements and transition to another system if required.

LESSON ONE	Materials to Be Learned

PART 1: PREFIXES FOR NUMBERS

Prefixes that denote numbers tell you whether something is one-half, one, two, three, or more; whether it is single or multiple; and whether it involves one side, two sides, or more. **Table 5-1** contains definitions and examples of some of the commonly used prefixes for numbers.

TABLE 5-1 Prefixes for Numbers

Prefix	Definition	Word Example	Pronunciation	Definition
uni- (mono-)	one	**uni**lateral	u´-ni-lat-er-al	affecting only one side
bi- (diplo-)	two (double), twice	**bi**lateral	bi-lat-er-al	having two sides; pertaining to both sides
		bicuspid	bi-kus-pid	having two points or cusps, e.g., bicuspid (mitral) valve; a bicuspid (premolar) tooth
gemin-	double, pair	**gemin**i	jim-in´-eh	twins
tri-	three	**tri**cuspid	tri-kus-pid	having three points or cusps, as a valve of the heart; the valve that guards the opening between the right atrium and right ventricle
		triceps	tri-seps	a muscle of the upper arm having three heads
quadri-	four	**quadri**plegic	kwod´-ri-ple-jic	paralysis of all four limbs
tetra-	four	**tetra**somic	tet-rah-some-ik	having four chromosomes where there should be only two
quint-	five	**quint**ipara	kwin-tip-ah-rah	a woman who has had five pregnancies that resulted in viable offspring (Para V)
sext-, sexti-	six	**sext**uplet	sexs-tu-plit	any one of six offspring produced at the same birth
sept-, septi-	seven	**sept**uplet	sep-tu-plit	one of seven offspring produced at the same birth
octa- (octo-)	eight	**octa**hedron	ok-ta-he-dron	an eight-sided solid figure
nona-	nine	**nona**n	no-nan	having symptoms that increase or reappear every ninth day; malarial symptoms are an example
deca-	ten	**deca**gram	dek-a-gram	a weight of 10 grams
multi-	many (more than one)	**multi**cellular	mul´-ti-sel-u-lar	composed of many cells
primi-	first	**primi**gravida	pri-mi-grav-i-dah	a woman pregnant for the first time
semi-	half (partially)	**semi**circular	sem´-i-ser-ku-lar	shaped like a half circle
hemi-	half, also one-sided	**hemi**anopsia	hem´-e-ah-nop-se-ah	defective vision or blindness in half of the visual field
ambi-	both or both sides	**ambi**dextrous	am´-bi-deks-trus	able to use either hand with equal dexterity
		ambivalence	am-biv-ah-lens	simultaneous existence of conflicting emotional attitudes toward a goal, object, or person
null-	None	**null**ipara	null-eh-pair-ah	a woman with no children
pan-	all	**pan**cytopenia	pan-site-oh-peen´-ee-ah	decreased number of all blood cells

PART 2: PREFIXES FOR POSITIONS AND DIRECTIONS

Prefixes that indicate directions describe a location. They tell you whether the location is above, below, inside, in the middle, around, near, between, or outside a body structure.

Figure 5-1 shows the movements of diarthrodial joints. Refer to this figure when studying **Table 5-2**, which contains definitions and examples of commonly used prefixes that describe positions and directions.

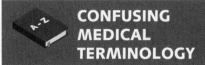

CONFUSING MEDICAL TERMINOLOGY

salping/o versus **salping/o**

salping/o – uterine (fallopian) tube, e.g., salpingitis (sal-pin-gi-tis) refers to inflammation of the fallopian tube

salping/o – auditory (Eustachian) tube, e.g., salpingitis (sal-pin-ji-tis) refers to inflammation of the Eustachian tube

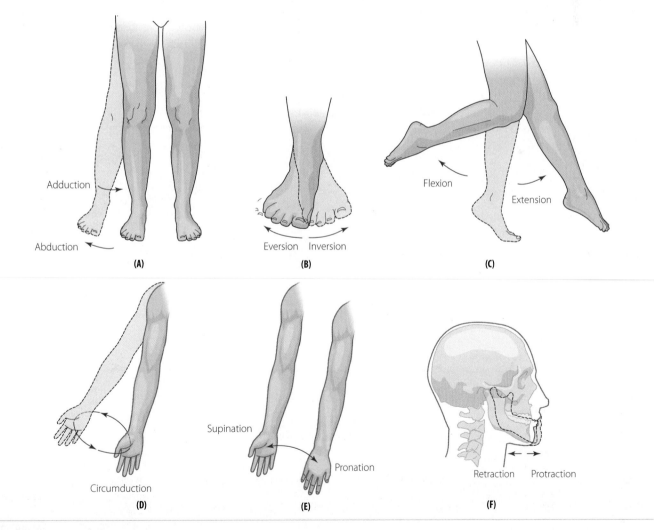

FIGURE 5-1 Movements of diarthrodial joints.

TABLE 5-2 Prefixes for Positions and Directions

Prefix	Definition	Word Example	Pronunciation	Definition
ab-	away from	**ab**duction	ab-<u>duk</u>-shun	to draw away from; the state of being abducted
ad-	toward	**ad**duction	ah-<u>duk</u>-shun	to draw toward a center or median line
ante-	before, in front	**ante**cubital	an-tee-<u>cu</u>-bi-tol	"The space" in front of the elbow
circum-	around	**circum**cision	ser´-kum-<u>sizh</u>-un	surgical removal of all or part of the foreskin, or prepuce, of the penis
contra-	opposition, against	**contra**indicated	kon´-tra-<u>in</u>-di-ka-ted	any condition that renders a particular line of treatment improper or undesirable
de-	down, away from	**de**cay	deh-<u>kay</u>´	waste away (from normal)
dia-	through	**dia**gnosis	dahy-uh-g-<u>noh</u>-sis	knowledge through testing
ecto-, exo-	outside	**ecto**pic	ek-<u>top</u>-ik	located away from normal position; arising or produced at an abnormal site or in a tissue where it is not normally found
		exogenous	ek-<u>soj</u>-e-nus	originating outside or caused by factors outside the organism
		exocrine	<u>ek</u>-so-krin	secreting externally via a duct; denoting such a gland or its secretion
endo-	within	**endo**crine	<u>en</u>-do-krin	pertaining to internal secretions; hormonal
		endogenous	en-<u>doj</u>-e-nus	produced within or caused by factors within the organism
epi-	upon, over	**epi**gastric	ep´-i-<u>gas</u>-tric	the upper and middle region of the abdomen
extra-	outside	**extra**uterine	ek´-strah-<u>u</u>-ter-in	situated or occurring outside the uterus
infra- (sub)	below, under	**infra**sternal	in´-frah-<u>ster</u>-nal	beneath the sternum
intra-	inside	**intra**cellular	in-tra-<u>sel</u>-u-lar	inside a cell
ipsi- (iso)	same (equal)	**ipsi**lateral	ip´-si-<u>lat</u>-er-al	situated on or affecting the same side
ir-	into, toward	**ir**rigate	ir´-reh-<u>gate</u>	wash into
meso-	middle, pertaining to mesentery	**meso**derm	<u>mez</u>-o-derm	the middle of the three primary germ layers of the embryo
meta- (supra)	after, beyond, over; change or transformation; following in a series	**meta**stasis	me-<u>tas</u>-tah-sis	the transfer of disease from one organ or part to another not directly connected with it
		metabolism	me-<u>tab</u>-o-lizm	the sum of the physical and chemical processes by which living organized substance is built up and maintained and by which large molecules are transformed into energy
		metamorphosis	met´-ah-<u>mor</u>-fo-sis	change of structure or shape; transition from one developmental stage to another

Prefix	Definition	Word Example	Pronunciation	Definition
para-	near, beside	**para**medical	par´-ah-<u>med</u>-i-kal	having some connection with or relation to the science or practice of medicine
		paranormal	par´-ah-<u>nor</u>-mal	near-normal function
peri-	around, surrounding	**peri**odontal	per´-e-<u>o</u>-don-tal	around a tooth
		pericardium	per´-i-<u>kar</u>-de-um	pertaining to the fibrous sac enclosing the heart and the roots of the great vessels
retro-	behind, backward	**retro**peritoneal	ret´-ro-<u>per</u>-i-to-<u>ne</u>-al	behind the peritoneum
sub-	under, near	**sub**merged	sub-<u>mer</u>-j-ĕd	under the surface
trans-	across, through	**trans**verse	trans´-<u>verz</u>	positioned across
		transvaginal	trans´-<u>vaj</u>-i-nal	through the vagina

PART 3: TERMS FOR DIRECTIONS AND POSITIONS

Table 5-3 contains both prefixes and suffixes, many of which are discussed in the preceding chapters and some of which are new. Both prefixes and suffixes are needed to describe body positions that indicate placement of a patient for procedures and/or treatments. Some words, such as Sims and Trendelenberg positions, are understood terms that denote the correct position without elaboration.

TABLE 5-3 Terms for Directions and Positions

Term	Pronunciation	Definition
anterior	an-<u>ter</u>-e-or	situated at or directed toward the front; opposite of posterior
posterior	pos-<u>ter</u>-e-or	directed toward or situated at the back; opposite of anterior
cephalic	se-<u>fal</u>-ik	pertaining to the head or the head end of the body
caudal	<u>kaw</u>-dal	situated toward the tail (coccygeal area)
decubitus	de-<u>ku</u>-bi-tus	the act of lying down; the position assumed in lying down
eversion	e-<u>ver</u>-zhun	a turning inside out; turning outward
extension	ek-<u>sten</u>-zhun	the movement bringing the members of a limb into or toward a straight condition
flexion	<u>flek</u>-zhun	the act of bending or the condition of being bent
Fowler's	<u>fow</u>-lerz	the head of the patient's bed is raised 18–20 inches above level
internal	in-<u>ter</u>-nal	situated or occurring within or on the inside
external	eks-<u>ter</u>-nal	situated or occurring on the outside

(continues)

TABLE 5-3 (*continued*)

Term	Pronunciation	Definition
knee-chest	<u>ne</u>-chest	the patient rests on his or her knees and chest; the head is turned to one side and the arms are extended on the bed, the elbows flexed and resting so that they partially bear the weight of the patient
lateral	<u>lat</u>-er-al	situated away from the midline of the body; pertaining to the side
bilateral	bi-<u>lat</u>-er-al	having two sides; pertaining to both sides
lithotomy	li-<u>thot</u>-o-me	position in which the patient lies on his or her back, legs flexed on the thighs, thighs flexed on the abdomen and abducted
medial	<u>me</u>-de-al	situated toward the midline
oblique	o-<u>blēk</u>	slanting; incline
peripheral	pe-<u>rif</u>-er-al	an outward structure or surface; the portion of a system outside the central region
proximal	<u>prok</u>-si-mal	toward the center or median line; the point of attachment or origin
distal	<u>dis</u>-tal	remote; farther from any point of reference
quadrant	<u>kwod</u>-rant	one of four corresponding parts or quarters, as of the surface of the abdomen or the field of vision
recumbent	re-<u>cum</u>-bent	lying down
rotation	ro-<u>ta</u>-shun	the process of turning around an axis
Sims'	simz	the patient lies on his or her left side and chest, the right knee and thigh drawn up, the left arm along the back
sinistro	<u>sin</u>-is-tro	left; left side
dextro	<u>dek</u>-stro	right; right side
superior	soo-<u>per</u>-e-or	situated above or directed upward
inferior	in-<u>fer</u>-e-or	situated below or directed downward
supine	<u>soo</u>-pīn	lying with the face upward or on the dorsal surface
supination	soo´-pi-<u>na</u>-shun	the act of placing or lying on the back
prone	prōn	lying face downward or on the ventral surface
pronation	prō-<u>na</u>-shun	the act of assuming the prone position
trans	trans	through; across; beyond
Trendelenburg's	tren-<u>del</u>-en-bergz	the patient is supine on a surface inclined 45 degrees, the head lower than the legs
upright	<u>up</u>-rit	perpendicular; vertical; erect in carriage or posture

UNITS OF WEIGHT AND MEASUREMENT

Units of weight and measure show more than what can be learned by looking at a number alone. For example, using the number 2 to denote the amount of blood taken from a patient means nothing if the unit or measure (the description) is not located immediately after the number. Is it 2 drops, 2 teaspoons, or 2 milliliters of blood? Including the unit of weight or measure informs another person of the exact amount involved and what measurement system is being used (e.g., metric).

This section contains weights and measures used most often in medicine. The transition between apothecary, avoirdupois, and metric is sometimes confusing to the learner. For the convenience of the learner, the units and equivalents are provided in **Table 5-4**, along with some symbols frequently encountered.*

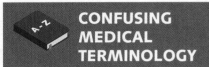

CONFUSING MEDICAL TERMINOLOGY

bi- versus bi/o

bi- – two, twice, double, e.g., bicuspid (bi-<u>kus</u>-pid) refers to the valve that is situated between the left atrium and the left ventricle of the heart

bi/o or bio- – life, pertaining to life, e.g., biology (bahy-<u>ol</u>-uh-jee) refers to the study of life

TABLE 5-4 Units of Weight and Measurement

Unit	Abbreviation(s)	Definition
Apothecaries' Weight (ah-<u>poth</u>-e-ka´-rez)		system used for measuring and weighing drugs and solutions, precious metals, and precious stones; fractions are used to designate portions of a unit and small Roman numerals are used to designate amounts (e.g., iss = one and one-half)
grains	gr	
minims	m	
drams	dr	
ounces	oz	
pounds	lb (12 oz = 1 lb)	
Avoirdupois Weight (aver-du-<u>poiz</u>)		the system of measuring and weighing used in English-speaking countries for all commodities except drugs, precious stones, and precious metals
drops	gtt	
teaspoon	tsp	
tablespoon	T	
ounces	oz	
pound	lb (16 oz = 1 lb)	

(continues)

TABLE 5-4 *(continued)*

Unit	Abbreviation(s)	Definition
Metric System (<u>met</u>-rik)		a system of weighing and measuring based on the meter and having all units based on the power of 10
Word Elements		
tera (10^{12})	T	monster: one trillion times the size of a unit
giga (10^9)	G	one billion times the size of a unit
mega (10^6)	M	one million times the size of a unit
kilo (10^3)	k	one thousand times the size of a unit
hecto (10^2)	h	one hundred times the size of a unit
deka (10)	dk	ten times the size of a unit
Unit Is One		
deci (10^{-1})	d	1/10 of a unit
centi (10^{-2})	c	1/100 of a unit
milli (10^{-3})	m	1/1000 of a unit
micro (10^{-6})	µ	1/1,000,000 of a unit
nano (10^{-9})	n	1/1,000,000,000 of a unit
pico (10^{-12})	p	1/1,000,000,000,000 of a unit
Metric Weight		
microgram	µg or mcg	1000 mcg = 1 milligram (mg)
milligram	mg	1000 mg = 1 gram (g or gm)
centigram	cg	100 cg = 1 g
decigram	dg	10 dg = 1 g
gram	g or gm	1 g = 1 g
dekagram	dkg	1 dkg = 10 g
hectogram	hg	1 hg = 100 g
kilogram	kg	1 kg = 1000 g
Metric Length		
millimeter	mm	1000 mm = 1 meter (m)
centimeter	cm	100 cm = 1 m
decimeter	dm	10 dm = 1 m

Unit	Abbreviation(s)	Definition
meter	m	1 m = 1 m
dekameter	dkm	10 m = 1 dkm
hectometer	hm	100 m = 1 hm
kilometer	km	1000 m = 1 km
Metric Volume		
cubic centimeter	cc	1 cc = 1 ml (milliliter)
milliliter*	ml or mL	1000 ml = 1 L (liter)
centiliter	cl	100 cl = 1 L
deciliter	dl	10 dl = 1 L
liter	l or L	1 L = 1 L
dekaliter	dkl	10 L = 1 dkl
hectoliter	hl	100 L = 1 hl
kiloliter	kl	1000 L = 1 kl
Equivalents (Equal to)		conversions from apothecary and avoirdupois to metric
weight	μg/mg	1000 μg = 1 mg
	mg/g	1000 mg = 1 g
	g/kg	1000 g = 1 kg
	kg/lb	1 kg = 2.2 lb
length	cm/in	2.5 cm = 1 in
volume	ml/cc/L	1000 ml = 1000 cc = 1 L
energy (joule)	J	1 J = 0.24 c
energy (calorie)	c	1 c = 4.18 J
Temperature (°T)		the degree (°) of sensible heat or cold expressed in terms of a specific scale
Celsius (or centigrade)	°C	scale at which the boiling point of water (H_2O) is 100° and the freezing point of H_2O is 0°
Fahrenheit	°F	scale at which the boiling point of H_2O is 212° and the freezing point of H_2O is 32°
conversion		to change from one scale or system to another
temperature		to convert Celsius to Fahrenheit, multiply by 9, divide by 5, and add 32: °F = ([°C × 9] ÷ 5) + 32 to convert Fahrenheit to Celsius, subtract 32, multiply by 5, and divide by 9: °C = ([°F − 32] × 5) ÷ 9

* Some textbooks in science and engineering use ML for milliliter while others use both mL and ml. We use both of the latter abbreviations.

Weights and Measures

Most members of the scientific community, including those in the medical field, depend upon the metric system because of the higher level of precision it offers in comparison to other systems. For example, scientific studies indicate that far fewer medication errors occur when dosages are delivered using milliliter units (the metric system) than by using teaspoon or tablespoon units (U.S. system). Prescription units are almost uniformly written in metric units. Confusion sometimes arises because of the need for scientists and medical staff to converse with patients and non-medical personnel who are not versed in the metric system. Misunderstandings and mistakes can be avoided if healthcare personnel possess a clear understanding of how to convert measurements between the two systems and convey that knowledge to patients and non-medical personnel. **Tables 5-5** is a conversion chart for length, mass, volume, and energy from the U.S. system to metric system, and vice versa.

TABLE 5-5 Conversion Tables for Length, Mass, Volume, and Energy

U.S. System to Metric		Metric to U.S. System	
U.S. Measure	Metric Measure	Metric Measure	U.S. Measure
Length		**Length**	
1 in	25.0 mm	1 mm	0.04 in
1 ft	0.3 m	1 m	3.3 ft
Mass		**Mass**	
1 gr (grain)	64.8 mg	1 mg	0.015 g
1 oz	28.35 g	1 gr (grain)	0.035 oz
1 lb	0.45 kg	1 kg	2.2 lb
Volume		**Volume**	
1 cu in	16.0 cm^3	1 cm^3	0.06 in^3
1 tsp	5.0 ml	1 ml	0.2 tsp
1 T	15.0 ml	1 ml	0.07 T
1 fl oz	30.0 ml	1 ml	0.03 oz
1 c	0.24 L	1 L	4.2 c
1 pt	0.47 L	1 L	2.1 pt
1 qt (liq)	0.95 L	1 L	1.1 qt
1 gal	0.004 m^3	1 m^3	264.0 gal
Energy		**Energy**	
1 cal (c)	4.18 J	1 J	0.24 cal (c)

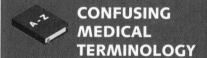

CONFUSING MEDICAL TERMINOLOGY

-tropia versus -tropin versus -trophy/trophia

-tropia – turning, e.g., anatropia (an-ah-<u>tro</u>-pe-ah) refers to upward deviation of the visual axis of one eye when the other eye is fixing

-tropin – an affinity for, stimulating, e.g., thyrotropin (thi-<u>rot</u>-rah-pin), a thyroid-stimulating hormone; a hormone of the anterior pituitary gland having an affinity for and specifically stimulating the thyroid gland

-trophy/trophia – a condition of nutrition or growth, e.g., cytotrophy (<u>si</u>-to-tro-fe), the nutrition of the fetus

Common Weights and Measures

Table 5-6 is a conversion table for some of the more common weights and measures in the U.S. system and their equivalents in the metric system.

TABLE **5-6** Conversion Tables for Common Weights and Measures	
Measure in U.S. System	**Equivalent in Metric System**
3 tsp	1 T
2 T	1 oz
4 T	1/4 c
8 T	1/2 c
16 T	1 c
2 c	1 pt
4 c	1 qt
4 qt	1 gal
1 tsp	5 g
1 T	15 g
1 oz	28.35 g
1 fl oz	30 g
1/2 c	120 g
1 c	240 g
1 lb	454 g
1 g	1 ml
1 tsp	5 ml
1 T	15 ml
1 fl oz	30 ml
1 c	240 ml
1 pt	480 ml
1 qt	960 ml
1 L	1000 ml

FREQUENTLY USED SYMBOLS

In addition to the many medical terms employed in the healthcare field, symbols are used for descriptive purposes. A symbol is a graphic portrayal of words, phrases, or sentences. **Table 5-7** contains the most frequently used symbols in medical fields of practice.

Symbol	Meaning	Symbol	Meaning
♂, □	male	↓	decreased, depressed
♀, ○	female	↑	increased, elevated
*	birth	Θ	absent
†	death	∧	diastolic blood pressure
ā	before	∨	systolic blood pressure
p̄	after	ʒ	dram
℞	take (prescription)	fʒ	fluidram
°T	degree (temperature)	∞	infinity
'	foot	±	indefinite (yes and no)
"	inch	#	number; weight; gauge
:	ratio (is to)	/	per
+	plus; positive; present	Ⓛ	left
−	minus, negative; absent	Ⓡ	right (also registered trademark)
ʒ	ounce	≥	greater than or equal to
fʒ	fluid ounce	≤	less than or equal to
µg	microgram	@	at
c̄	with	%	percent
s̄	without		

ED Note

Patient is a 68-year-old Asian male with complaint of **angina** with shortness of breath. Patient states he has had a "chest cold" for 3 weeks with no improvement. Symptoms include a productive cough with some greenish colored mucus, low-grade fever with highest temp of 102.4 today. Increasing **malaise** and some **diaphoresis** caused patient to seek medical attention. **EKG** at bedside is normal.
Impression: R/O pneumonia.

Plan: **CXR AP/Lateral**. CBC, Chem Panel, **cardiac enzymes x 3** over 3 hours.

Direction: For the portions of the clinical note shown by a colored font, provide the definition and/or words for abbreviation.

LESSON TWO	Progress Check

COMPARE AND CONTRAST

Explain the *differences* in the following prefixes:
Example: ab/ad ab-: away from; ad-: toward (center or median)

1. circum/contra _____

2. ecto/endo _____

3. infra/ipsi _____

4. para/peri _____

5. uni/bi/tri _____

6. prima/multi _____

7. semi/hemi _____

8. ambi/quadri _____

9. meso/meta _____

10. retro/trans _____

IDENTIFY THE LOCATION

Identify these locations by writing in the correct medical term:

1. Toward the front _____

2. Situated at the back _____

3. Toward the head _____

4. Toward the tail _____

5. Lying down position _____

6. Turned inside out _____

7. Straightening a limb _____

8. Slanting/inclined _____

9. Middle of the body _____

10. Part of the body that is attached to another part _____

DEFINE THE TERM

Define the following terms:

1. Apothecaries' _____

2. Avoirdupois _____

3. Metric _____

4. Tera _____

5. Micro _____

6. Temperature _____

7. Celsius _____

8. Fahrenheit _____

9. Conversion _____

10. Equivalent _____

MATCHING: POSITIONS

Match the position at the left to its correct direction:

Position	Direction
1. Fowler's	**a.** One of four parts
2. Flexion	**b.** Lying on left side and chest; right knee and thigh up, left arm to back
3. Lithotomy	**c.** To the left; left side
4. Peripheral	**d.** On top; above
5. Quadrant	**e.** Lying face up
6. Recumbent	**f.** Lying face down
7. Sims'	**g.** Through; across; beyond
8. Sinistro	**h.** Lying with head lower than legs
9. Dextro	**i.** Bottom; below
10. Superior	**j.** Outside; outward
11. Inferior	**k.** Right side; to the right
12. Supine	**l.** Lying down
13. Prone	**m.** Head and knees elevated
14. Trendelenburg's	**n.** Back position with legs bent or flexed and thighs abducted
15. Trans	**o.** Bending; being bent

MATCHING: METRIC UNITS

Match the metric unit prefix at the left to their description on the right:

Metric Prefix	Description
1. Milli	**a.** Ten times the size of the unit
2. Pico	**b.** One thousand times the size of the unit
3. Kilo	**c.** One hundred times the size of the unit
4. Deka	**d.** One-tenth of a unit
5. Deci	**e.** One-hundredth of a unit
6. Centi	**f.** One-thousandth of a unit
7. Hecto	**g.** One-trillionth of a unit

FILL IN

Fill in the blanks to make a complete, accurate sentence:

1. A milligram equals _____ micrograms.

2. A gram equals _____ milligrams.

3. A gram equals _____ centigrams.

4. A gram equals _____ decigrams.

5. A hectogram equals _____ grams.

6. A kilogram equals _____ grams.

7. One meter equals _____ millimeters.

8. One cubic centimeter equals _____ milliliter(s).

9. One kilogram equals _____ pounds.

10. One inch equals _____ centimeters.

11. One liter equals _____ milliliters or _____ cubic centimeters.

12. To convert Celsius to Fahrenheit, multiply by _____, divide by _____, and add _____.

13. To convert Fahrenheit to Celsius, subtract _____, multiply by _____, and divide by _____.

14. One calorie equals _____ joules.

15. One tablespoon equals _____ teaspoon(s).

16. One fluid ounce equals _____ milliliters.

17. One cup equals _____ milliliters.

18. One liter equals _____ cups.

19. One joule equals _____ calories.

SHORT ANSWER

Write the term for the following abbreviations and symbols:

1. mg _____

2. μg _____

3. kg _____

4. gtt _____

5. ℥ _____

6. f℥ _____

7. G _____

8. L _____

9. J _____

10. T _____

11. °C _____

12. g _____

13. ↑ _____

14. ℞ _____

15. s̄ _____

16. c̄ _____

17. ∞ _____

18. ā _____

19. p̄ _____

20. ♀, ○ _____

Medical and Health Professions

© teekid/iStock/Getty Images

OBJECTIVES

After completing this chapter and the exercises, the student should be able to:

1. Identify and define the medical terms and their word components for the major scientific health disciplines in medicine.
2. Identify and define the terms and their word components for physicians and professionals for each major medical specialty.
3. Identify and define the terms of other health professions who deliver patient care.
4. Identify and define the terms of other health professions with limited or no direct patient care contact.

LESSON ONE	Materials to Be Learned

Scientific studies are a hallmark of medicine, ushering in new treatment modalities and changes in clinical practice on a routine basis. Many of the decisions reached in treating patients are based on the results of scientific research studies, as are decisions related to how to address public health emergencies. Healthcare professionals across multiple disciplines rely upon the methods of scientific inquiry to acquire new knowledge and correct prior knowledge. Young scientists working in a lab under the direction of a senior doctor are seen in **Figure 6-1**.

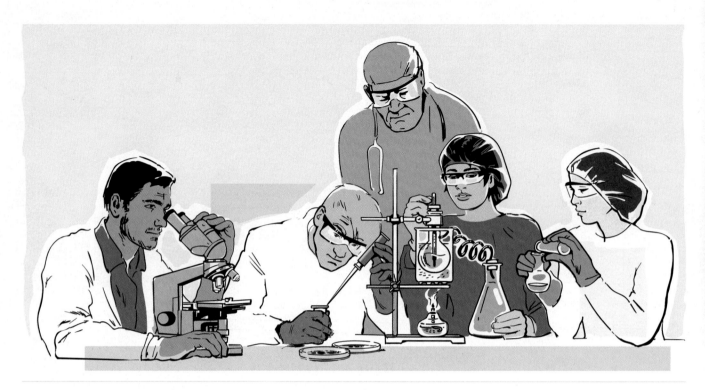

FIGURE 6-1 A research laboratory team.
© Uncle Leo/Shutterstock.

SCIENTIFIC STUDIES

The bases for many scientific studies pursued in today's healthcare environment are
listed in **Table 6-1**.

TABLE **6-1** Scientific Studies

Root	Word Example	Pronunciation	Definition
Suffux: -logy			
audi/o	**audio**logy	aw´-de-<u>ol</u>-o-je	the science concerned with the sense of hearing, especially the evaluation and measurement of impaired hearing and the rehabilitation of those with impaired hearing
bacteri/o	**bacterio**logy	bak-te´-re-<u>ol</u>-o-je	scientific study of bacteria
bi/o	**bio**logy	bi-<u>ol</u>-o-je	scientific study of living organisms
cardi/o	**cardio**logy	kar´-de-<u>ol</u>-o-je	study of the heart and its functions
dermat/o	**dermat**ology	der´-mah-<u>tol</u>-o-je	the medical specialty concerned with the diagnosis and treatment of skin diseases
endocrine/o	**endocrin**ology	en´-do-krin-<u>nol</u>-o-je	study of the endocrine system

Root	Word Example	Pronunciation	Definition
gastr/ oenter/o	**gastroenter**ology	gas´-tro-en´-ter-<u>ol</u>-o-je	study of the stomach and intestine and their diseases
gynec/o	**gynec**ology	gi´-ne-<u>kol</u>-o-je	the branch of medicine dealing with diseases of the genital tract in women
hemat/o	**hemat**ology	he´-mah-<u>tol</u>-o-je	the science dealing with the morphology of blood and blood-forming tissues and with their physiology and pathology
neur/o	**neur**ology	nu-<u>rol</u>-o-je	the branch of medical science that deals with the nervous system, both normal and diseased
onc/o	**onc**ology	ong-<u>kol</u>-o-je	the sum of knowledge regarding tumors; the study of tumors
ophthalm/o	**ophthalm**ology	of´-thal-<u>mol</u>-o-je	the branch of medicine dealing with the eye
path/o	**path**ology	pah-<u>thol</u>-o-je	the branch of medicine treating the essential nature of disease, especially changes in body tissues and organs that cause or are caused by disease
physi/o	**physi**ology	fiz´-e-<u>ol</u>-o-je	the science that treats the functions of the living organism and its parts, and the physical and chemical factors and processes involved
proct/o	**proct**ology	prok-<u>tol</u>-o-je	the branch of medicine concerned with disorders of the rectum and anus
psych/o	**psych**ology	si-<u>kol</u>-o-je	the science dealing with the mind and mental processes, especially in relation to human and animal behavior
radi/o	**radi**ology	ra´-de-<u>ol</u>-o-je	the branch of medical science dealing with the use of X-rays, radioactive substances, and other forms of radiant energy in the diagnosis and treatment of disease
ur/o	**ur**ology	u-rol-o-je	the branch of medicine dealing with the urinary system in the female and the genitourinary system in the male
Suffix: -iatry			
phys	**phys**iatry	<u>fiz</u>-e-ah-tree	the branch of medicine that deals with the physical restoration, rehabilitation, and maintenance of the body structures
psych	**psych**iatry	si-<u>ki</u>-ah-tree	the branch of medicine that deals with the study, treatment, and prevention of mental illness

SPECIALTIES AND SPECIALISTS

Healthcare facilities today are run by teams of medical personnel, including doctors, nurses, aides, pharmacists, laboratory personnel, health information managers, technicians, dietary personnel, and social service workers. All these professionals and others, named later in this chapter, play important roles in patient care and recovery. Additionally, some members of the healthcare team do not provide patient care directly, but are integral to the successful delivery of patient care through their support efforts. Further details of these professions, and others not named in this text, can also be found in *Stanfield's Introduction to Health Professions, 7th ed.* (2017) by Nanna Cross and Dana McWay.

Physicians and Medical Specialties

One of the most readily identifiable health professions is that of the physician. This profession requires formal training that is among the most demanding and rigorous of any occupation. Training typically includes four years of undergraduate study, four years of medical school, one year of internship, and two to seven years of residency and fellowship. Numerous variations exist within the discipline of medicine and **Table 6-2** provides a listing of the specialties.

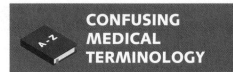

CONFUSING MEDICAL TERMINOLOGY

psychiatry versus physiatry

psychiatry – treatment of mental disorders, e.g., psychiatry (si-ki-ah-tre) refers to the branch of medicine that deals with the treatment of mental disorders

physiatry – treatment of physical disorders, e.g., physiatry (fiz´-i-ah-tre) refers to the branch of medicine that deals with prescribing and providing physical therapy and rehabilitation for patients

TABLE 6-2 Specialties and Specialists: Physicians and Medical Specialties

Root	Word Example	Pronunciation	Definition
Suffix: -ologist			
cardi/o	**cardi**ologist	kar´-de-<u>ol</u>-o-jist	a physician skilled in the diagnosis and treatment of heart disease
derm/o (dermat/o)	**dermat**ologist	der´-mah-<u>tol</u>-o-jist	a physician who specializes in the treatment of infections, growths, and injuries related to the skin
esthesia	an**esthesi**ologist	an´-es-the´-ze-<u>ol</u>-o-jist	a physician who specializes in anesthesiology; an anesthesiologist administers anesthetics, of which there are two types: *general* anesthetics, which produce sleep, and *regional* anesthetics, which render a specific area insensible to pain
endocrine/o	**endocrin**ologist	en´-do-kri-<u>nol</u>-o-jist	a physician skilled in the diagnosis and treatment of disorders of the glands of internal secretion
gastr/ oenter/o	**gastroenter**ologist	gas-tro-en´-ter-<u>ol</u>-o-jist	a physician who specializes in the study of the stomach and intestines and their diseases
gynec/o	**gynec**ologist	gi´-ne-<u>kol</u>-o-jist	a physician who specializes in the diseases of the genital tract in women
hemat/o	**hemat**ologist	he´-mah-<u>tol</u>-o-jist	a physician who specializes in the science of blood and blood-forming tissues
immun/o	allergist/**immun**ologist	al-ler-jist /im´-u-nol-o-jist	a physician who specializes in addressing allergic reactions and immunologic disorders
nephr/o	**nephr**ologist	ne´-fral-o-jist	a physician who specializes in the science of the kidneys
neur/o	**neur**ologist	nu-<u>rol</u>-o-jist	a physician who specializes in the science of the central nervous system
onc/o	**onc**ologist	ong-<u>kol</u>-o-jist	a physician who specializes in the study of tumors
ophthalm/o	**ophthalm**ologist	of´-thal-<u>mol</u>-o-jist	a physician who specializes in diagnosing and prescribing treatment for defects, injuries, and diseases of the eye

Root	Word Example	Pronunciation	Definition
ot/orhin/ olaryng/o	**otorhinolaryng**ologist	o´-to-ri´-no-lar-ing-<u>gol</u>-o-jist	a physician who specializes in the diseases of the ear, nose, and throat
path/o	**path**ologist	pah-<u>thol</u>-o-jist	a physician who specializes in diagnosing changes in body tissues and organs that cause or are caused by disease
proct/o	**proct**ologist	prok-<u>tol</u>-o-jist	a physician who specializes in the diagnosis and treatment of diseases of the rectum and anus
radi/o	**radi**ologist	ra´-de-<u>ol</u>-o-jist	a physician who specializes in the interpretation of X-rays and other radioactive substances used for diagnostic purposes
Suffix: -ian			
obstetric	**obstetric**ian	ob´-ste-<u>trish</u>-an	a physician who specializes in pregnancy, labor, and the puerperium
pediatric	**pediatric**ian	pe´-de-ah-<u>trish</u>-an	a physician who specializes in the diagnosis and treatment of children's diseases
Suffix: -ician			
geriatric	**geriatric**ian	jer´-e-a-<u>trish</u>-an	a physician who specializes in the diagnosis and treatment of the diseases of the aging and elderly
phys	**phys**ician	fi-<u>zish</u>-an	one who studies body function; an authorized practitioner of medicine
Suffix: -iatrist			
psych	**psych**iatrist	si-<u>ki</u>-a-trist	a physician who specializes in the diagnosis and treatment of mental disorders
Suffix: -ist			
intern	**intern**ist	in-<u>ter</u>-nist	a physician who specializes in internal organs of the body and their function
orth/o	**orth**opedist	<u>or</u>-tho-pe´-dist	a surgeon who specializes in the preservation and restoration of the function of the skeletal system, its articulation, and associated structures
phys	**phys**iatrist	fiz´-i-<u>a</u>-trist	a physician who specializes in prescribing and providing physical therapy and rehabilitation for patients requiring it
Suffix: -itioner			
practice	**prac**titioner (family practice [MD, Doctor of Medicine] or general practice [DO, Doctor of Osteopathy])	prak-<u>tish</u>-a-ner	a physician who is schooled in six basic areas: internal medicine, obstetrics and gynecology, surgery, psychiatry, pediatrics, and community medicine; the practitioner can treat the whole family and coordinate specialty care if necessary

Other Health Professions Delivering Patient Care

Many health professionals are integral players in diagnosing and treating diseases and illnesses. Changes in the healthcare industry, combined with innovations in technology, have created new and expanded existing allied health professions. Many of these professions deliver care directly to patients, often under the supervision of a physician. The listing in **Table 6-3**, while not exhaustive, provides an expansive inventory of the many allied health professionals in the healthcare industry today. Many of these same professions are highlighted in more detail in later chapters of this text. Pronunciations are provided for some but not all professions, as some professional titles include terms commonly used beyond the healthcare environment.

TABLE 6-3 Other Health Professions

Specialty	Title	Pronunciation	Definition
chiropractic (ki´-ro-prak-tik)	chiropractor (DC)	ki´-ro-prak-tor	a person trained in the manipulation of the vertebral column
communication	audiologist	aw-dee-ol-uh-jist	a professional who works with people with hearing, balance, and related ear problems
	speech-language pathologist		a professional who assesses, diagnoses, treats, and helps prevent disorders related to speech, language, cognitive communication, voice, swallowing, and fluency
dentistry (den-tis-tre)	dentist (DDS, DMD)	den-tist	a physician who is concerned with the teeth and associated structures
subspecialties of dentistry	endodontist	en´-do-don-tist	a dentist who specializes in conditions of the tooth pulp and root and the periapical tissues
	oral surgeon		a dentist who specializes in surgery of the mouth
	orthodontist	or´-tho-don-tist	a dentist who specializes in the treatment of irregularities of the teeth, malocclusion, and associated facial problems
	pedodontist	pe´-do-don-tist	a dentist who treats children's teeth
	periodontist	per´-e-o-don-tist	a dentist who treats diseases of the gums
	prosthodontist	pros´-tho-don-tist	a dentist who constructs artificial appliances designed to restore and maintain oral function
related fields of dentistry	dental hygienist (RDH)	den-tal hi´-je-nist	a dental specialist (not an MD) whose primary concern is maintenance of dental health and prevention of oral disease
	dental assistant		a person who assists the dentist
diagnostic technology	cardiovascular technologist	kar-di-o-vas-cu-lar tek-nol-o-jist	a person who specializes in invasive procedures of the heart
dietetics	diagnostic medical sonographers	son-o-graf-ers	a person who uses specialized equipment to direct nonionizing, high-frequency sound waves into areas of a patient's body
	electroencephalograph technician (EEG)	e-lek-tro-en-cef-a-lo-graf tek-ni-shin	a person whose area of practice includes recording electrical activity of the brain
	electrocardiograph technician (ECG or EKG)	e-lek-tro-kar-di-o-graf tek-ni-shin	a person whose area of practice includes taking electrocardiograms and conducting stress testing

Specialty	Title	Pronunciation	Definition
	nuclear medicine technologist	noo-klee-er tek-nol-o-jist	a person who operates cameras that detect and map a radioactive drug contained in a patient's body in order to create diagnostic images
	surgical technologist		one who assists in surgical operations under the supervision of surgeons, registered nurses, or other surgical personnel
	registered dietitian (RD, MS, PhD)	reg-is-ter-ed di´-e-tish-an	a specialist schooled in the use of proper diet for the promotion of health, prevention of disease, and therapy for the treatment of disease
	dietetic technician (DTR)		a person with a science degree trained to work under the guidance of a dietitian; can plan menus and/or nutritional care for patients
emergency care	emergency medical technician (EMT)		a person who cares for people at the scene of an accident and transports them to hospital under medical direction
	paramedic		a person who cares for people at the scene of an accident by administering drugs orally and intravenously, performs intubations, and monitors and uses complex equipment
foot care	podiatrist (DMP)	po-di-ah-trist	a specialist who deals with the study and care of the foot
genetics	genetic counselor (CGC)	ge-ne-tik koun-se-lor	a person who provides advice and counseling to healthcare providers, individuals, and families concerning the risk of inherited conditions
health education	behavioral analyst		a professional who designs and implements treatment plans for patients with autism spectrum disorder
	community health worker		one who serves as a link between health educators/professionals and the community by developing and implementing strategies to improve community health
	health educator		one who teaches people about behaviors that promote and improve wellness
	orientation and mobility instructor for the blind		a specialist who teaches people with blindness or visual impairments to move about effectively, efficiently, and safely
	vision rehabilitation therapist		one who provides to persons with visual impairments instruction and guidance concerning assistive technology and community resources
medical assisting	medical assistant		a person trained to assist physicians in examining and treating patients, routine laboratory testing, and assigned clerical duties
	home health aide		a person who works under the direct supervision of a medical professional and provides basic health-related services in the patient's home
medical technology	medical technologist or clinical laboratory scientist (ASCP)		a person skilled in performing tests in a laboratory to identify and track diseases

(continues)

TABLE 6-3 (*continued*)

Specialty	Title	Pronunciation	Definition
mental health	psychologist (PhD, MS)	si-<u>kol</u>-o-jist	a person with advanced degrees who specializes in the treatment of disturbed mental processes and abnormal behavior; does not prescribe medications/drugs
	behavioral disorder counselor		a person who advises individuals how to modify their behavior to deal with specific aspects of their life
	substance abuse counselor		a person who advises individuals dealing with alcoholism, illegal drug addiction, and other addictions such as tobacco, gambling, and painkillers
	psychiatric technician		a person who provides therapeutic care to patients who are mentally impaired or emotionally disabled
nursing	registered nurse (RN) or advanced practice nurse (APN)		a specialist licensed to work directly with patients, administering treatments as ordered by the physician
	nurse: midwife (RN, APN)	<u>mid</u>-wīf	a professional nurse with additional training who specializes in the care of women throughout pregnancy, delivery, and the postpartum period
	nurse practitioner (RN, APN)		a registered nurse who has completed required additional training and certification; a nurse practitioner with physician referral is able to offer patients personal attention and follow-up care
	public health nurse (PHN)		a registered nurse concerned with the prevention of illness and care of the sick in a community setting rather than a healthcare facility
nursing, practical	licensed practical nurse/licensed vocational nurse (LPN, LVN)		a person who has completed a one-year program in a state-recognized school and has taken and passed the state licensing test; works under the supervision of an RN
	nursing assistant (CNA)		a person trained to help the RN and LPN in a clinical situation
occupational therapy	occupational therapist (OTR)		a professional person schooled in the rehabilitation of fine motor skills who coordinates patient activities
	occupational therapy assistant		a person who helps patients with rehabilitative activities and exercises outlined in a treatment plan developed by an occupational therapist
	occupational therapy aide		a person who prepares materials and assembles equipment for use during an occupational therapy session
optometry	optometrist (OD)	op-<u>tom</u>-e-trist	a professional person trained to examine the eyes and prescribe corrective lenses when there are irregularities in vision
	optician	op-tish-an	one who helps select and fit eyeglasses and contact lenses for people with eye problems

Specialty	Title	Pronunciation	Definition
pharmacy	pharmacist (RPh, PharmD)	<u>far</u>-mah-sist	one who is licensed to prepare, sell, or dispense drugs, compounds, and prescriptions
	pharmacy technician		a person responsible for receiving prescription requests, counting tablets, and labeling bottles
physical therapy	physical therapist (RPT)		a professional person skilled in the techniques of physical therapy and qualified to administer treatment prescribed by a physician or referred by a physician
	orthotist	or-thot-ist	a person who designs and fits corrective braces, inserts, and supports for body parts that need straightening or other curative functions
	physical therapy assistant		a person who provides care to patients under the direction of a physical therapist; for example, helping patients exercise or learn to use crutches
	physical therapy aide		a person who helps make physical therapy sessions productive, working under the direct supervision of a physical therapist or physical therapist assistant
	prosthetist	pros-the-tist	one who designs, measures, fits, and adjusts artificial limbs for amputees and devices for people with musculoskeletal or neurological conditions
physician assistant	physician assistant (PA)		a professional person trained in some medical procedures (not a physician) who performs limited duties under physician guidance
radiology	radiologic technologist (ARRT)		one who specializes in the use of X-rays and radioactive isotopes in the diagnosis and treatment of disease and who works under the supervision of a radiologist
	radiologic technician		one who produces X-ray images of the human body for use in diagnosing medical problems
	radiation therapist		one who uses highly complex machines, named linear accelerators, to administer radiation to cancer patients
respiratory care	respiratory therapist (RRT & CRT)		one who holds at least an associate's degree in respiratory therapy and who assists patients to improve impaired respiratory functions under a physician's direction
	respiratory therapy technician		one who administers oxygen and breathing treatments to patients
social work	healthcare social worker (MSW, PhD)		a professional skilled in helping patients and their families handle personal problems that result from long-term illness or disability
	psychiatric social worker (MSW, PhD, ACSW)		a professional skilled in maintaining contact among patients with mental illness, their psychiatrist, and families and facilitating patients' return to community life
	social and human services assistant		a person who helps people get through difficult times or get additional support

(continues)

TABLE **6-3** (*continued*)			
Specialty	**Title**	**Pronunciation**	**Definition**
sports medicine	athletic trainer		a professional trained in the prevention, diagnosis, assessment, treatment, and rehabilitation of muscle injuries, bone injuries, and illnesses
	exercise physiologist	fiz-ee-ol-uh-jist	a professional who provides health education and develops exercise plans to reduce risk for disease
Therapists, alternative	art therapist		a person who employs the visual art forms to improve human development
	corrective therapist		a person who applies medically prescribed physical exercises and activities to strengthen body functions and prevent muscle degeneration
	dance therapist		a person who uses movement to further emotional, cognitive, physical, and social integration
	horticulture therapist		a person who trains others in gardening and plant-based activities to achieve treatment goals
	manual arts therapist		a person who instructs patients in prescribed manual arts activities to prevent anatomical and physiological deconditioning
	massage therapist		a person who treats patients by using touch to manipulate the soft tissues
	music therapist		a person who employs music to accomplish treatment goals
	recreational therapist		a person who plans, directs, and coordinates recreation-based treatment programs

Additional Health Professions with Limited to No Patient Care Contact

Vital members of the healthcare team often support patient care without delivering care to the patient directly. Space limitations prohibit a complete presentation of known health professionals recognized by state and federal health authorities who provide this support. Instead, **Table 6-4** lists other health professions that are not covered previously and who support patient care through limited to no patient care contact.

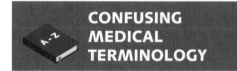

CONFUSING MEDICAL TERMINOLOGY

culd/o versus colp/o

culd/o: Rectouterine (blind) pouch, culde-sac, e.g., culdoscopy (cull-<u>dohs</u>-cope) refers to the visual examination of the rectovaginal pouch and pelvic viscera by the introduction of an endoscope through the posterior vaginal wall

colp/o: Vagina, e.g., colporrhaphy (kol-<u>po</u>-rah-fe) refers to the suture of the vagina

TABLE 6-4 Additional Health Professions with Limited to No Patient Care Contact

Specialty	Title	Description
dietetics	dietetic assistant or aide	a person who works to prepare and serve meals in hospitals and other healthcare facilities
environment	environmental scientist/specialist	a person who protects human health by analyzing environmental problems and developing solutions
	environmental science and protection technician	one who protects human health by monitoring and investigating sources of pollution and contamination
	occupational health and safety specialist	a person who protects human health by analyzing work environment and processes and designing programs to prevent disease or injury
	occupational health and safety technician	a person who protects human health by conducting tests and collecting samples and measurements as part of workplace inspections
healthcare administration	healthcare administrators	a person who plans, directs, coordinates, and supervises the delivery of healthcare
health information personnel	health information administrator (RHIA)	a person skilled in managing an information system that meets medical, ethical, and legal requirements; compiling statistics; and directing and controlling health record staff
	health information technician (RHIT)	a person who organizes, handles, and evaluates patient health records
related health information fields	medical librarian (MLA)	a professional person skilled in providing large volumes of current information to professional staff and personnel in medicine, dentistry, nursing, pharmacy, and other allied health professions
	medical secretary	a person with responsibility for orderly and efficient operation of a medical office
	medical transcriptionist (RHDS and CHDS)	a person who translates and edits recorded dictation by physicians and other healthcare providers regarding patient assessment and treatment
illustration	biologic photographer	a person who produces still and motion pictures of subjects for the health profession and natural sciences
	medical and scientific illustrator	a person who draws illustrations of human anatomy and surgical procedures
laboratory	dental laboratory technician	a person specially trained to prepare prosthetics such as dentures, crowns, bridges, and partials
	ophthalmic laboratory technician	a person who grinds and inserts lenses into a frame
pharmacy	pharmacy aide	a person who performs administrative functions in a pharmacy such as answering phones, stocking shelves, and operating cash registers
veterinary medicine	veterinarian (DVM)	a doctor trained and authorized to practice veterinary medicine and perform surgery on animals; may also do research
related fields of veterinary medicine	veterinarian technologist and technician	a person with credentials who works directly with animals, administering treatments as ordered by the veterinarian
	animal care and service workers	people who feed, water, groom, bathe, and exercise pets and other nonfarm animals

CLINICAL
Note

Dermatology Consultation Report

Patient identification: James Smith

Physician requesting consult: Dr. William Johnson

Consultation physician: Dr. Henri Adams

Reason for consultation: Abnormal appearing lesion on right thigh.

Impressions: R/O melanoma.

Recommendations: **Bx** and pathology of lesion with continued treatment plan according to findings.

H&P

History of present illness: A 33-year-old Caucasian male construction worker admitted for symptoms of heat stroke.

Allergies: NKA

Present illness: Patient was working in the heat (outside T of 105° F today) without adequate shade or hydration. Patient began to feel dizzy and developed severe stomach cramps with vomiting. Patient became unconscious, at which time an ambulance was called and patient was transported to the ED and subsequently admitted for **IV** fluid therapy for rehydration with isotonic saline and observation.

Past History Family Medical History/Social History:

ROS: Negative

HEENT: Negative

Neuro: WNL

Neck: Supple without swelling, masses, or adenopathy.

Skin: Hot, dry, and assessment of **skin turgor** indicates dehydration. Noted is an irregular **lesion** on the right thigh measuring approximately 3 cm by 5 cm. Reddish to black in color with undifferentiated margins. Suspicious for **melanoma in situ**.

Cardio/Pulmonary: WNL, no arrhythmia, wheezing, **rales**.

Abdominopelvic: WNL No tenderness or masses.

Genitalia: Deferred

BP/Temp – 120/80 T: 100.2 F/37.9 C

Review of lab results: Electrolytes increased indicating dehydration.

Findings discussed with the attending and plan is to schedule biopsy of the lesion as an outpatient upon discharge.

Thank you, Dr. Johnson for referring this interesting patient to me for evaluation.

Dr. Henri Adams, Dermatologist

<electronic Signature on file>

Direction: For the portions of the clinical note shown by a colored font, provide the definition and/or words for abbreviation.

LESSON TWO   **Progress Check**

MULTIPLE CHOICE: SCIENTIFIC STUDIES

Circle the letter of the correct answer:

1. The science concerned with the evaluation and measurement of hearing is
   a. Neurology
   b. Biology
   c. Anesthesiology
   d. Audiology

2. The scientific study of living organisms is
   a. Bacteriology
   b. Biology
   c. Pathology
   d. Hematology

3. The study of conditions of the blood and blood-forming organs is called
   a. Endocrinology
   b. Cardiology
   c. Hematology
   d. Bacteriology

4. Oncology is the study of
   a. Tumors
   b. Kidneys
   c. Diseases
   d. Eyes

5. The science that specializes in diseases of the stomach and intestines is
   a. Gynecology
   b. Enterology
   c. Gastroenterology
   d. Radiology

6. The branch of medicine dealing with the mind and its diseases is
   a. Neurology
   b. Physiatry
   c. Proctology
   d. Psychiatry

7. The branch of medicine dealing with disorders of the rectum and anus is
   a. Neurology
   b. Physiatry
   c. Proctology
   d. Psychiatry

MATCHING

Match the specialist with the field of practice:

Specialist
1. Anesthesiologist
2. Dermatologist
3. Gastroenterologist
4. Internist
5. Gynecologist
6. Otorhinolaryngologist
7. Immunologist
8. Ophthalmologist
9. Nephrologist
10. Radiologist
11. Geriatrician
12. Pediatrician

Field of Practice
a. Children's diseases
b. Diseases of the elderly
c. Interpretation of diagnostic X-ray studies
d. Skin diseases
e. Diseases of stomach and intestines
f. Diseases of female genital tract
g. Diseases of the ear, nose, and throat
h. Administration of therapeutic measures for pain insensibility
i. Diseases and functions of body organs
j. Diseases of the eye
k. Diseases of the kidney
l. Diseases involving allergic reactions

SHORT ANSWER

Describe these *specialties* related to the medical profession and *name* the specialist, including his or her title:

1. Dentistry _____

2. Dietetics _____

3. Podiatry _____

4. Midwifery _____

5. Practical nursing _____

6. Psychology _____

7. Pharmacy _____

8. Nursing _____

9. Veterinary medicine _____

COMPLETION

Complete the statements by filling in the name of the *specialist*:

1. The specialist who performs surgery of the mouth is called a(n) _____ .

2. The specialist who treats diseases of the gums is called a(n) _____ .

3. A specialist whose primary concern is prevention of oral disease is a(n) _____ .

4. A person who assists in the nutritional care of patients in a healthcare facility is called a(n) _____ .

5. A person who treats problems and maintains the health of the foot is a(n) _____ .

6. A professional person who performs specialized tests in a laboratory is a(n) _____ .

7. A professional person who helps to restore and rehabilitate a patient to the physical use of body parts is a(n) _____ .

8. The specialist who treats behavior and mental disturbances with communication therapies is a(n) _____ .

9. The specialist who dispenses medications is a(n) _____ .

10. The specialist who examines the eyes and prescribes corrective lenses is a(n) _____ .

11. The specialist who protects human health by analyzing environmental problems and developing solutions is a(n) _____ .

12. The person who provides health education and develops exercise plans to reduce risk for disease is a(n) _____ .

13. The person who provides advice and counseling to healthcare providers, individuals, and families concerning the risk of inherited conditions is a(n) _____ .

14. The person who works with people with hearing, balance, and related ear problems is a(n) _____ .

MULTIPLE CHOICE: PROFESSIONS

For the following professions, circle *all* the correct answers:

1. A nurse may be
  a. licensed
  b. certified
  c. registered
  d. a PhD

2. A physician may be
  a. an MD
  b. a DDS
  c. certified
  d. licensed

3. A dentist may be
   a.   an MD
   b.   a DDS
   c.   licensed
   d.   certified

4. A chiropractor may be
   a.   licensed
   b.   certified
   c.   an MD
   d.   registered

ABBREVIATIONS

List the appropriate letters (abbreviations) for the following professional titles:

1. Occupational therapist _____

2. Physical therapist _____

3. Public health nurse _____

4. Registered dietitian _____

5. Vocational nurse _____

6. Professional nurse _____

7. Medical technician _____ or _____

8. Radiology technician _____

9. Dentist _____

10. Veterinarian _____

11. Optometrist _____

12. Ophthalmologist _____

13. Psychologist _____

14. Psychiatrist _____

15. Pharmacist _____

16. Respiratory therapist _____

17. Osteopathy practitioner _____

18. Family practitioner _____

19. Health information technician _____

DESCRIBE THE SPECIALTY

Describe the specialty of the following practitioners:

1. Anesthesiologist _____

2. Endocrinologist _____

3. Hematologist _____

4. Radiologist _____

5. Pathologist _____

6. Bacteriologist _____

7. Biologist _____

8. Geriatrician _____

9. Pediatrician _____

10. Podiatrist _____

11. Dietitian _____

12. Obstetrician _____

13. Veterinarian _____

14. Healthcare social worker _____

15. Behavioral analyst _____

16. Biological photographer _____

17. Prosthetist _____

18. Athletic trainer _____

Abbreviations

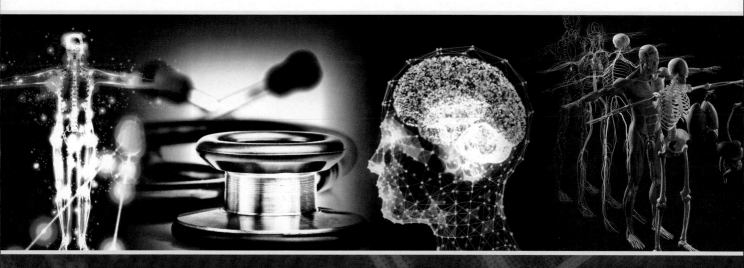

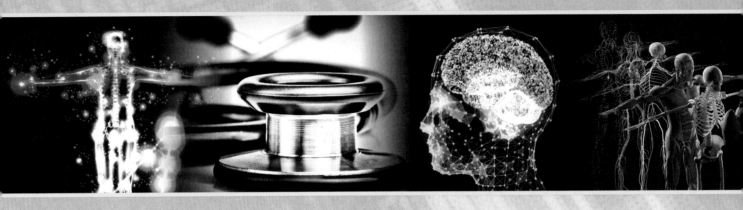

CHAPTER

7

© teekid/iStock/Getty Images

Medical Abbreviations

OBJECTIVES

After completing this chapter and the exercises, the student should be able to:

1. Summarize why healthcare professionals use medical abbreviations.
2. Explain the dangers of using nonstandard abbreviations.
3. Recognize medical abbreviations used by various services in a healthcare facility.
4. Identify abbreviations used when charting diet orders, activities, and medications for a patient.

LESSON ONE	Materials to Be Learned

The following information will help you in your study of medical abbreviations:

1. There are numerous medical abbreviations (only samples are given in this chapter).
2. The necessity to learn certain medical abbreviations is directly related to a student's health career plan. For example, laboratory abbreviations and terms are essential for students planning to be Clinical Laboratory Technologists.
3. A physician's handwriting, especially abbreviations, is difficult to read.
4. Purchase a medical abbreviations book recommended by your instructor.

Healthcare professionals frequently use abbreviations in their work as a means to communicate information in a succinct manner. For those healthcare professionals involved in documenting the delivery of patient care, abbreviations improve workflow and efficiency, allowing more work to be performed in less time. The danger in using abbreviations is that some healthcare professionals may not rely upon a standard compilation of abbreviations or may even be unfamiliar with standard abbreviations, thereby causing confusion. This confusion can lead to misinterpretation, which in turn may lead to negative consequences for a patient.

Learning abbreviations as part of a future healthcare professional's education is time well spent. By learning abbreviations early in training, the future healthcare professional is able to apply this knowledge to multiple science classes and practical learning experiences. Further, time is made available so the student can focus on other matters, such as clinical rotations, knowing that medical abbreviations are understood thoroughly.

Some abbreviations are considered acronyms, meaning the initial letters of words in a sequence are combined together and pronounced as a single word. While an individual may wish to pronounce each word in the sequence separately, it is often easier to pronounce the acronym. Some examples of acronyms are included in the tables in this chapter.

ABBREVIATIONS FOR SERVICES OR UNITS IN A HEALTHCARE FACILITY

Some of the various abbreviations for the services and units in a healthcare facility are listed in **Table 7-1**.

TABLE **7-1** Abbreviations for Services or Units in a Healthcare Facility	
Abbreviation	**Definition**
A & D	admitting and discharge
CS	central service (or supply)
OR	operating room (surgery); MOR, minor surgery
RR	recovery room
PT & OT	physical therapy and occupational therapy (may be under PM & R, physical medicine and rehabilitation)
X-ray	radiology
Lab	medical laboratory
MR	medical records
peds	pediatrics
Med-Surg	ward for medical and surgical patients (may be combined or separate)
OB	obstetrics (includes labor and delivery rooms, postpartum ward, and newborn nursery for healthy babies)
ICN or NICU	intensive care nursery or newborn intensive care unit (for premature or unhealthy babies)
OPD	outpatient department
ER	emergency room; ED, emergency department

Abbreviation	Definition
ENT	ear, nose, and throat
GU	genitourinary
NP	neuropsychiatric
SS	social service
CCU or ICU	coronary care unit or intensive care unit
DOU	definitive observation unit (less than intensive care, but more than "floor" care)
dietary (FS)	food service/dietary department
housekeeping	janitorial service
pharmacy	drugstore
morgue	unit for autopsies/holding the deceased
pathology (path)	laboratory for study of diseased tissues, including blood

ABBREVIATIONS COMMONLY USED IN HEALTH RECORDS

Abbreviations that are commonly found in health records of patients are listed in **Table 7-2**.

TABLE **7-2** Abbreviations Commonly Used in Health Records	
Abbreviation	**Definition**
CC	chief complaint of patient
EHR	electronic health record
H&P	history and physical
HPI	history of present illness
NKDA	no known drug allergies
PE	physical examination
PMHx	past medical history
PSHx	past surgical history
ROS	review of systems
SHx & FHx	social history and family history

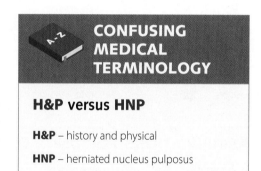

CONFUSING MEDICAL TERMINOLOGY

H&P versus HNP

H&P – history and physical

HNP – herniated nucleus pulposus

ABBREVIATIONS FOR FREQUENCIES

Abbreviations used to indicate the frequency of administering a treatment (drugs, etc.) are listed in **Table 7-3**.

TABLE **7-3** Abbreviations for Frequencies	
Abbreviation	**Definition**
q	every
qd	once a day
qod	every other day
q ___ h	every ___ hours (insert hours)
bid	twice a day
tid	three times a day
qid	four times a day
hs	at bedtime (hour of sleep)
ac	before meals
pc	after meals
prn	when needed
ad lib	as desired
stat	immediately

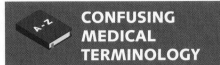

CONFUSING MEDICAL TERMINOLOGY

phren/o versus phren/o

phren/o – (phreno, phren, phreni, phrenic) – mind, e.g., phrenology (fri-<u>nol</u>-uh-jee) refers to a psychological theory or analytical method based on the belief that certain mental faculties and character traits (the mind) are indicated by the configurations of the skull

phren/o – (phreno, phren, phreni, phrenic) – diaphragm, e.g., phrenogastric (fre-<u>no</u>-gas-trik) refers to the diaphragm and stomach

ABBREVIATIONS FOR UNITS OF MEASURE

Abbreviations that are used as units of measure are as shown in **Table 7-4**.

TABLE **7-4** Abbreviations for Units of Measure	
Abbreviation	**Definition**
tabs.	tablets, pills
g, gm	grams
gr.	grains
cc	cubic centimeters
mL, ml	milliliters
L	liter (1,000 cc or ml)
mEq	milliequivalent
U	units

Abbreviation	Definition
gtts	drops
oz	ounces
dr.	drams

ABBREVIATIONS FOR MEANS OF ADMINISTERING SUBSTANCES INTO THE BODY

Abbreviations for the means of administering substances into the body of a patient are listed in **Table 7-5**.

TABLE **7-5** Abbreviations for Means of Administering Substances into the Body	
Abbreviation	**Definition**
PO	by mouth (*per os*)
IV	intravenously (into a vein; usually a peripheral vein)
IM	intramuscularly (into a muscle)
H	hypodermically (with a needle)
subcu, subq	subcutaneously (through the skin, into the fatty tissue)
subling	sublingually (under the tongue)
R	rectally (by rectum)
parenteral	a solution given intravenously
enteral	tube feeding (into stomach or small intestine)
D_5W	5% glucose in distilled water; use IV
caps.	capsules
supp	suppository
ss	one-half
mg	milligrams
N.S.	normal saline solution: isotonic solution
clysis	fluids given by needle, under skin (not in vein)
TKO	to keep open (vein)
KVO	keep vein open

ABBREVIATIONS FOR DIET ORDERS

Abbreviations that are used in diet orders for patients are listed in **Table 7-6**.

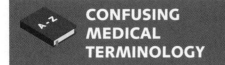

CONFUSING MEDICAL TERMINOLOGY

phall/o versus phalang/o

phall/o – penis, e.g., phalloplasty (fal-lo-plas-te) refers to the reparative or plastic surgery of the penis

phalang/o – bone in the finger or toe; phalanges, finger and toe, e.g., phalangectomy (fal-an-jek-to-me) refers to excision of a finger or toe bone

TABLE 7-6 Abbreviations for Diet Orders

Abbreviation	Definition
NPO	nothing *per os* (nothing to eat or drink orally)
I & O	intake and output (measured)
Cl Liq	clear liquids only: ginger ale, tea, broth, Jell-O, 7-Up, coffee
F Liq	full liquid: addition of milk and milk products; liquid at body temperature
Lo Salt, Low Na, Salt Free	restricted in sodium: ordered by mg or g of sodium desired, e.g., 2 g Na, 500 mg Na
NAS	no added salt packet; usually 4–6 g Na (mild restriction)
reg	regular diet ("house" or "normal" sometimes used); a balanced diet without restrictions as to the type of food texture, seasoning, or preparation method
mech soft	mechanical soft; a regular diet with alteration in texture only; sometimes called "edentulous"
med soft	medical soft; alterations in texture, preparation methods, and seasonings
bland	a medical soft diet further altered to omit acid-producing beverages and restrict seasonings; altered feeding intervals
Lo res	low residue; alteration in texture and a limited food selection to yield little intestinal residue
high fiber	a regular diet with increased amounts of foods containing dietary fiber
FF or PF	force or push fluids; increasing the liquid intake by addition of extra fluids
int fdg or int nour	interval feeding; supplemental nourishment served between meals
DAT	diet as tolerated
dysphagia pureed	regular diet pureed to a smooth, homogeneous, and cohesive consistency like pudding
consistent or controlled carbohydrate (CCHO)	consistent amounts of carbohydrate at meals and snacks to regulate blood glucose levels primarily for diabetes
Lo Fat, Lo Chol	low saturated fat, low cholesterol; a "Healthy Diet," based on *The Dietary Guidelines for Americans, 2010,* to reduce the risk of heart disease

ABBREVIATIONS FOR ACTIVITY AND TOILETRY

Abbreviations related to activity and toiletry are listed in **Table 7-7**.

TABLE 7-7 Abbreviations for Activity and Toiletry

Abbreviation	Definition
CBR	complete bed rest; ABR, absolute bed rest
dangle	sit at edge of bed, legs over the side
ambulate	walk
OOB	out of bed
BRP	bathroom privileges; may be up to bathroom only
commode	bedside toilet

ABBREVIATIONS FOR LABORATORY TESTS, X-RAY STUDIES, AND PULMONARY FUNCTION

Abbreviations related to laboratory tests, X-ray studies, and pulmonary function are included in **Table 7-8**.

TABLE 7-8 Abbreviations for Laboratory Tests, X-Ray Studies, and Pulmonary Function

Abbreviation	Definition
AP and Lat	routine X-ray picture of chest (front to back and side view)
up	upright X-ray picture
decub	decubitus (lying) position
IVP	intravenous pyelogram (kidney)
BE	barium enema (colon)
2GI series	upper (barium swallow): X-ray of stomach/duodenum; lower (same as BE): X-ray of lower bowel/colon
GB series	gallbladder X-ray picture
MRI	magnetic resonance imaging; noninvasive procedure using a magnetic field that yields images for diagnosis
RAI, RAIU	radioactive iodine (uptake) for diagnosing thyroid function
SCAN	CT, CAT: computed tomography, computerized axial tomography
CBC	complete blood count
UA	urinalysis
VC	vital capacity (lungs)

ABBREVIATIONS FOR MISCELLANEOUS TERMS

Abbreviations of some miscellaneous terms used in the field of medicine are listed in **Table 7-9**.

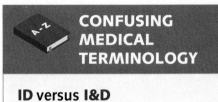

CONFUSING MEDICAL TERMINOLOGY

ID versus I&D

ID – intradermal

I&D – incision and drainage

TABLE **7-9** Abbreviations for Miscellaneous Terms	
Abbreviation	**Definition**
qns	quantity not sufficient (lab requires a larger specimen); also refers to insufficient food/liquid intake
c̄	with (con)
s̄	without (sans)
dc	discontinue
TLC	tender loving care
stat	immediately
ASAP	as soon as possible
CPR	cardiopulmonary resuscitation
EUA	examination under anesthesia
DOA	dead on arrival
OD	overdose; also means right eye (refer to context where used)
prep	prepare
V/S	vital signs
ECG, EKG	electrocardiogram
EEG	electroencephalogram
Dx	diagnosis
Tx	treatment
Rx	prescription
Sx	symptoms
Na^+	natrium: sodium (chemical symbol for)
K^+	potassium (chemical symbol for)
Ca^{++}	calcium (chemical symbol for)
P^{+++}	phosphorus (chemical symbol for)
Cl^-	chloride (chemical symbol for)

Abbreviation	Definition
I⁻	iodine (chemical symbol for)
Fe⁺⁺	iron (chemical symbol for)
Hg⁺⁺	mercury (chemical symbol for)
DS	double strength
O.S.	left eye
PDR	Physicians' Desk Reference

CLINICAL Note

Hospital Progress Note

Ninety-two-year-old Asian female with dehydration appears slightly improved today.

Patient continues to improve on I.V. Fluids **D5W** @ 100cc/hr for hydration.

Patient continues on current meds:

Biaxin 500 **mg** PO **q**12 hr for sinusitis

Omeprazole 20 mg. **PO** daily for **GERD**

Xalatan 2 **gtt OS** daily for Glaucoma

Xalatan 2 gtt **OD** daily for Glaucoma

Will reassess tomorrow. If improvement continues, will **D/C** to **LTC**.

Direction: For the portion of the clinical note shown by a colored font, provide the definition and/or words for abbreviation.

LESSON TWO | Progress Check

IDENTIFY THE DEPARTMENT

As a new employee of the hospital, you are given a list of departments that you will tour. Identify these units that are on your list:

1. A & D _____

2. CS _____

3. OR _____

4. PM & R _____

5. X-ray _____

6. Lab _____

7. OB _____

8. peds _____

9. OPD _____

10. ER _____

11. SS _____

12. ICU _____

13. FS_ _____

IDENTIFY THE PRESCRIPTION

Medications are given in many different forms and dosages and at scheduled times. They are administered into the body in various ways. In the following questions, identify (a) the form, (b) the type of administration, (c) the scheduled time of the dose, and (d) the dosage amount:

1. 2 g PO tid _____

2. 60 mEq R supp hs _____

3. gtts vi subling 4h _____

4. 2 L IV d _____

5. 30 U IM ac _____

6. 10 ml subcu prn _____

7. gr. ii in 10 cc n.s. clysis d _____

8. ss mg PO _____

IDENTIFY THE DIET ORDER

Identify the following *diet orders* from their abbreviations:

	Room	Name	Diet
1.	123	Mr J	NPO _____
2.	231	Mrs K	DAT _____
3.	301	Ms B	CCHO _____
4.	111	Mr H	2 g Na med soft _____
5.	112	Mr P	mech soft _____
6.	321	Mrs L	cl liq _____
7.	222	Mr K	Reg Hi Fiber FF _____
8.	232	Mrs R	f. liq c̄ int. nour.10-2-HS. I&O _____
9.	125	Mr M	pc _____
10.	119	Mrs F	prn _____

MATCHING

Match the abbreviation to its description:

Abbreviation	**Description**
1. AP and Lat	**a.** Diagnostic for thyroid function
2. IVP	**b.** Hepatitis A virus
3. BE	**c.** Diagnostic for gastric diseases
4. GB series	**d.** Four times a day
5. Upper GI	**e.** Analysis of kidney excretion
6. UA	**f.** Routine chest X-rays
7. VC	**g.** Diagnostic for colon diseases
8. RAI	**h.** Diagnostic for cholecystic diseases
9. HAV	**i.** Measuring lung capacity
10. qid	**j.** Kidney function test

SPELL OUT THE ABBREVIATION

In the following sentences, write in the complete words for the abbreviations given:

1. The nurse told the aide to *prep* the patient *pre-op*. _____

2. That man was *DOA*. _____

3. They checked his *TPR*. _____

4. She required *CPR*. _____

5. *BP* was 110/80 *mm Hg*. _____

6. What I need is *TLC*. _____

7. *DC* the *IV ASAP*. _____

8. End products of respiration are CO_2 and H_2O. _____

9. The *Tx* was more painful than the *Sx*. _____

10. Her serum NA^+ was elevated, but the K^+ was low. _____

11. The *Dx* was Fe^{++} deficiency anemia. _____

12. The patient reported *NKDA*. _____

13. The patient's *PMHx* revealed asthma. _____

14. When admitted to the ER, chest pain was his *cc*. _____

CHAPTER

8

Diagnostic and Laboratory Abbreviations

OBJECTIVES

After completing this chapter and the exercises, the student should be able to:

1. Use appropriate abbreviations for diagnostic, laboratory, and X-ray procedures.
2. Describe some abbreviations specific to a particular medical facility or specialty unit.

LESSON ONE	Materials to Be Learned

While many words are used to name and describe medical terms, certain terms are sometimes confusing and repetitive. That is especially true for those terms dealing with diagnosing patients and the results of tests and experiments conducted in a laboratory setting. In order to simplify any confusion, healthcare professionals employ standard abbreviations to specify exactly what is being talked about or conveyed in patient documentation. Recognizing and understanding these abbreviations should assist learners in communicating with healthcare professionals, both through taking notes and reading the notes of others.

DIAGNOSTIC ABBREVIATIONS

Abbreviations related to diagnostics are listed in **Tables 8-1**.

TABLE 8-1 Diagnostic Abbreviations with Definition

Abbreviation	Definition
A & P	auscultation and percussion
ABG	arterial blood gases
ACE	angiotensin converting enzyme
ASHD	arteriosclerotic heart disease
CA	carcinoma (cancer)
CBS	chronic brain syndrome
CC	chief complaint
CHD	coronary heart disease; congenital heart disease
CHF	congestive heart failure
c/o	complains of
COPD/COLD	chronic obstructive pulmonary (lung) disease
CP	cerebral palsy
CVA	cerebrovascular accident (stroke)
CVD	cardiovascular disease
DJD	degenerative joint disease (osteoarthritis)
Dx	diagnosis
FH	family history
FUO	fever of undetermined origin
GC	gonorrhea
HEENT	head, eyes, ears, nose, throat
Hx	history
(S)LE	(systemic) lupus erythematosus
m	murmur
MD	muscular dystrophy
MI	myocardial infarction
MS	multiple sclerosis

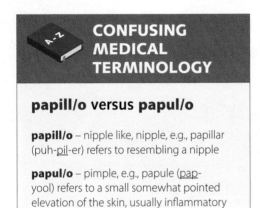

CONFUSING MEDICAL TERMINOLOGY

papill/o versus papul/o

papill/o – nipple like, nipple, e.g., papillar (puh-<u>pil</u>-er) refers to resembling a nipple

papul/o – pimple, e.g., papule (<u>pap</u>-yool) refers to a small somewhat pointed elevation of the skin, usually inflammatory but nonsupportive

Abbreviation	Definition
P & A	percussion and auscultation
PE	physical examination
PERRLA	pupils equal, round, react to light, and accommodation (eyes)
PH	past history
PI	present illness
PID	pelvic inflammatory disease
PTSD	post-traumatic stress disorder
RA	rheumatoid arthritis
R/O	rule out
Rx	recipe, take, prescription
SOB	short of breath
SR or ROS	systemic review or review of systems
Sx	symptoms
T & A	tonsillectomy and adenoidectomy
TIA	transient ischemic attack
TPR	temperature, pulse, respiration
URI	upper respiratory infection
UTI	urinary tract infection

LABORATORY ABBREVIATIONS

Abbreviations used in a laboratory are listed in **Tables 8-2**.

TABLE **8-2** Laboratory Abbreviations	
Abbreviation	**Definition**
AFB	acid-fast bacillus (tuberculosis organism)
C & S	culture and sensitivity
CATH	catheterize
CBC	complete blood count
Crit, Hct	hematocrit

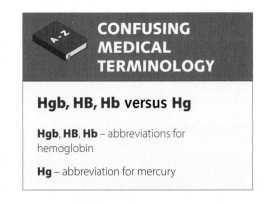

CONFUSING MEDICAL TERMINOLOGY

Hgb, HB, Hb versus Hg

Hgb, **HB**, **Hb** – abbreviations for hemoglobin

Hg – abbreviation for mercury

(continues)

TABLE **8-2** (continued)

Abbreviation	Definition
diff	differential
ESR	erythrocyte sedimentation rate
FBS	fasting blood sugar
GTT	glucose tolerance test
Hb, Hgb	hemoglobin
RA	rheumatoid arthritis
RBC	red blood (cell) count (erythrocytes); red blood cells
STS	serologic test of syphilis
VDRL	venereal disease research laboratory
WBC	white blood (cell) count (leukocytes); white blood cells

A LIST OF COMMON DIAGNOSTIC AND LABORATORY ABBREVIATIONS

Some of the more commonly used abbreviations in diagnostics and in the laboratory are listed in **Tables 8-3**.

TABLE **8-3** A List of Common Diagnostic and Laboratory Abbreviations*

Name of Test, Screening, Procedure, or Others	Explanatory Notes
cardio CRP™ (high-sensitivity C-reactive protein)	as stated in name
cervical biopsy	as stated in name
chlamydia tests	sexually transmitted diseases (STDs)
chloride (Cl)	blood/chemistry tests
cholesterol and triglycerides tests	blood/chemistry tests
chromosome analysis	as stated in name
CK (creatine kinase)	as stated in name
colon biopsy	as stated in name
colorectal cancer screen	as stated in name
complete blood count (CBC)	blood/chemistry tests
creatinine and creatinine clearance	blood/chemistry tests

Name of Test, Screening, Procedure, or Others	Explanatory Notes
C-reactive protein	as stated in name
cystic fibrosis test	screening
esophageal biopsy	as stated in name
fecal occult blood test	as stated in name
ferritin	blood/chemistry tests
folic acid	blood/chemistry tests
follicle-stimulating hormone (FSH)	as stated in name
glycohemoglobin (GHb)	as stated in name
gonorrhea test	sexually transmitted diseases (STDs)
Helicobacter pylori (H. pylori) tests	as stated in name
hemoglobin (part of CBC)	as stated in name
hepatitis B antigen and antibody tests	sexually transmitted diseases (STDs)
hepatitis C genotype	as stated in name
hepatitis C viral load	as stated in name
hepatitis C virus test	as stated in name
herpes test	sexually transmitted diseases (STDs)
HIV testing	sexually transmitted diseases (STDs)
HIV viral load	as stated in name
homocysteine	as stated in name
HPV test (human papillomavirus)	sexually transmitted diseases (STDs)
human chorionic gonadotropin (hCG)	blood/chemistry tests
iron tests	blood/chemistry tests
lactic dehydrogenase (LDH)	blood/chemistry tests
lead	as stated in name
luteinizing hormone (LH)	as stated in name
magnesium (Mg)	blood/chemistry tests
maternal serum screening: alpha-fetoprotein (AFP) in blood estrogens, human chorionic gonadotropin (hCG), and maternal serum triple test	blood/chemistry tests

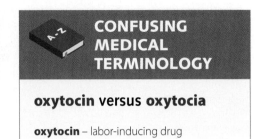

CONFUSING MEDICAL TERMINOLOGY

oxytocin versus oxytocia

oxytocin – labor-inducing drug

oxytocia – rapid birth

(continues)

TABLE **8-3** (continued)

Name of Test, Screening, Procedure, or Others	Explanatory Notes
osteoporosis/bone mineral density testing	as stated in name
ovarian cancer	as stated in name
Pap test	as stated in name
parathyroid hormone (bio-intact PTH)	as stated in name
partial thromboplastin time (PTT)	as stated in name
phosphorus: phosphate in blood and in urine	blood/urine chemistry tests
potassium (K)	blood/chemistry tests
progesterone	as stated in name
prolactin	as stated in name
prostate biopsy	as stated in name
prostate-specific antigen (PSA)	as stated in name
prothrombin time (PT)	as stated in name
rheumatoid factor (RF)	as stated in name
rubella test	as stated in name
sedimentation rate	as stated in name
sickle cell testing	as stated in name
skin biopsy	as stated in name
sodium (Na)	blood/chemistry tests
stomach biopsy	as stated in name
syphilis tests	sexually transmitted diseases (STDs)
testosterone	as stated in name
thyroid hormone tests (T-3 total; T-3 uptake; T-4 total [thyroxine])	blood/chemistry tests
total serum protein and/or albumin	blood/chemistry tests
TSH	blood/chemistry tests
uric acid: uric acid in blood and in urine	blood/chemistry tests
urine test	as stated in name
vitamin B12	as stated in name

* This list is provided here for reference only. The instructor may choose examples for discussion or testing.

CLINICAL
Note

Radiology Report

Patient: Betty Street

Age: 79 years

Sex: F

Diagnosis: Cervical **FX**

Date: 09/15/2017

Bone Scan: Total body

Whole body skeletal survey on the A/P views 3 hours after intravenous injection of 20 mCi of Tc99m-MDP in a 79-year-old woman with a **Hx** of a fall and back pain.

Findings: On the whole body survey, there are some degenerative changes in the **lower T-spine** and **lower L-vertebrae**. A **bony focus** distinctive of metastatic disease or recent compression FX is not seen. There is abnormality of the right **superior** and **inferior** pubic rami consistent with traumatic fractures.

Summary: Bone scan demonstrating degenerative changes and abnormality of the right superior and inferior pubic rami consistent with traumatic fractures.

Read by Radiologist/M. Arter MD
09/15/2017

Direction: For the portions of the clinical note shown by a colored font, provide the definition and/or words for abbreviation.

LESSON TWO   **Progress Check**

IDENTIFY THE DISEASE

Identify the following diseases or conditions from the diagnostic abbreviations given:

1. ASHD _____

2. CHD _____

3. CHF _____

4. CVD _____

5. CVA _____

6. CBS _____

7. COPD _____

8. MI _____

9. PTSD _____

10. RA _____

11. TIA _____

12. STDs _____

SHORT ANSWER

To what *procedure* do the following abbreviations refer?

1. A & P _____

2. PERRLA _____

3. P & A _____

4. R/O _____

5. SR _____

6. T & A _____

7. PE _____

8. Rx _____

9. HEENT _____

10. Dx _____

11. RBC _____

MATCHING

Match the laboratory abbreviation to its descriptive term:

Abbreviation	Description
1. Hct	**a.** Test for abnormal blood sugar levels
2. C & S	**b.** Test for blood sugar level before eating
3. ESR	**c.** Test for volume of packed red cells
4. FBS	**d.** Test for iron-containing red blood cells
5. GTT	**e.** Count of both white and red blood cells
6. CBC	**f.** Determination of rate of settling of red blood cells
7. AFB	**g.** Test for tuberculosis organism
8. Hb	**h.** Culture for organism sensitivity
9. EEG	**i.** Bathroom privileges
10. qns	**j.** Right eye
11. dc	**k.** Examination under anesthesia
12. decubitus	**l.** Out of bed
13. CAT	**m.** Electroencephalogram
14. OD	**n.** Computerized axial tomography
15. DOA	**o.** X-ray study taken in a lying position
16. OOB	**p.** Inadequate quantity
17. BRP	**q.** Discontinue
18. EUA	**r.** Dead on arrival

DEFINE THE ABBREVIATION

Define the following abbreviations commonly used by medical personnel to speed up their charting in the patient's record:

1. CC _____

2. c/o _____

3. FH _____

4. FUO _____

5. Hx _____

6. SOB _____

7. URI _____

8. UTI _____

9. m _____

10. PI _____

11. Sx _____

12. PH _____

Review

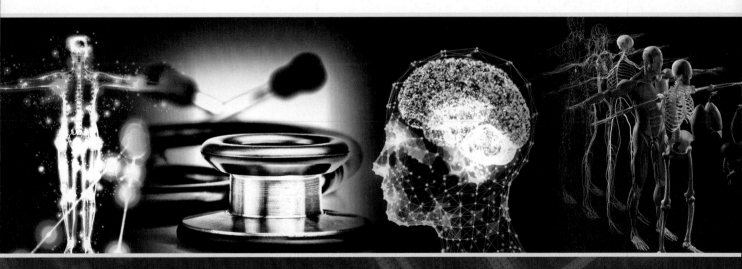

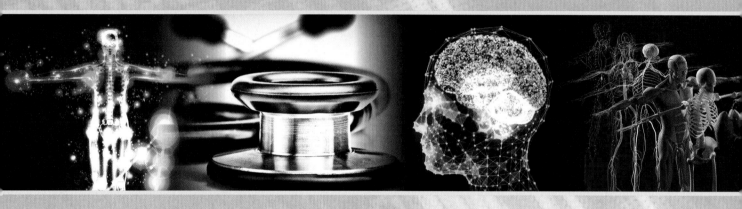

© teekid/iStock/Getty Images

Review of Word Parts from Units I, II, and III

OBJECTIVES

After completing this chapter and the exercises, the student should be able to:

1. Define the meaning of given word elements.
2. Define whole medical terms by applying knowledge gained from previous study.
3. Recognize the meaning of new terms by dividing them into their respective elements.

This chapter is designed to assist you by pulling together the terminology to reinforce your learning. These exercises are designed as learning tools. They give you the opportunity to write in your answers and test yourself. Check your answers carefully against the information contained in the previous three units. You also may use your medical dictionary. Check your spelling of the terms because spelling is very important to the meaning of medical words.

If you have audiotapes with your text, listen to each term for the correct pronunciation and repeat the word out loud several times so you will be comfortable using it in conversation.

LESSON ONE	Materials to Be Learned

REVIEW A: SUFFIXES

Write the meaning of each suffix in the space provided in **Table 9-1**.

TABLE 9-1 Review A: Suffixes

Suffix	Meaning
-algia	
-ceie	
-dynia	
-ectasis	
-emia	
-gen	
-gram	
-graph	
-graphy	
-gravid	
-iasis	
-it is	
-logy	
-malacia	
-megaly	
-oid	
-oma	
-pathy	
-penia	
-phagia	
-phasia	
-phobia	
-plegia	

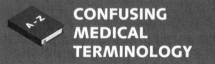

CONFUSING MEDICAL TERMINOLOGY

trop/o versus troph/o

trop/o or tropo – turn, turning, change, e.g., tropocollagen (tro-po-<u>col</u>-la-gen) refers to the molecular component of a collagen fiber, consisting of three polypeptide chains coiled around each other; e.g., tropism (troh-piz-<u>uhm</u>) refers to an orientation (movement or bending) of an organism to an external stimulus (i.e., light, heat, gravity) especially by growth rather than by movement

troph/o – relation to nutrition, nourishment, development, growth, e.g., trophoplasm (<u>tra</u>-fo-plae-zem) refers to a type of protoplasm that provides nourishment to a cell

Suffix	Meaning
-ptosis	
-rrhage	
-rrhexis	
-sclerosis	
-scopy	
-sis	
-spasm	
-stasis	

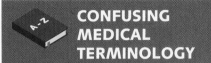

CONFUSING MEDICAL TERMINOLOGY

per- versus peri- versus pre-

per- – excessive, through, e.g., pertussis (per-<u>tus</u>-is) refers to the medical form for whooping cough, a respiratory infection caused by the bacteria *Bordetella pertussis*, marked by a peculiar cough ending in a prolonged crowing or whooping respiration

peri- – around, surrounding, e.g., periatrial (per-re-<u>a</u>-tre-al) refers to the area surrounding or around the atrium of the heart

pre- – before, in front of, e.g., premenstrual (pre-<u>men</u>-stroo-uh-al) refers to the one or two days before the menstrual period

REVIEW B: PREFIXES

Write the meaning of each prefix in the space provided in **Table 9-2**.

TABLE **9-2** Review B: Prefixes	
Prefix	**Meaning**
a-, an-	
ab-	
ad-	
aero-	
aniso-	
bi-	
brady-	
de-	
di-	
dia-	
dif-, dis-	
dys-	
ec-, ecto-	

(continues)

TABLE **9-2** (continued)	
Prefix	**Meaning**
end-, endo-	
ep-, epi-	
eu-	
ex-, exo-	
extra-	
hemi-	
hemo-	
hetero-	
homo-	
hyper-	
hypo-	
in-	
iso-	
lip-	
mal-	
mega-	
megalo-	
meno-	
meta-	
noct-	
nyct-	
pan-	
para-	
per-	
peri-	
poly-	
post-	
pre-	

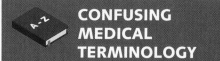

CONFUSING MEDICAL TERMINOLOGY

peritone/o versus perone/o versus perine/o

peritone/o – membrane that lines the abdominal cavity, peritoneum, e.g., peritoneal (per-rih-<u>to</u>-ne-al) refers to pertaining to peritoneum

perone/o – fibula, e.g., perone (puh-<u>rohn</u>) refers to the small bone of the arm or leg, the fibula

perine/o – the space between the anus and external reproductive organs, perineum, e.g., episioperineoplasty (<u>ep</u>-iz-e-o-peh-rih-ne-o-plas-te) refers to plastic repair of the vulva and perineum

Prefix	Meaning
pro-	
pyo-	
pyro-	
re-	
super-	
supra-	
syn-	
tachy-	

REVIEW C: ROOT WORDS FOR BODY PARTS

Many of the words in this section have been introduced in previous chapters. They should serve as a small review of root words.

Cover the definitions in the last column of **Table 9-3** and try to define the term before looking at the answer by using your previous knowledge of word parts. A short definition is okay. The answer column contains a more detailed definition, but your answer may contain just the essential meaning of the word at this time.

TABLE 9-3 Review C: Root Words for Body Parts

Root Word	Meaning	Word Example	Pronunciation	Definition
carp/o	wrist	metacarpal	met´-ah-kar-pal	the bones between the wrist and fingers
celi/o	abdomen			see *lapar/o*
cervic/o	neck	cervical	serv-i-cal	pertaining to the neck or to the cervix
		cervix (of uterus)	ser-viks	the narrow lower end (neck) of the uterus
chondr/o	cartilage	chondritis	kon-dri-tis	inflammation of a cartilage
colp/o	vagina	colpitis	kol-pi-tis	inflammation of the vagina; vaginitis
dent/o-odont	teeth	dentist	den-tist	a person who has received a degree in dentistry and is authorized to practice dentistry
		orthodontia	or-tho-don-ti-a	the branch of dentistry concerned with correcting and preventing irregularities of the teeth
esophag/o	esophagus	esophagitis	e-sof´-ah-ji-tis	inflammation of the esophagus
lapar/o	abdominal wall	laparotomy	lap´-ah-rot-o-me	incision through the flank or, more generally, through any part of the abdominal wall

(continues)

TABLE 9-3 (*continued*)

Root Word	Meaning	Word Example	Pronunciation	Definition
laryng/o	larynx	**laryng**itis	lar´-in-<u>ji</u>-tis	inflammation of the larynx
myring/o	myringo (eardrum)	**myring**otomy	mir´-ing-<u>got</u>-o-me	incision of the tympanic membrane; tympanotomy
onych/o	nail	par**onych**ia	par´-o-<u>nik</u>-e-ah	inflammation in the folds of the tissue around the fingernail
oophor/o	ovary	**oophor**ectomy	o´-of-o-<u>rek</u>-to-me	excision of one or both ovaries
ophthalm/o	eye	**ophthalm**ologist	of´-thal-<u>mol</u>-o-jist	a physician who specializes in diseases of the eyes
pancreat/o	pancreas	**pancreat**itis	pan´-kre-ah-<u>ti</u>-tis	inflammation of the pancreas
pelv/i	pelvis	**pelv**imeter	pel-<u>vim</u>-e-ter	an instrument for measuring the pelvis
phleb/o	vein	**phleb**itis	fle-<u>bi</u>-tis	inflammation of a vein
pleur/o	pleura	**pleur**isy	<u>ploor</u>-i-se	inflammation of the pleura
pod/o	foot	**pod**iatry	po-<u>di</u>-ah-tre	specialized field dealing with the treatment and care of the foot
psych/o	mind	**psych**iatrist	si-<u>ki</u>-ah-trist	a physician who specializes in treatment of the mind
pub/o	pubes (pubic bones)	supra**pub**ic	soo´-prah-<u>pu</u>-bik	above the pubes
rhin/o	nose	**rhin**oplasty	<u>ri</u>-no-plas´-te	plastic surgery of the nose
salping/o	fallopian tube or Eustachian tube	**salping**itis	sal´-pin-<u>ji</u>-tis	inflammation of the uterine or auditory tube
soma	body	psycho**soma**tic	si´-ko-so-<u>mat</u>-ik	pertaining to the mind–body relationship; having bodily symptoms of psychic, emotional, or mental origin
splen/o	spleen	**splen**ectomy	sple-<u>nek</u>-to-me	excision of the spleen
spondyl/o	vertebra	**spondyl**itis	spon´-di-<u>li</u>-tis	inflammation of the vertebrae
stomat/o	mouth	**stomat**itis	sto´-mah-<u>ti</u>-tis	generalized inflammation of the oral mucosa
tars/o	ankle	meta**tars**al	met´-ah-<u>tar</u>-sal	bones between the ankle and toes
thorac/o	thorax (chest)	**thorac**entesis	tho´-rah-sen-<u>te</u>-sis	surgical puncture of the chest wall into the parietal cavity for aspiration of fluids
tympan/o	tympanum (eardrum or middle ear)	**tympan**otomy	tim´-pah-<u>not</u>-o-me	incision of the tympanic membrane
ureter/o	ureter	**ureter**itis	u-re´-ter-<u>i</u>-tis	inflammation of a ureter

Root Word	Meaning	Word Example	Pronunciation	Definition
urethr/o	urethra	**urethr**itis	u´-re-<u>thri</u>-tis	inflammation of the urethra
vas/o	vessel	cardio**vas**cular	kar´-de-o-<u>vas</u>-ku-lar	pertaining to the heart and blood vessels
ven/o	vein	intra**ven**ous	in´-trah-<u>ve</u>-nus	within a vein

REVIEW D: DESCRIPTIVE WORD ELEMENTS

Cover the definitions in the last column of **Table 9-4** and try to define the term before looking at the answer by using your previous knowledge of descriptive word elements. A short definition is okay. The answer column contains a more detailed definition, but your answer may contain just the essential meaning of the word at this time.

TABLE 9-4 Review D: Descriptive Word Elements

Root Word	Meaning	Word Example	Pronunciation	Definition
ankyl/o	stiffening or fusion	**ankyl**osis	ang´-ki-<u>lo</u>-sis	immobility and consolidation of a joint from disease, injury, or surgical procedure
carcin/o	cancer (malignancy)	**carcin**oma	kar´-si-<u>no</u>-mah	a malignant new growth made up of epithelial cells that may infiltrate surrounding tissues
cry/o	cold	**cry**osurgery	kri´-o-<u>ser</u>-jer-e	the destruction of tissue by application of extreme cold
crypt/o	hidden (small hidden sac)	**crypt**orchidism	krip-<u>tor</u>-ki-dism	failure of one or both testes to descend into the scrotum
esthesia	feeling	an**esthesia**	an´-es-<u>the</u>-ze-ah	loss of feeling or sensation, especially the loss of pain sensation induced to permit surgery
gravid/o	pregnant	primi**gravid**a	pri´-mi-<u>grav</u>-i-dah	a woman pregnant for the first time, gravida I
lip/o	fat	**lip**oma	li-<u>po</u>-mah	a benign fatty tumor
lith/o	stone	chole**lith**iasis	ko´-le-li-<u>thi</u>-ah-sis	the presence or formation of gallstones
necr/o	dead (decayed)	**necr**osis	ne-<u>kro</u>-sis	cell death: it may affect groups of cells or part of a structure or an organ
par-	to bear (children)	multi**par**a	mul-<u>tip</u>-ah-rah	a woman who has had two or more pregnancies
path/o	disease state	osteo**path**y	os´-te-<u>op</u>-ah-the	any disease of a bone
phag/o-phagia	eating, swallowing	dys**phag**ia	dis-<u>fa</u>-je-ah	difficulty in swallowing

(continues)

TABLE 9-4 (continued)

Root Word	Meaning	Word Example	Pronunciation	Definition
-phasia	speech	a**phasia**	ah-<u>fa</u>-zhe-ah	defect or loss of the power of expression by speech, writing, or signs or of comprehending spoken or written language, caused by injury or disease of the brain centers
phon/o	voice	a**phon**ia	a-<u>fo</u>-ne-ah	loss of voice; inability to produce vocal sounds
schiz/o	split	**schiz**ophrenia	skit´-so-<u>fre</u>-ne-ah	any of a group of severe emotional disorders characterized by withdrawal from reality, delusions, hallucinations, and bizarre behavior
scler/o	hardening	arterio**scler**osis	ar-te´-re-o´-skle-<u>ro</u>-sis	hardening and thickening of the walls of arterioles
sta	slowed, halted, controlled	hemo**sta**sis	he´-mo-<u>sta</u>-sis	the arrest of bleeding, either by vasoconstriction and coagulation or by surgical means
therap	treatment	psycho**therapy**	si-ko-<u>ther</u>-ah-pe	treatment designed to produce a response by mental rather than physical effects
therm/o	heat	**therm**ometer	ther-<u>mom</u>-e-ter	an instrument for determining temperatures
thromb/o	clot, lump	**thromb**osis	throm-<u>bo</u>-sis	the formation or presence of a thrombus (clot)
traumat/o	injury, wound, damage from an external source	**traumat**openea	<u>traw</u>-ma-top-ne´-ah	passage of air through a wound in the chest wall

REVIEW E: ADDITIONAL MEDICAL TERMS

Review E, on additional medical terms, contains some words with which you will not be familiar. Test your ability to recognize the meaning of new medical terms by covering the definition column on the right side of **Table 9-5**, dividing the word into its respective parts, and seeing if you can define it before you look at the answer.

TABLE 9-5 Review E: Additional Medical Terms

Word	Pronunciation	Definition
abdomen	<u>ab</u>-do´-men	that part of the body lying between the thorax and the pelvis and containing the abdominal cavity and viscera
abdominal	ab-<u>dom</u>-i-nal	pertaining to the abdomen
abortion	ah-<u>bor</u>-shun	expulsion from the uterus of the products of conception before the fetus is viable
abscess	<u>ab</u>-ses	a localized collection of pus in a cavity formed by disintegration of tissues
acute	ah-<u>kut</u>	sharp; having severe symptoms and a short course
adhesion	ad-<u>he</u>-zhun	stuck together; abnormal joining of parts to one another

Word	Pronunciation	Definition
adnexa	ad-<u>nek</u>-sah	accessory structures of an organ: of the eye, including the eyelids and tear ducts; of the uterus, including the uterine tubes and ovaries
anomaly	ah-<u>nom</u>-ah-le	marked deviation from normal, especially as a result of congenital or hereditary defects
auscultation	aws´-kul-<u>ta</u>-shun	listening for sounds within the body, chiefly to detect conditions of the thorax, abdominal viscera, or a pregnancy
autoclave	<u>aw</u>-to-klav	a self-locking apparatus for sterilization of materials by steam under pressure
axilla (axillary)	ak-<u>sil</u>-ah	the armpit
biopsy	<u>bi</u>-op-se	removal and examination, usually microscopic, of tissue from the living body, performed to establish precise diagnosis
catgut	<u>kat</u>-gut	an absorbable, sterile strand obtained from collagen derived from healthy mammals used to suture
catheter	<u>kath</u>-e-ter	a tubular, flexible instrument passed through body cavities for withdrawal of fluids from (or introduction of fluids into) a body cavity
cervical	<u>ser</u>-vi-kal	pertaining to the neck or to the cervix
chronic	<u>kron</u>-ik	persisting for a long time
coccyx	<u>kok</u>-siks	triangular bone formed usually by fusion of last four vertebrae; the "tailbone"
congenital	kon-<u>jen</u>-i-tal	existing at the time of birth
defibrillator	de-fib´-ri-<u>la</u>-tor	an electronic apparatus used to produce defibrillation by application of brief electric shock to the heart directly or through electrodes placed on the chest wall
dilatation	dil´-ah-<u>ta</u>-shun	the condition of being stretched open beyond normal dimensions
dilation	di-<u>la</u>-shun	the act of dilating or stretching
edema	e-<u>de</u>-mah	an abnormal accumulation of fluid in intercellular spaces of the body (**Figure 9-1**)
embolus	<u>em</u>-bo-lus	a clot or other plug brought by the blood from another vessel and forced into a smaller one, thus obstructing the circulation
emesis	<u>em</u>-e-sis	the act of vomiting; also used as a word termination, as in hematemesis
enema	<u>en</u>-e-mah	introduction of fluid into the rectum for evacuation of feces or as a means of introducing nutrient or medicinal substances, or the opaque material used in roentgenographic examination of the lower intestinal tract (BE)
exacerbation	eg-zas´-er-<u>ba</u>-shun	increase in severity of a disease or any of its symptoms
excretion	eks-<u>kre</u>-shun	the act of eliminating waste
fascia	<u>fash</u>-e-ah	a sheet or band of fibrous tissue that lies deep in the skin or binds muscles and various body organs
febrile	<u>feb</u>-ril	pertaining to fever; feverish

(continues)

TABLE 9-5 (continued)

Word	Pronunciation	Definition
fibrillation	fib´-ri-la-shun	a small, local, involuntary muscular contraction caused by activation of muscle cells or fibers
hemorrhage	hem-o-rij	the escape of blood from the vessels; bleeding
icterus	ik-ter-us	jaundice
immunization	im´-u-ni-za-shun	the process of providing immunity to disease processes
incontinence	in-kon-ti-nens	inability to control bowel and bladder functions
inflammation	in´-flah-ma-shun	a protective tissue response to injury or destruction of tissues
ischemia	is-ke-me-ah	deficiency of blood in a part caused by functional constriction or actual obstruction of a blood vessel
jaundice	jawn-dis	icterus; yellowness of the skin, sclerae, mucous membranes, and excretions (**Figure 9-2**)
metastasis	me-tas-tah-sis	transfer of disease from one organ or body part to another not directly connected with it
mucus	mu-kus	the free slime of the mucous membranes composed of secretions of the glands, various salts, desquamated cells, and leukocytes
obese	o-bes	very fat; stout; corpulent
obesity	o-bes-i-te	an increase in body weight beyond the limitation of skeletal and physical requirements: the result of excessive accumulation of body fat
palpable	pal-pah-bul	felt by touching
paralysis	pah-ral-i-sis	loss or impairment of voluntary motor function
paralyzed	par-e-lizd	a condition of helplessness caused by inability to move; being ineffective or powerless
parietal	pah-ri-e-tal	pertaining to the walls of a cavity or located near the parietal bone
percussion	per-kush-un	the act of striking a part with short, sharp blows as an aid in diagnosing the condition of the underlying parts by the sound obtained
perineum	per´-i-ne-um	the pelvic floor and associated structures occupying the pelvic outlet
peritoneum	per´-i-to-ne-um	the serous membrane lining the walls of the abdominal and pelvic cavities and the contained viscera
pleura (pleural, adj.)	pleu-ra (pleu-ral)	serous membrane enveloping the lungs and lining the walls of the thoracic cavity
prolapse	pro-laps	the falling down or downward displacement of a part
prophylaxis	pro-fi-lak-sis	prevention of disease; preventive treatment
purulent	pur-roo-lent	containing or forming pus
remission	re-mish-un	having periods of abatement or of exacerbation

Word	Pronunciation	Definition
rheumatic	roo-<u>mat</u>-ik	a state of inflammation; inflammatory diseases
serous	<u>se</u>-rus	pertaining to or resembling serum
sputum	<u>spu</u>-tum	matter ejected from the trachea, bronchi, and lungs through the mouth
suture	<u>su</u>-chur	a stitch or series of stitches made to secure the edges of a surgical or traumatic wound; used also as a verb to indicate application of such stitches (**Figure 9-3**)
virus	<u>vi</u>-rus	a minute infectious agent that, with certain exceptions, is too small to be seen by microscope and is able to reproduce only within a living host cell
viscera, viscus	<u>vis</u>-er-ah, <u>vis</u>-kus	any large interior organ in any of the four great body cavities, especially those in the abdomen
void (voided)	void	to urinate

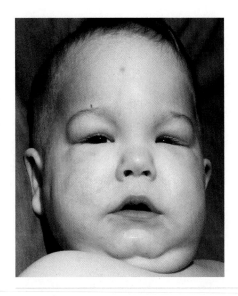

FIGURE 9-1 Edema as a result of increased capillary permeability. Note the swelling of the eyelids and face.
Courtesy of Leonard V. Crowley, MD, Century College.

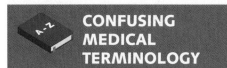

CONFUSING MEDICAL TERMINOLOGY

py/o versus pyel/o

py/o – pus, e.g., pyuria (pi-u-<u>re</u>-ah) refers to pus in the urine

pyel/o – renal pelvis, bowl of kidney, e.g., pyelostomy (<u>pi</u>-el-os-to-me) refers to the creation of an artificial opening in the renal pelvis

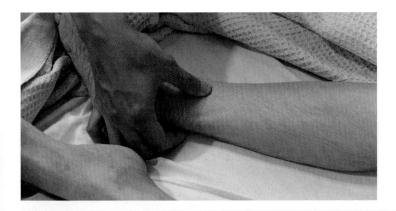

FIGURE 9-2 Jaundice
© Casa nayafana/Shutterstock.

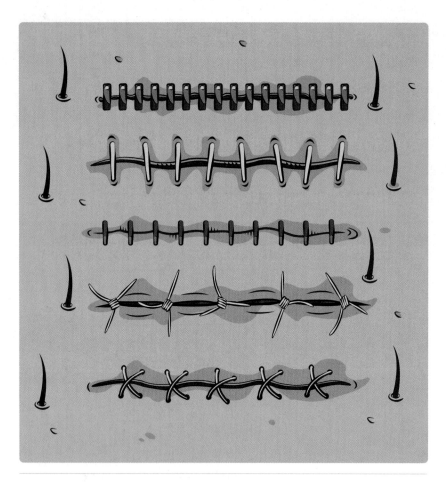

FIGURE 9-3 Sutures

© Gal Csilla/Shutterstock.

CLINICAL
Note

Review: Hospital Discharge Summary

HISTORY OF PRESENT ILLNESS: The patient is a 28 year old black male with a one week history of pain and swelling of the right index finger **distal phalanx**. The patient is a right handed copier technician. The patient had his right index distal interphalangeal joint **aspirated** earlier the day of admission. He was admitted through the **ED** as a direct admission for intravenous antibiotics

PHYSICAL EXAMINATION: This was notable for soft tissue swelling and **erythema** of the right index finger primarily over the distal phalanx but also including the middle phalanx. He was distally neurovascular intact.

LABORATORY VALUES: His **WBC** on admission was 13,600.

HOSPITAL COURSE: The patient was admitted for intravenous Oxacillin. He was discharged on March 23, 2017, after being switched to oral antibiotic. At that time, he had no erythema or **edema**. **C&S** through his stay remained negative

DISCHARGE MEDICATIONS: Augmentin, one **p.o.** q. 8 hours for seven days.

FOLLOW UP: This was scheduled with the hand clinic on Monday, March 26, 2017

Direction: For the portions of the clinical note shown by a colored font, provide the definition and/or words for abbreviation.

LESSON TWO	Progress Check

COMPARE AND CONTRAST

In the following sets of words, explain the differences by contrasting the meaning of each word:
Example: cry/o—crypto <u>cry/o means *cold*, but crypto is a term meaning *hidden*</u>

1. lipo—litho _____

2. para—pathy _____

3. phagia—phasia—phonia _____

4. schizo—sclera _____

5. thrombo—thermo—trauma _____

6. abscess—adnexa _____

7. axilla—anomaly _____

8. cervical—coccyx _____

9. edema—embolus _____

10. emesis—enema _____

11. icterus—ischemia _____

12. palpable—parietal _____

13. prolapse—prophylaxis _____

14. suture—sputum _____

15. viscera—virus _____

BUILDING MEDICAL TERMS

Recall the rule for combining vowels and the suffix that means inflammation.
Build a medical word meaning *inflammation of*:

1. A cartilage _____

2. The vagina _____

3. The larynx _____

4. Folds of tissue around a fingernail _____

5. The pancreas _____

6. A vein _____

7. An uterine tube _____

8. An Eustachian tube _____

9. The pleura _____

10. The vertebrae _____

11. The mouth and oral mucosa _____

12. A ureter _____

13. A urethra _____

14. The esophagus _____

15. A nerve _____

Build a medical word that means:

16. Loss of the power of speech _____

17. Difficulty swallowing _____

18. A malignant new growth _____

19. Cell death _____

20. A fat _____

21. Thickening of the skin _____

22. Controlling the blood flow _____

23. Any injury _____

24. Severe but short duration _____

25. A congenital defect _____

26. Persisting for a long time _____

27. A clot or a plug in the bloodstream _____

28. Vomiting _____

29. Urinating _____

30. Abnormal fluid accumulation _____

31. "Tailbone" _____

32. Vertebrae in the neck _____

33. Eliminating waste _____

34. Increased severity of disease symptoms _____

35. Inability to control bowel and bladder function _____

36. A protective tissue response to injury or destruction _____

37. Deficiency of blood in a part _____

38. Escape of blood from vessels _____

39. Transfer of a disease from one part or organ to another not directly connected _____

40. Excessive accumulation of adipose tissue _____

41. Felt by touching _____

42. Preventive treatment _____

43. Matter ejected from lungs through the mouth _____

44. An infectious agent too small to be seen by an ordinary microscope _____

45. Securing the edges of a wound with stitches _____

FILL IN

Fill in the blanks to make a complete, accurate sentence:

1. The bones between the wrist and fingers are the _____.

2. An incision through part of the abdominal wall is a(n) _____.

3. Excision of the ovaries is called a(n) _____
or a(n) _____.

4. The specialty dealing with care of the foot is called _____.

5. Plastic surgery of the nose is _____.

6. The bones between the ankle and the toes are the _____.

7. Surgical puncture of the chest wall to aspirate fluid is known as a(n) _____.

8. Failure of the testes to descend is called _____.

9. A woman pregnant for the first time is a(n) _____.

10. A woman who has had two or more pregnancies is a(n) _____.

11. Inflammation of the uterine tube is _____.

MATCHING

Match the body parts at the left to their medical terms on the right:

Body Part	**Medical Term**
1. Mind	**a.** cervical
2. Body	**b.** ophthalm/o
3. Neck	**c.** thorax
4. Wrist	**d.** soma
5. Teeth	**e.** psyche
6. Abdomen	**f.** myring/o
7. Eye	**g.** vas/o
8. Chest	**h.** carpal
9. Eardrum	**i.** celi/o
10. Blood vessel	**j.** odont

DEFINE THE TERM

Define the following terms:

1. Abortion _____

2. Auscultation _____

3. Catgut _____

4. Catheter _____

5. Dilatation _____

6. Embolus _____

7. Exacerbation _____

8. Fascia _____

9. Metastasis _____

10. Percussion _____

11. Congenital _____

SHORT ANSWER: ROOT WORDS

State the *root* word for the following body parts:

1. Wrist _____

2. Neck _____

3. Teeth _____

4. Esophagus _____

5. Abdomen _____

6. Fingernail _____

7. Eye _____

8. Pancreas _____

9. Body _____

10. Foot _____

11. Pubic bone _____

12. Nose _____

13. Mouth _____

14. Ankle _____

15. Chest _____

SHORT ANSWER: BODY PARTS

State the *body part or organ* involved in the following conditions:

1. Colpitis _____

2. Phlebitis _____

3. Pleurisy _____

4. Spondylitis _____

5. Stomatitis _____

UNIT V

Medical Terminology and Body Systems

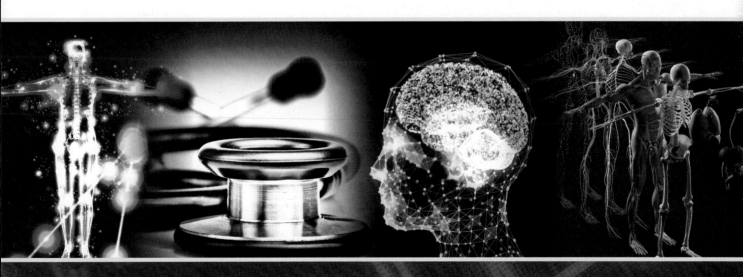

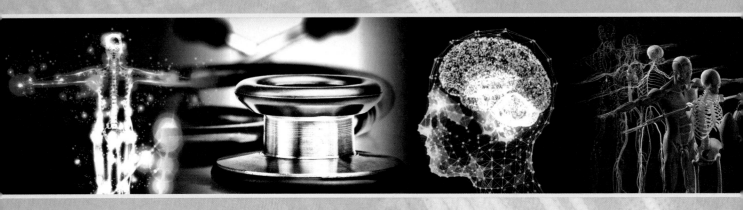

© teekid/iStock/Getty Images, © Anatomy Insider/Shutterstock, © Adrian Grosu/Shutterstock, © Hubis/Shutterstock, © Kamira/Shutterstock.

CHAPTER

10

© teekid/iStock/Getty Images

Body Organs and Parts

OBJECTIVES

After completing this chapter and the exercises, the student should be able to:

1. Identify the parts of a cell and the specialized functions of tissues.
2. Identify the body systems.
3. Describe the functions of the body systems and how they work together.
4. Define the anatomic positions of the body and directional terms used to indicate them.
5. List the body cavities and the organs contained within them.
6. Identify nine body regions.
7. Use appropriate medical terms when describing locations of various parts of the body.

This chapter focuses on the way medical terms (that you have previously learned) relate to the body as a whole. To accurately understand and communicate data from medical reports, medical personnel use topographic anatomy. *Topographic* refers to the surface landmarks of the body. They are used as guides to the internal structures that lie beneath them, as well as the major regions of the body and their locations.

To describe the position of a structure or locate one structure in relation to another, medical professionals start with a position called the anatomical position. In this position, a person is standing erect, facing you, with hands at sides and palms forward, and feet and head pointed straight ahead. This is the position you will use to find the landmarks of the body. We begin with a discussion of cells, the structural and functional unit of all living matter.

ALLIED HEALTH PROFESSIONS

Dietitians and Dietetic Technicians

Registered dietitians nutritionists (RDN) are professionals trained in applying the principles of nutrition to food selection and meal preparation. They help prevent and treat illnesses by promoting healthy eating habits, scientifically evaluating clients' diets, and suggesting diet modifications. They advise people what to eat in order to lead a healthy lifestyle or achieve a specific health-related goal. They counsel individuals and groups; set up and supervise food service systems for institutions such as schools, hospitals, and prisons; promote sound eating habits through education; and conduct research. Major areas of specialization include clinical, management, community, business and industry, and consultant dietetics. Dietitians also work as educators and researchers.

A dietetic technician, registered (DTR) works as a member of the food service, management, and healthcare team independently or in consultation with a registered dietitian. The dietetic technician supervises support staff, monitors cost control procedures, interprets and implements quality assurance procedures, counsels individuals or small groups, screens patients/clients for nutritional status, and develops nutrition care plans. The dietetic technician helps to supervise food production and service; plans menus; tests new products for use in the facility; and selects, schedules, and conducts orientation programs for personnel. The technician may also be involved in selecting personnel and providing on-the-job training. The dietetic technician obtains, evaluates, and uses dietary histories to plan nutritional care for patients. Using this information, the technician guides families and individuals in selecting food, preparing it, and planning menus based on nutritional needs. The dietetic technician has an active part in calculating nutrient intakes and dietary patterns.

INQUIRY

The Academy of Nutrition and Dietetics: www.eatright.org
Data from Cross, Nanna, and McWay, Dana. *Stanfield's Introduction to the Health Professions*, 7th ed. Burlington, MA: Jones & Bartlett Learning; 2017.

LESSON ONE | **Materials to Be Learned**

STRUCTURAL UNITS OF THE BODY

Structural units of the body can be divided into four categories: cells, tissues, organs, and systems (**Table 10-1**). *Cells* are the most basic structural unit of all living organisms, with new cells formed from preexisting cells. A group of specialized cells that are structurally and functionally similar is called *tissue*. An *organ* is a group of tissues joined in a structural unit to perform a specific function or group of functions. A *system* is a group of organs and tissues that work together to perform important functions of the body.

TABLE 10-1 Structural Units of the Body

Unit	Pronunciation	Definition
Cells		
cell	sel	minute protoplasmic masses making up organized tissue, consisting of the nucleus surrounded by cytoplasm enclosed in a cell or plasma membrane. Fundamental, structural, and functional unit of living organisms. Each cell performs functions necessary for its own life. Cells multiply by dividing; this is called mitosis
nucleus	nu-kle-us	cell nucleus; a spheroid body within a cell consisting of a thin nuclear membrane and genes or chromosomes
chromosomes	kroh´-moh-sohms	thread-like structures in the cell nucleus that control growth, repair, and reproduction of the body

Unit	Pronunciation	Definition
cytoplasm	<u>si</u>-to-plasm	the protoplasm of a cell exclusive of that of the nucleus (nucleoplasm)
cell membrane	sel <u>mem</u>-bran	a thin layer of tissue serving as the wall of a cell; selectively allows substances to pass in and out of the cell and refuses passage to others

Tissues

Unit	Pronunciation	Definition
tissue	<u>tish</u>-u	a group of similarly specialized cells that together perform certain special functions
epithelial tissue	ep´-i-<u>the</u>-le-al <u>tish</u>-u	the skin and lining surfaces that protect, absorb, and excrete
connective tissue	ko-<u>nek</u>-tiv <u>tish</u>-u	the fibrous tissue of the body that binds together and is the ground substance of the various parts and organs of the body; examples are bones, tendons, and so on
muscle tissue	<u>mus</u>-el <u>tish</u>-u	tissue that contracts; consists of striated (striped), cardiac, and smooth muscle
nerve tissue	nerv <u>tish</u>-u	a collection of nerve fibers that conduct impulses that control and coordinate body activities

Organ

Unit	Pronunciation	Definition
organ	<u>or</u>-gan	tissues arranged together to perform a specific function; these internal structures are contained within the body cavities. Some examples include the heart, lungs, and organs of digestion, such as the liver and gallbladder, and the organs of reproduction

Systems

Unit	Pronunciation	Definition
system	<u>sis</u>-tem	a set of body organs that work together for a common purpose
integumentary system	in-teg´-u-<u>men</u>-ter-e <u>sis</u>-tem	skin serves as the external covering of the body; accessory organs of this system are nails, hair, and oil and sweat glands
musculoskeletal system	mus´-ku-lo-<u>skel</u>-e-tal <u>sis</u>-tem	skeleton and muscles: the 206 bones, the joints, cartilage, ligaments, and all the muscles of the body
cardiovascular system	kar´-de-o-<u>vas</u>-ku-lar <u>sis</u>-tem	heart and blood vessels; blood pumped and circulated through the body
gastrointestinal system	gas´-tro-in-tes-ti-nal <u>sis</u>-tem	a long tube commonly called the GI tract; consists of mouth, esophagus, stomach, and intestines; accessory organs are pancreas, liver, gallbladder, and salivary glands
respiratory system	re-spi-rah-to´-re <u>sis</u>-tem	nose, pharynx, larynx, trachea, bronchi, and lungs; furnishes oxygen, removes carbon dioxide (respiration)
genitourinary system	jen´-i-to-u-re-ner´-e <u>sis</u>-tem	reproductive and urinary organs, also called urogenital system (GU or UG). The urinary organs are the kidneys, ureters, bladder, and urethra; the reproductive organs are the gonads and various external genitalia and internal organs
endocrine system	en-do-krin <u>sis</u>-tem	glands and other structures that make hormones and release them directly into the circulatory system; ductless glands
nervous system	ner-vus <u>sis</u>-tem	brain and spinal cord make up the central nervous system (CNS); the autonomic nervous system (ANS) or the peripheral nervous system consists of 12 pairs of cranial nerves and 31 pairs of spinal nerves
lymphatic system	lim-<u>fa</u>-tik <u>sis</u>-tem	includes lymphatic vessels which permeate the body and serve to fight infection

BODY CAVITIES AND PLANES

Body cavities are hollow spaces containing body organs. Refer to **Figures 10-1, 10-2, 10-3** and **Table 10-2** when studying body cavities and planes. The body has two main large cavities that contain the internal body organs—the *ventral* and *dorsal* cavities. Each of these cavities is further divided into smaller cavities that contain specific organs. *Ventral* refers to the front or belly portion of the body and *dorsal* refers to the back portion of the body. *Body planes* are imaginary flat surfaces that divide and are used in anatomic diagrams.

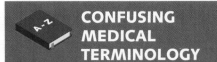

CONFUSING MEDICAL TERMINOLOGY

palpebrate versus palpate versus palpitate

palpebrate – blink or wink, e.g., palpebrate (pal-pee-<u>brit</u>) refers to winking

palpate – touch, e.g., palpate (<u>pal</u>-peyt) refers to the examination or exploring by touching (an organ or area of the body), usually as a diagnostic aid

palpitate – pulsate, quiver, throb, tremble, e.g., palpitate (<u>pal</u>-pi-teyt) as in "his heart palpitates wildly"

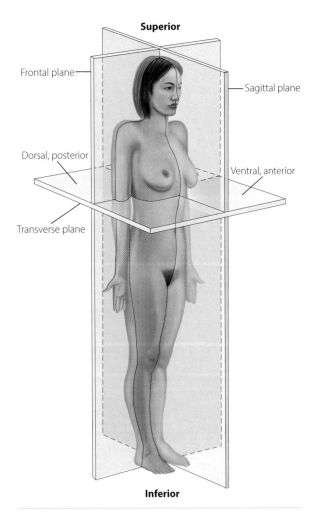

FIGURE 10-1 Body planes and directions

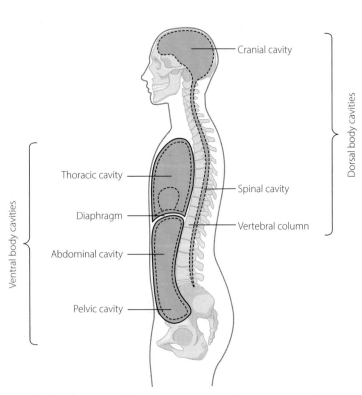

FIGURE 10-2 Sagittal section of the body, showing the dorsal and ventral body cavities

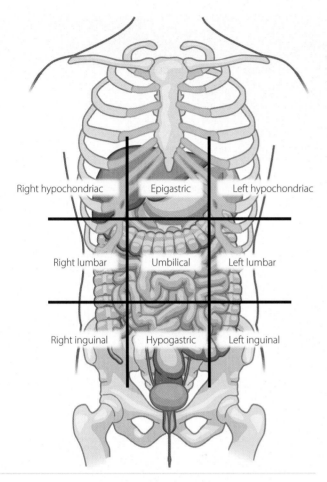

Right hypochondriac   Epigastric   Left hypochondriac

Right lumbar   Umbilical   Left lumbar

Right inguinal   Hypogastric   Left inguinal

FIGURE 10-3 Abdominal regions

A-Z **CONFUSING MEDICAL TERMINOLOGY**

cyt/o versus cyst/o

cyt/o – cell, e.g., cytoplasm (<u>sahy</u>-tuh-plazuhm) refers to the gelatinous fluid outside the nucleus

cyst/o – bladder of a sac, urinary bladder, cyst, sac of fluid, e.g., cystoplasty (sis-to-<u>plas</u>-te) refers to plastic repair of the bladder

TABLE 10-2 Body Cavities and Planes

Term	Pronunciation	Definition
Body Cavities		
body cavities		hollow spaces containing body organs
abdominal cavity	ab-<u>dom</u>-uh-nl <u>kav</u>-i-te	the cavity beneath the thoracic cavity that is separated from the thoracic cavity by the diaphragm; contains the liver, gallbladder, spleen, stomach, pancreas, intestines, and kidneys
pelvic cavity	<u>pel</u>-vik <u>kav</u>-i-te	the lower front cavity of the body located beneath the abdominal cavity; contains the urinary bladder and reproductive organs
pleural cavity	<u>pleu</u>´-ral <u>kav</u>-i-te	the thoracic cavity containing the lungs, trachea, esophagus, and thymus gland
thoracic cavity	tho-<u>rass</u>-ik <u>kav</u>-i-te	the chest cavity, which contains the lungs, heart, aorta, esophagus, and trachea
mediastinum	me´-de-ah-<u>sti</u>-num	the mass of tissues and organs separating the sternum in front and the vertebral column behind, containing the heart and its large vessels

(continues)

TABLE **10-2** (continued)

Term	Pronunciation	Definition
peritoneal cavity	per´-i-to-<u>ne</u>-al <u>kav</u>-i-te	the space containing the stomach, intestines, liver, gallbladder, pancreas, spleen, reproductive organs, and urinary bladder
cranial cavity	<u>kra</u>-ne-al <u>kav</u>-i-te	space enclosed by skull bones containing the brain
spinal cavity	<u>spi</u>-nal <u>kav</u>-i-te	cavity containing the spinal cord
diaphragm	<u>di</u>-ah-fram	dome-shaped muscle separating the abdominal and thoracic cavities
Body Planes		
body planes		imaginary flat surfaces that divide (used in anatomic diagrams)
sagittal	<u>saj</u>-i-tal	a sagittal plane divides the body into right and left portions
midsagittal	mid-<u>saj</u>-i-tal	a plane that vertically divides the body or some part of it into equal right and left portions (medial)
coronal	ko-<u>ro</u>-nal	also called frontal; a plane that divides the body into anterior and posterior sections (front and back)
transverse	trans-<u>vers</u>	a plane that divides the body into superior and inferior sections (top and bottom)

METABOLISM AND HOMEOSTASIS

There are two important terms in medicine that have general application (**Table 10-3**). A metabolism is important because it releases the energy required for a body to function. Homeostasis allows the body to maintain a stable internal environment despite changes in external conditions.

TABLE **10-3** Metabolism and Homeostasis

Term	Pronunciation	Definition
metabolism	me-<u>tab</u>-o-lizm	sum of the body's physical and chemical processes that convert food into elements for body growth, energy, building body parts (anabolism), and degrading body substances for recycling or excretion (catabolism)
homeostasis	ho´-me-o-<u>sta</u>-sis	a steady state: the tendency of stability in the normal physiologic systems of the organism to maintain a balance optimal for survival. Body temperature, osmotic pressure, normal cell division rate, and nutrient supply to cells are a few examples

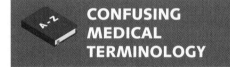

CONFUSING MEDICAL TERMINOLOGY

perionychium versus paronychia

perionychium – structure that surrounds the nail, e.g., perionychium (per-ee-oh-<u>nik</u>-ee-uhm) refers to the epidermis surrounding the base and sides of a fingernail or toenail

paronychia – infection of the nail, e.g., paronychia (par-uh-<u>nik</u>-ee-uh) refers to inflammation of the epidermis (folds of skin) bordering a nail of a finger or toe, usually characterized by infection and pus formation

CLINICAL
Note

Dietician Note

As per the **gastroenterologist's** request, I examined today a 23-year-old Caucasian female who has tested positive for **celiac disease** and **anemia**. The patient has abdominal bloating and pain, chronic **diarrhea** with pale, foul-smelling stool. Low **BMI** 17.5. I have reviewed the dietary restrictions with the patient to include a strict **GFD**. Patient has been given information for celiac disease support groups as well as a schedule for gluten-free meal planning at this hospital. Patient acknowledges instructions and appears to understand the severity of her condition as well as the need for strict dietary changes. Will schedule an outpatient follow-up visit for 6 weeks from now to review progress and persistence of symptoms.

Barbara Shear, **RDN**
<electronic Signature on file>

Direction: For the portions of the clinical note shown by a colored font, provide the definition and/or words for abbreviation.

LESSON TWO   Progress Check

SPELLING AND DEFINITION

Spell and *list* the parts of each of these body systems:

1. Serves as a covering:

   _____ system. Consists of _____

   _____ .

2. Pumps and circulates blood:

   _____ system. Consists of _____ .

   _____

3. Bones and muscles:

   _____ system. Consists of _____ .

   _____

4. A long tube for input of nutrients and excretion of solid wastes:

   _____ system. Consists of _____

   _____ .

5. Furnishes oxygen and removes carbon dioxide:

   _____ system. Consists of _____

   _____ .

6. Permeates the body and serves to fight infection:

   _____ system. Consists of _____ .

   _____ .

7. Reproductive organs and liquid waste disposal:

_____ system. Consists of _____

_____ .

8. Makes hormones and releases them directly into the blood:

_____ system. Consists of _____

_____ .

9. Controls all thought and movement:

_____ system. Consists of _____

_____ .

FILL IN

Fill in the blanks to make a complete, accurate sentence:

1. The _____ is the functional unit of all living organisms.

2. The function of the nucleus is to furnish _____ material.

3. Cell division is called _____ .

4. When cells divide, they are really _____ .

5. The wall of the cell is called a(n) _____ .

6. When groups of cells have specialized functions they are called _____ .

7. The skin and lining surfaces that protect, absorb, and excrete are _____ .

8. The fibrous bonds that are the ground substance of various parts are called _____ .

9. Groups of cells that contract are _____ .

10. Those fibers that conduct impulses are _____ .

11. A body part that performs special functions is called a(n) _____ .

12. When a set of body parts works together for a common purpose it is called _____ .

13. The space that contains body organs is called a(n) _____ .

14. Imaginary flat surfaces that divide the human anatomy are called _____ .

15. The _____ separates the abdomen from the lungs.

16. Thread-like structures in the cell nucleus that control growth, repair, and reproduction are called _____ .

17. Accessory organs of the GI tract are the _____, _____,
_____ , and _____ .

DEFINITIONS

1. Metabolism _____

_____

2. Homeostasis _____

_____

SHORT ANSWER

1. Name the four types of specialized body tissues and one major function of each:

a. _____

b. _____

c. _____

d. _____

2. What is the function of a *cell membrane*?

_____

3. Of what does a *cell nucleus* consist?

_____

4. Why is a *metabolism* important?

_____

5. What does *homeostasis* do?

_____

CHAPTER 11

© teekid/iStock/Getty Images

Integumentary System

OBJECTIVES

After completing this chapter and the exercises, the student should be able to:

1. Identify the structures of the skin and accessory organs.
2. List and describe the five functions of the skin.
3. Identify and describe the lesions and pathologic conditions that affect the integumentary system.
4. Describe clinical procedures used in diagnosing and treating skin disorders.
5. Identify and define commonly used vocabulary terms that pertains to the skin.

THE INTEGUMENTARY SYSTEM

The skin and its accessory organs are called the *integumentary system*. The *integument* (skin) is a vital organ serving as a protective barrier that responds to internal and external stimuli and contributes to the maintenance of homeostasis. The integument forms the outer covering of the body. It consists of the skin and certain specialized tissues. Specialized tissues are hair, nails, *sebaceous* (oil) and *sudoriferous* (sweat) glands, and mammary glands.

The skin is the largest organ of the body, weighing about 9 pounds and covering approximately 18 square feet in an adult. It consists of two layers of tissue, the *epidermis* and *dermis*, and a layer of *subcutaneous* tissue. Embedded in these layers are various accessory appendages. Skin components are defined in the section titled Parts of the Skin in Lesson One of this chapter. A brief discussion of the components and functions of the integument follows.

The epidermis is the skin's outer layer. It contains no blood vessels and receives its nourishment from the dermis. The cells are packed closely together, being thickest on the palms of the hands and soles of the feet. The epidermis is firmly attached to the dermis, the deeper layer of skin that lies below it. In turn, the dermis is attached through subcutaneous tissue to

ALLIED HEALTH PROFESSIONS

Registered Nurses, Licensed Practical Nurses, Licensed Vocational Nurses and Home, Personal and Psychiatric Aides

Registered nurses (RNs), regardless of specialty or work setting, treat patients and educate patients and the public about various medical conditions, and provide advice and emotional support to patients' family members. RNs record patients' medical histories and symptoms, help perform diagnostic tests and analyze results, operate medical machinery, administer treatment and medications, and assist with patient follow-up and rehabilitation.

RNs teach patients and their families how to manage their illness or injury, explaining posttreatment home care needs; diet, nutrition, and exercise programs; and self-administration of medication and physical therapy. Some RNs work to promote general health by educating the public on warning signs and symptoms of disease. RNs also might run general health screening or immunization clinics, blood drives, and public seminars on various conditions.

Under the direction of physicians and RNs, licensed practical nurses (LPNs) or licensed vocational nurses (LVNs) care for people who are sick, injured, convalescent, or disabled. The nature of direction and supervision required varies by state and job setting.

LPNs care for patients in many ways. Often, they provide basic bedside care. Many LPNs measure and record patients' vital signs such as height, weight, temperature, blood pressure, pulse, and respiration. They also prepare and give injections and enemas, monitor catheters, dress wounds, and give alcohol rubs and massages. To help keep patients comfortable, they assist with bathing, dressing, and personal hygiene, and turning in bed, standing, and walking. They might also feed patients who need help eating. Experienced LPNs may supervise nursing assistants and aides.

Nursing and psychiatric aides help care for physically or mentally ill, injured, disabled, or infirm individuals in hospitals, nursing care facilities, and mental health settings. Home health aides have duties that are similar, but they work in patients' homes or residential care facilities. Nursing aides and home health aides are among the occupations commonly referred to as direct care workers because of their role in working with patients who need long-term care. The specific care they give depends on their specialty.

INQUIRY

National League for Nursing: www.nln.org
American Association of Colleges of Nursing: www.aacn.nche.edu
American Nurses Association: nursingworld.org
National Association for Practical Nurse Education and Service: www.napnes.org
National Federation of Licensed Practical Nurses: www.nflpn.org
National Association for Home Care and Hospice: www.nahc.org
Visiting Nurse Associations of America: www.vnaa.org
Center for the Health Professions: www.futurehealth.ucsf.edu

Data from Cross, Nanna and McWay, Dana. *Stanfield's Introduction to the Health Professions*, 7th ed. Burlington, MA: Jones & Bartlett Learning; 2017.

underlying structures such as muscle and bone (see Table 11-1). The appendages of fingernails and toenails are found only in humans and other primates, and hair is characteristic only of mammals (**Figure 11-1**).

A strand of hair is a tightly fused meshwork of horny cells filled with keratin. It has a root embedded in the hair follicle and a shaft, which is the visible part of hair. Each hair develops in the hair follicle as new growth forms from keratin located at the bottom of the follicle. Cutting the hair does not affect its rate of growth. Melanocytes located at the root of the hair follicle gives hair its color, and the color is dependent on the amount of melanin produced. As people age, melanocytes stop producing melanin, and the hair turns gray or white.

Fingernails and toenails are composed of hard keratin plates that cover the dorsal surface of the tip of each toe and finger. The horny cells are tightly packed and cemented together and continue to grow indefinitely unless cut or broken. Fingernails can be replaced in 3–5 months; toenails grow more slowly, requiring 12–18 months to be completely replaced.

The visible part of the nail is the nail body. At the base of the nail body and around the sides is a fold of skin called *cuticle*. The *lunula* is a half-moon crescent at the base of

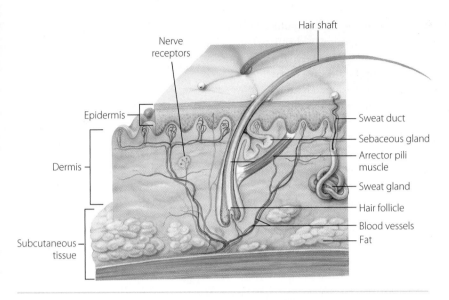

FIGURE 11-1 Components of the epidermis, dermis, and subcutaneous tissue.

the nail plate. Underneath the cuticle, the nail body extends into the root of the nail. It is nourished by the nail bed, an epithelial layer lying just beneath it, which contains a supply of blood vessels and gives the nails their pinkish coloring. Alterations in the growth and appearance can give an indication of systemic disease. For example, a flattened or spoon-shaped nail plate can result from iron deficiency anemia.

Skin glands in humans include sebaceous glands, sudoriferous glands, and *mammary* glands, which are modified sweat glands. The glands of the ear canal that produce *cerumen* (ear wax) are also modified sweat glands, as are the specialized glands found in the *axilla* (armpit) and the *anogenital* area. A modified type of sweat gland, active only from puberty onward, is concentrated near the reproductive organs and in the armpits. These glands secrete an odorless sweat that contains substances that are quickly decomposed by bacteria on the skin. The end products of this breakdown are responsible for human body odor. Mammary glands are another type of modified sweat gland. They only secrete milk after a female has given birth. The skin performs five essential functions: protection, temperature regulation, communication, metabolism, and excretion (see Table 11-2).

1. ***Protection***: The skin protects the body from microorganisms, fluid loss or gain, and other mechanical and chemical irritants. Melanin pigment provides some protection against the sun's ultraviolet rays.
2. ***Temperature regulation***: The blood supply to the skin nourishes the skin and helps regulate body temperature. Sweat glands also assist in the maintenance and regulation of body temperature.
3. ***Communication***: All stimuli from the environment are received through the skin by receptors that detect temperature, touch, pressure, and pain. Skin is the medium of facial expression (e.g., smiles, frowns, grimaces).
4. ***Metabolism***: In the presence of sunlight (ultraviolet radiation), the synthesis of vitamin D, essential for bone growth and development, is initiated from a precursor molecule (7-dehydrocholesterol) found in the skin.
5. ***Excretion***: Fatty substances, water, and salts (mainly the Na^+ ion) are eliminated from the skin.

Conditions and diseases of the skin can be temporary and self-limiting, for example, a sunburn, or can be a symptom of a contagious disease, e.g., chicken pox (see Table 11-4) or a chronic disease such as psoriasis or an undiagnosed diabetes

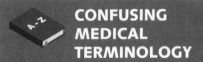

CONFUSING MEDICAL TERMINOLOGY

dermatome versus
dermatome versus
dermatome

dermatome (<u>dur</u>-muh-tohm) as in anatomy – an area of skin that is supplied with the nerve fibers of a single, posterior, spinal root

dermatome (<u>dur</u>-muh-tohm) as in surgery – an instrument that cuts thin slices of skin for grafting

dermatome (<u>dur</u>-muh-tohm) as in embryology – a mesodermal layer in early development, which becomes the dermal layers of the skin

mellitus (see Table 11-6). Skin exposure to insect bites and bee stings can be painful and cause an allergic reaction in susceptible individuals. Chronic exposure to chemicals and even water can cause a skin rash (contact dermatitis) (see Table 11-5). The most serious cause of skin injury is burns, especially second- and third-degree burns that extend below the top skin layer because of loss of fluid and exposure to bacteria (**Figure 11-2**). Cuts of the skin cause bleeding. Although new skin fills in during healing, there may be a permanent scar (**Figure 11-3**).

The study of the skin is called *dermatology*, and the medical doctor who specializes in the study of the diseases and disorders of the skin is called a *dermatologist*. *Plastic surgeons* do reconstructive surgery, including skin grafts after burns or cancer. *Podiatrists* treat skin ulcers of the lower leg, often secondary to complications of diabetes mellitus or peripheral vascular disease. Patients may be referred to a dermatologist by primary care physicians—pediatricians, family practice physicians, or general internal medicine—after an initial evaluation. Details of the integumentary system are provided in succeeding sections of this chapter.

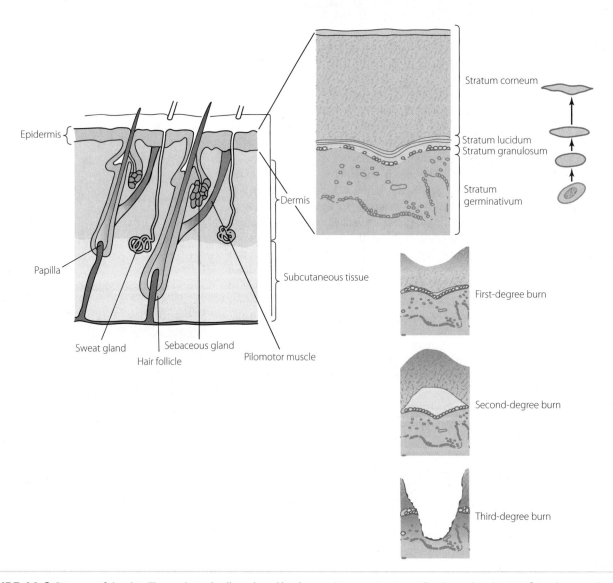

FIGURE 11-2 Diagram of the skin. The nucleated cell produced by the stratum germinativum dies (granulates) as it is forced outward to become the dead, scaly stratum corneum. The number of layers of the epidermis affected by the three types of skin burns is also shown. Only corneum cells are involved in first-degree burns. Damage to the upper three layers occurs in second-degree burns, forming a blister between layers 3 and 4. A third-degree burn involves all epidermal layers and, therefore, usually requires a skin graft to replace the stratum germinativum.

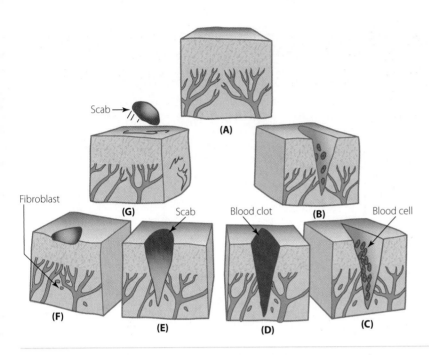

FIGURE 11-3 If normal skin **(A)** is injured deeply **(B)**, blood escapes from dermal blood vessels **(C)**, and a blood clot soon forms **(D)**. The blood clot and dried tissue form a scab **(E)**, which protects the damaged region. Later, blood vessels send out branches, and fibroblasts migrate into the area **(F)**. The fibroblast produce new connective tissue fibers, and when the skin is largely repaired, the scab sloughs off **(G)**.

LESSON ONE   **Materials to Be Learned**

PARTS OF THE SKIN

Table 11-1 describes the major parts of the skin.

TABLE **11-1** Parts of the Skin		
Part	**Pronunciation**	**Definition**
skin	skin	the outer covering of the body
epidermis (cuticle)	ep´-i-<u>der</u>-mis (<u>ku</u>-ti-kul)	the outermost, nonvascular layer of the skin; composed of, from within outward, five layers: basal layer, prickle-cell layer, granular layer, clear layer, and horny layer
dermis corium	<u>der</u>-mis <u>ko</u>-re-um	layer of the skin deep in the epidermis, consisting of a dense bed of vascular connective tissue and containing the nerves of terminal organs or sensation, the hair roots, and sebaceous and sweat glands
hair, nails	hare, nales	appendages of the skin
subcutaneous	sub´-ku-<u>ta</u>-ne-us	beneath the skin, containing adipose tissue, connective tissue, blood vessels, and nerves

(continues)

Part	Pronunciation	Definition
breasts	brests	mammary glands; in female mammals, the breast contains milk-secreting elements for nourishing the young
squamous epithelium	skway-mus ep-ih-thee-lee-um	a layer of flattened plate-like cells that cover internal and external body surfaces
stratum basale	strat-um bay-sil	in this layer of skin, new cells are formed and push older cells to the outermost surface of the skin
stratum corneum	strat-um cor-nee-um	outermost layer of skin where dead cells are converted to keratin, which flakes away

*TABLE **11-1** (continued)*

FUNCTIONS OF THE SKIN

Table 11-2 describes the major functions of the skin.

TABLE **11-2** Functions of the Skin

Function	Pronunciation	Definition
protection	pro-tek-shun	from microorganisms, injuries, and excessive exposure to ultraviolet rays of the sun
sensory organ (receptor)	sen-so-re (re-cep-tor)	for the body to feel pain, cold, heat, touch, and pressure
temperature regulator	tem-per-ah-tur reg-u-la´tor	insulation against heat and cold, e.g., perspiration for cooling
metabolism	me-tab-o-lizm	in the presence of sunlight, synthesize vitamin D from a precursor molecule found in the skin
waste elimination	wast e-lim-i-na-shun	eliminate body wastes in the form of perspiration

SKIN GROWTHS

Table 11-3 lists common skin growths. The chapter on cancer medicine (Chapter 20) will discuss in detail growths that are cancerous.

TABLE **11-3** Skin Growths

Growth	Pronunciation	Definition
Carcinoma	kahr-suh-noh-muh	a malignant new growth made up of epithelial cells tending to infiltrate surrounding tissues and give rise to metastases (**Figure 11-4**)
Keratosis	ker´-ah-to-sis	any horny growth such as a wart or callosity
malignant melanoma	ma-lig-nant mel-a-no-ma	cancerous tumor of melanin-forming cells of the skin; changes in the appearance of a mole may indicate melanoma

Growth	Pronunciation	Definition
nevus (plural: nevi)	ne-vus	a mole or growth, e.g., birthmark; there are many types (**Figure 11-5**)
steatoma	ste´-ah-to-mah	lipoma; a fatty mass retained within a sebaceous gland; sebaceous cyst
verruca (plural: -ae)	ve-roo-kah	a wart caused by viruses; a plantar wart is on the sole or plantar surface of the foot

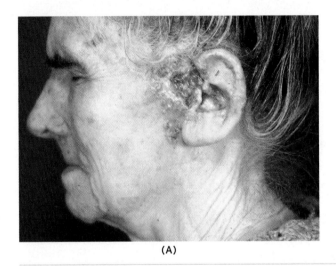
(A)

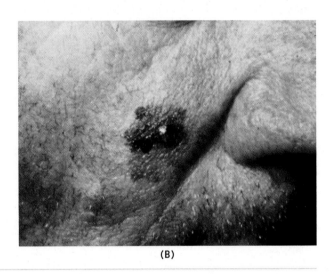
(B)

FIGURE 11-4 Common skin cancers caused by excessive sun exposure. **(A)** Cancer arising from keratinocytes (basal cell carcinoma). **(B)** Cancer arising from melanocytes (malignant melanoma).

Courtesy of Leonard V. Crowley, MD, Century College

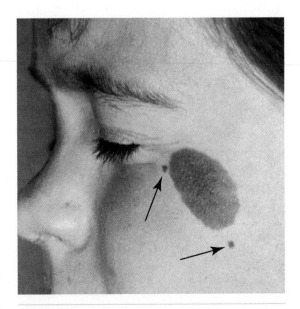

FIGURE 11-5 Benign nevi of skin; a large nevus is near the eye, and two smaller adjacent nevi are shown.

Courtesy of Leonard V. Crowley, MD, Century College

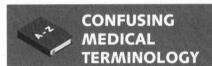
CONFUSING MEDICAL TERMINOLOGY

milia versus miliaria

milia – a condition of the skin resulting from oil-filled ducts (mil-ee-uh)

miliaria – a condition of the skin resulting from sweat-filled ducts (mil-ee-air-ee-uh)

BIOLOGIC AGENTS AND SKIN INFECTION

Skin infections are caused by viruses, bacteria, fungi and parasites. Common examples are listed in **Table 11-4**.

TABLE **11-4** Biologic Agents and Skin Infection

Infection	Pronunciation	Definition
Bacteria		
acne vulgaris	<u>ak</u>-ne vul-<u>ga</u>-ris	develops when skin pores become clogged with dead skin cells because of excess production of sebum (oil) causing dead skin cells to stick together and clog the pore. Bacteria in the clogged pore causes inflammation and the formation of a cyst
carbuncle, furuncle	<u>kar</u>-bung-k´-l <u>fu</u>-rung-k´-l	furuncles (boils) are painful, pus-filled bumps that form under the skin when staphylococcal bacteria infect hair follicles; a carbuncle is a cluster of furuncles that form a connected area (track) of infection under the skin
cellulitis	sel´-u-<u>li</u>-tis	inflammation of the skin and subcutaneous tissue caused by streptococcal or staphylococcal bacteria as a result of a break in the skin from injury, surgery, or an insect bite; may lead to ulceration and abscess
impetigo	im-pe-<u>ti</u>-go	a streptococcal or staphylococcal skin infection marked by vesicles or bullae that become pustular, rupture, and form yellow crusts, especially around the mouth and nose
Methicillin-Resistant Staphylococcus Aureus (MRSA)	Meth-i-<u>cil</u>-lin Re-<u>sis</u>-tant Staph-y-lo-<u>coc</u>-cus <u>Aur</u>-e-us	skin infection caused by bacteria resistant to treatment with methicillin and other antibiotics
Rosacea	rose-<u>ay</u>-sha	common skin condition with redness and visible blood vessels of the nose and cheek that slowly spread to the forehead and chin, and eventually form small pus-filled bumps similar to acne. More common in those with fair skin or a history of acne
Virus		
herpes	<u>her</u>-pez	inflammatory skin disease caused by a herpes virus; acute symptoms are small blisters that appear in clusters; can be a chronic condition with periods of remission
herpes genitalis	<u>her</u>-pez jen´-i-<u>tal</u>-is	herpes infection (HSV-2) of the genitals; may harm an infant if the mother is infected at the time of delivery
herpes ophthalmicus	<u>her</u>-pez oph-<u>thal</u>-mi-cus	severe herpes zoster involving the ophthalmic nerve (eye)
herpes simplex virus (HSV)	<u>her</u>-pez <u>sim</u>-plex	herpes infection (HSV-1) on the borders of the lips or nares (cold sores)
herpes zoster (shingles)	<u>her</u>-pez <u>zos</u>-ter	painful rash on one side of the body caused by varicella zoster virus (VZV), the virus that causes chickenpox; virus is dormant in those who have had chickenpox but often reappears as shingles in those over 60 years of age or those who are immunocompromised
roseola (sixth disease)	ro-<u>se</u>-o-la	illness common in children from birth to 2 years of age; symptoms begin with a high fever followed by a red-colored skin rash; caused by herpesvirus 6 (HHV-6) and possibly herpesvirus 7 (HHV-7)

Infection	Pronunciation	Definition
verruca (wart)	ve-<u>ru</u>-kah	growth of the outer layer of the skin (the epidermis) caused by the human papillomavirus (HPV) and transmitted by human contact. *Common* warts occur on the hands or feet; *plantar* warts occur on the sole of the foot and *genital* warts are found in the genital area
Fungus		
tinea (ringworm)	<u>tin</u>-e-ah	called ringworm because of the circular shape of the rash (shaped like a ring); a name applied to many different superficial fungal infections of different parts of the body
tinea barbae	<u>tin</u>-e-ah <u>bar</u>-bae	infection of the bearded parts of the face by ringworm
tinea capitis	<u>tin</u>-e-ah <u>kap</u>-i-tis	infection of the scalp by ringworm
tinea corporis	<u>tin</u>-e-ah <u>cor</u>-por-is	skin infection of the entire body by ringworm
tinea cruris	<u>tin</u>-e-ah <u>cru</u>-ris	infection of the groin area by ringworm ("jock itch")
tinea pedis	<u>tin</u>-e-ah <u>pe</u>-dis	athlete's foot; a chronic superficial infection of the skin of the foot by ringworm
tinea unguium	<u>tin</u>-e-ah <u>un</u>-guium	infection of the fingernails by ringworm; the nails become opaque, white, thickened, and friable
Parasites		
pediculosis	pe-dik´-u-<u>lo</u>-sis	body infestation with lice, usually of the scalp and pubic area; lice suck blood from humans causing itching and infection secondary to scratching
pediculosis capitis	pe-dik´-u-<u>lo</u>-sis <u>kap</u>-i-tis	head lice
pediculosis corporis	pe-dik´-u-<u>lo</u>-sis cor-por-is	body lice
pediculosis pubis	pe-dik´-u-<u>lo</u>-sis <u>pu</u>-bis	pubic lice or crabs
scabies	<u>ska</u>-bez	caused by a mite, a small parasite that burrows under the skin; symptoms are an itchy rash

ALLERGY AND THE SKIN

Table 11-5 describes responses of the skin to different negative stimuli, both internal and external.

TABLE 11-5 Allergy and the Skin

Term	Pronunciation	Definition
allergic contact dermatitis	a-<u>ler</u>-gic contact der-ma-<u>ti</u>-tis	itchy, blistering rash after contact with poison ivy, oak, or sumac; other causes are latex gloves or jewelry containing nickel
atopic dermatitis (AD; eczema)	a-<u>top</u>-ic der-ma-<u>ti</u>-tis <u>ek</u>-ze-ma	common skin condition in children during the first year of life; dry, scaly, and itchy patches appear on the scalp, forehead, and face
contact dermatitis	contact der-ma-<u>ti</u>-tis	skin reaction which appears as an itchy rash in response to contact with a skin irritant, e.g., diaper rash or dry, cracked hands because of frequent contact with water, e.g., bartenders, hairdressers, and housekeeping workers
neurodermatitis	nu´-ro-der´-mah-<u>ti</u>-tis	skin condition that begins with itching related to emotional causes or psychological factors

SKIN DISORDERS FROM SYSTEMIC DISEASES

Table 11-6 lists systemic diseases that include symptoms involving the skin.

TABLE **11-6** Skin Disorders from Systemic Diseases		
Disease	**Pronunciation**	**Definition**
Coccidioidomycosis (Valley Fever)	coc-cid-i-oi-do-my-<u>co</u>-sis	fungal infection of the lungs caused by inhaling spores of the fungus, *Coccidioides*, which lives in the soil; symptoms include flu-like symptoms and red bumps on the skin
erysipelas (St. Anthony's fire)	er´-i-<u>sip</u>-e-las	a contagious disease of the skin and subcutaneous tissues caused by infection with Group A Streptococci organisms; complication of strep throat, surgical wound, or skin injury; redness and swelling of affected areas
histoplasmosis	his´-to-plaz-<u>mo</u>-sis	a systemic fungal disease caused by inhalation of dust contaminated by spores of the fungus, *Histoplasma*, which lives in soil that contains large amounts of bird or bat droppings. Symptoms include flu-like symptoms; red bumps appear on the lower legs in some patients
Lyme Disease	līm di-<u>zēz</u>	inflammatory disease with early symptoms of a characteristic circular red rash and flu-like symptoms; caused by bacteria and transmitted by deer tick bites. Later complications can be arthritis and neurological and cardiac disorders
psoriasis	so-<u>ri</u>-ah-sis	a chronic, hereditary, recurrent dermatosis marked by discrete vivid red macules, papules or plaques covered with silvery laminated scales
Rocky Mountain Spotted Fever (RMSF)	Rock-y Moun-tain	symptoms are small, flat, pink, non-itchy spots (macules) on the wrists, forearms, and ankles which can spread to the trunk, palms and soles. Transmitted by tick bites and caused by bacterium *Rickettsia rickettsia*; if untreated, complications include organ failure and death
rubella (German measles)	roo-<u>bel</u>-ah	early symptoms are a rash that starts on the face and spreads to the rest of the body; later symptoms can include a low-grade fever, cough, runny nose, sore throat, and pink eye
rubeola (measles)	ru-<u>be</u>-o-la	symptoms are fever, runny nose, cough, red eyes, and sore throat, followed by a rash that spreads over the body. The disease is very contagious and is spread through air from coughing and sneezing
syphilis	<u>sif</u>-i-lis	a sexually transmitted bacterial disease; early skin symptoms are ulcers on the genital area, followed by white patchy skin
systemic lupus erythematosus (SLE)	si-<u>stem</u>-ik <u>loo</u>-pus er-i´-<u>the</u>-ma-to-sus	autoimmune disease that can affect all organs; common symptom is a rash that forms a butterfly pattern over the bridge of the nose and cheeks
varicella (chickenpox)	var´-i-<u>sel</u>-ah	a very contagious disease caused by the varicella-zoster virus (VZV); symptoms are blister-like rash, itching, fatigue, and fever

Some common skin conditions among children are listed in **BOX 11-1**.

Box 11-1 Common Skin Conditions in Children

Common skin conditions in infants and children are:

- Atopic dermatitis or eczema
- Contact dermatitis
- Hives
- Heat rash or prickly heat
- Impetigo
- Lice
- Ringworm
- Roseola
- Warts

Childhood immunizations for some common communicable diseases among children are listed in **BOX 11-2**.

Box 11-2 Childhood Immunizations

Common communicable diseases in children that affect the skin can be prevented with immunizations:

- Varicella (chickenpox)
- Rubella
- Measles

MMRV (measles, mumps, rubella, varicella) vaccine is part of the immunization program for children to prevent these communicable disease and serious complications.

TERMS USED IN THE DIAGNOSIS AND TREATMENT OF DISEASES OF THE SKIN

Table 11-7 describes terms used to describe the symptoms, diagnosis, and treatment of diseases of the skin.

TABLE 11-7 Terms Used in the Diagnosis and Treatment of Diseases of the Skin

Term	Pronunciation	Definition
History and Physical Exam		
actinic keratosis (AK)	ak-<u>tin</u>-ik ker-uh-<u>toe</u>-sis	precancerous patch of thick, scaly, or crusty skin; usually forms when skin is damaged by ultraviolet (UV) radiation exposure from the sun or indoor tanning beds
albinism	<u>al</u>-bi-nizm	no body pigment; white skin and hair
alopecia	al´-o-<u>pe</u>-she-ah	baldness; hereditary or caused by chemotherapy
bulla (plural: -ae)	<u>bul</u>-ah	large blisters, as in burns
burn	bern	thermal injury to tissues: first-degree burns are often caused by sunburn, affect the top skin layer (corneum) and show redness; second-degree burns affect the upper three skin layers (corneum, lucidum, and granulosum) and produce blisters between the third and fourth skin layer; third-degree burns affect the top three layers plus the fourth layer (germinativum) with fluid loss, risk for infection, and require skin grafting (see Figure 11-2)
callus	<u>kal</u>-us	localized hyperplasia of the horny layer of the epidermis (skin) caused by pressure or friction; most common sites are the hands and feet
cicatrix	<u>sik</u>-ah-triks	a scar
cyst	sist	a closed epithelium-lined cavity or sac, normal or abnormal, usually containing liquid or semisolid material
ecchymosis	ek´-i-<u>mo</u>-sis	bruise, caused by bleeding under the skin
erosion	e-<u>ro</u>-shun	eating or gnawing away, e.g., an early ulcer
eruption	e-<u>rup</u>-shun	breaking out; a rash

(continues)

TABLE 11-7 *(continued)*

Term	Pronunciation	Definition
erythema	er´-i-<u>the</u>-mah	redness of the skin
eschar	<u>es</u>-kar	a slough (hard crust) produced by a thermal burn
exanthem	eg-<u>zan</u>-them	an eruptive (rose colored) skin rash caused by disease or fever
excoriation	eks-ko´-re-<u>a</u>-shun	a superficial loss of skin, e.g., by scratching
exfoliation	eks-fo´-le-<u>a</u>-shun	skin falling off in scales or layers
fissure	<u>fish</u>-er	a narrow slit on the skin surface, e.g., anal fissure, athlete's foot lesion
gangrene	<u>gang</u>-gren	necrotic or dead tissue (**Figure 11-6**)
hemangioma	he-man-gi-<u>o</u>-ma	network of small blood-filled capillaries near the surface of the skin forming a reddish or purplish birthmark; may appear in newborn infants
hirsutism	<u>her</u>-soot-ism	abnormal hairiness on the body and face, especially in women
keloid	<u>ke</u>-loid	a sharply elevated, progressively enlarging scar that does not fade with time
laceration	las´-e-<u>ra</u>-shun	cut; tearing; a torn wound
lesion	<u>le</u>-zhun	any pathologic or traumatic discontinuity of tissue, e.g., a sore
macule	<u>mak</u>-ul	a spot or thickening, e.g., freckle, flat mole. Area is not raised above the surface
miliaria (prickly heat; heat rash)	mil-i-<u>ar</u>-i-a	inflammatory disorder of the skin characterized by redness, eruption, and burning or itching due to blockage of the ducts of the sweat glands; common in hot and humid climates
nodule	<u>nod</u>-ul	a small node that is solid and can be detected by touch; a rounded prominence, e.g., a boss
nummular	<u>num</u>-u-lar	coin-shaped skin sores; often appear after a burn or skin injury
papulae	<u>pap</u>-u-le	a small, circumscribed, solid elevated lesion of the skin, e.g., wart, acne, mole
paronychia	par´-o-<u>nik</u>-e-ah	inflammation of the folds of tissue around the fingernail
petechia	pay-<u>tee</u>-kee-ee	small pinpoint hemorrhages of the skin, red or purple in color
plaque	plak	any patch or flat area; used to describe the silvery scales of psoriasis
pruritus	proo-<u>ri</u>-tus	itching
pustule	<u>pus</u>-tul	a small, elevated, pus-containing lesion of the skin
scales, crusts	scalz, krusts	an outer layer formed by drying of a bodily exudate or secretion; flaking type of lesion, e.g., psoriasis, fungus
scar, cicatrix	sk-<u>ahr</u>, sik-<u>ah</u>-triks	a mark remaining after the healing of a wound or break in the skin
superfluous hair	soo-<u>pur</u>-floo-es har	excessive hair on the face of women
ulcer	<u>ul</u>-cer	Local destruction of tissue from sloughing of necrotic inflammatory tissue, e.g., varicose ulcer, decubitus ulcer

Term	Pronunciation	Definition
urticaria (hives)	er´-ti-<u>ka</u>-re-ah	transient elevated patches (wheals); an allergic response
vesicle	<u>ves</u>-i-k´-l	a small blister containing liquid
vitiligo	vit´-i-<u>li</u>-go	loss of pigment; white, patchy areas
wheal	hwel	a localized area of swelling on the body surface, e.g., produced by a skin test reaction
xanthoderma	zan-thoh-<u>der</u>-mah	yellow coloration of the skin, e.g., from jaundice
xeroderma	zee-roh-<u>der</u>-mah	rough and dry skin, a clinical and chronic condition especially in a cold climate

Diagnostic Tools: Skin Tests

Term	Pronunciation	Definition
allergy skin test	<u>al</u>-er-jee skin test	used to determine an allergy to food items, pollen, or animal dander; a small drop of a suspected allergen is placed on the skin, which is then scratched; a rash or itching indicates an allergic response
coccidioidin	kok-sid´-e-<u>oi</u>-din	a sterile preparation injected intracutaneously as a test for present or past infection of valley fever (respiratory fungal disease)
Mantoux or PPD	man-<u>too</u>	a skin test for tuberculosis (TB), a bacterial disease; PPD: purified protein derivative
Dick test	dik test	an intracutaneous test for susceptibility to scarlet fever; redness at the injection site indicates susceptibility
Schick test	shik test	an intracutaneous test for susceptibility to diphtheria; a redness at the injection site indicates susceptibility

Diagnostic Tools: Laboratory Tests

Term	Pronunciation	Definition
enzyme-linked immunosorbent assay (ELISA or EIA)	<u>en</u>-zahym linked im-mu-no-<u>sor</u>-bent a-<u>sey</u>	blood test to measure the presence and amount of allergen-specific antibodies

Surgery for the Diagnosis and Treatment of Skin Disorders

Term	Pronunciation	Definition
biopsy	<u>bi</u>-op-se	removal of skin or tissue from the body for examination; used to make a diagnosis
cautery	<u>kaw</u>-ter-e	tissue destruction by electricity
debridement	da-<u>bred</u>-ment	removal of contaminated or devitalized tissue from a traumatic or infected lesion, e.g., a decubitus ulcer
dermabrasion	der-mah-<u>bra</u>-shun	the surface of the epidermis of the skin is removed by abrasion, typically to remove scarring or sun-damaged skin
dermatome	<u>der</u>-mah-tom	an instrument for cutting thin skin slices for grafting
electrodesiccation	e-lek´-tro-des´-i-<u>ka</u>-shun	destruction of tissue by dehydration with high-frequency electric current
escharotomy	es-kah-<u>rot</u>-omy	removal of burn scar tissue

(continues)

TABLE **11-7** (continued)		
Term	**Pronunciation**	**Definition**
graft	graft	a piece of donor skin transplanted to replace skin damaged by burns, pressure ulcers, infection, or trauma
hyfrecator	hi-fra-<u>cate</u>-or	single-electrode, low-powered device that destroys tissue using electrosurgery

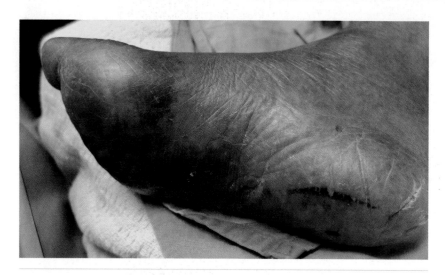

FIGURE 11-6 Gangrene of right foot as a result of arterial obstruction.

© Casa nayafana/Shutterstock.

THE ORIGIN OF MEDICAL TERMS

Table 11-8 explains the origin of several terms used in this chapter.

TABLE **11-8** The Origin of Medical Terms		
Word	**Pronunciation**	**Origin and Definition**
actinic	ak-<u>tin</u>-ik	Greek, *aktis, aktin*, ray + Latin, *icus*, or Greek, *ikos*, pertaining to
dermabrasion	der-mah-<u>bra</u>-shun	Greek, *derm*, for skin Latin, *ab*, away from + Latin, *radere*, to scrape
exanthem	eg-<u>zan</u>-them	Greek, *exanthema*, a breaking out
melanocyte	muh-<u>lan</u>-uh-sahyt	Greek, *melas, melan*, "black" + Greek, *kytos*, cell
keloid	<u>ke</u>-loid	Greek, *khēlē*, crab's claw + Greek, *oeidēs*, form
pediculosis	pe-dik´-u-<u>lo</u>-sis	Latin, *pediculus*, "louse" + English, *osis*, condition
macule	<u>mak</u>-ul	Latin, *macula*, "spot"
Rubeola (measles)	ru-<u>be</u>-o-la (mea-sles)	Latin, *rubeus*, red Middle Dutch, *masule*, pustule
miliaria	mil-i-<u>ar</u>-i-a	Latin, *milium*, millet (millet seeds)
pruritus	pru-<u>ri</u>-tus	Latin, *prurire*, to itch

ABBREVIATIONS

The abbreviations listed in **Table 11-9** are frequently used to describe the integumentary system, including clinical disorders and diagnostic tools.

TABLE 11-9 Abbreviations

Abbreviation	Definition	Abbreviation	Definition
AD	atopic dermatitis	PPD	purified protein derivative
AK	actinic keratosis	RMSF	Rocky Mountain Spotted Fever
ELISA/EIA	enzyme-linked immunosorbent assay	SLE	systemic lupus erythematosus
HPV	human papillomavirus	TB	tuberculosis
HSV	herpes simplex virus	UV	ultraviolet
MRSA	Methicillin-resistant *Staphylococcus aureus*	VZV	Varicella-zoster virus

The following box lists three different categories of medications that may be prescribed by a physician treating the integumentary system.

PHARMACOLOGY AND MEDICAL TERMINOLOGY

Drug Classification	antihistamine (an-tih-<u>hiss</u>-tah-meen)	antifungal (an-ti-fun-gal)	anesthetic (an-ess-<u>thet</u>-ik)
Function	opposes the action of histamine, which is released in allergic reactions	limits or prevents the growth of fungal organisms	partially or completely numbs or eliminates sensitivity with or without loss of consciousness
Word Parts	**anti-** = against; **histamine** = a chemical responsible for allergic reactions in human	**anti-** = against; **fungal** = single-celled or multicellular organism	**an-** = without; **esthesi**/o = feeling or sensation; -tic = pertaining to
Active Ingredients (Samples)	diphenhydramine hydrochloride (Benadryl); brompheniramine maleate (Dimetane)	fluconazole (Diflucan); clotrimazole (Lotrimin)	lidocaine (Xylocaine)

CLINICAL PEDIATRIC OFFICE NOTE

Healthy, active 10-month-old female presents with mother in the office today with patches of **eruption**. The eruptions are causing **erythema** and **pruritus** on the cheeks and scalp indicative of **AD**. One area in particular may be slightly infected. Mother reports no new exposures to bath soap, laundry soap, or new clothing. Patient has a history of asthma and parents are both positive for a history of AD. Will prescribe **OTC** cortisone cream to be used sparingly twice daily on current lesions in the morning and after bathing. In addition, use OTC Neosporin **b.i.d.** on infected or severely inflamed areas. Mother is advised to call with worsening of symptoms or if improvement is not seen within 7 days. Will consider future **allergy testing** if incidents increase or fail to improve.

Direction: For the portions of the clinical note shown by a colored font, provide the definition and/or words for abbreviation.

| LESSON TWO | Progress Check |

LIST: SKIN FUNCTIONS

List the five major functions of the skin:

1. _____

2. _____

3. _____

4. _____

5. _____

SPELLING AND DEFINITIONS: SKIN TERMS

Circle the correct spelling for the following terms and then define the term:

1. **(a)** Epidermis   **(b)** Epidermosis   **(c)** Epedermis   **(d)** Epodermasis
   Definition: _____

2. **(a)** Subcutenous   **(b)** Subcortenus   **(c)** Subcuteneous   **(d)** Subcutaneous
   Definition: _____

3. **(a)** Biopse   **(b)** Biopsy   **(c)** Biospy   **(d)** Bispoy
   Definition: _____

4. **(a)** Debraidment   **(b)** Debrisment   **(c)** Debridement   **(d)** Derbrement
   Definition: _____

5. **(a)** Escharotomy   **(b)** Scarotomy   **(c)** Eschrotomy   **(d)** Secharotomy
   Definition: _____

6. **(a)** Keratinous   **(b)** Keratosis   **(c)** Karatosis   **(d)** Karathosis
   Definition: _____

7. **(a)** Steatanoma   **(b)** Steteanoma   **(c)** Steatoma   **(d)** Stetusoma
   Definition: _____

8. **(a)** Verracula   **(b)** Verookah   **(c)** Veracola   **(d)** Verruca
   Definition: _____

9. **(a)** Impitigo   **(b)** Impetigo   **(c)** Impecito   **(d)** Imtipego
   Definition: _____

10. **(a)** Pediculosis   **(b)** Pedicleiosis   **(c)** Pedicullosis   **(d)** Pediculasis
    Definition: _____

11. **(a)** Exema   **(b)** Exczema   **(c)** Eczema   **(d)** Ekzema
    Definition: _____

12. **(a)** Posorasis   **(b)** Psoriasis   **(c)** Posorosis   **(d)** Poriaahis

    Definition: _____

13. **(a)** Erisepilas   **(b)** Erysipolus   **(c)** Erisipilas   **(d)** Erysipelas

    Definition: _____

14. **(a)** Varicella   **(b)** Variccela   **(c)** Variccella   **(d)** Varecella

    Definition: _____

15. **(a)** Actomic   **(b)** Actinic   **(c)** Actinus   **(d)** Actonus

    Definition: _____

COMPLETION: SKIN TERMS

Write in the medical terms for the following definitions:

1. _____ : White skin and hair

2. _____ : Baldness

3. _____ : Medical specialty that deals with skin diseases

4. _____ : Redness of the skin

5. _____ : A hard crust produced by a thermal burn

6. _____ : Coin-sized or coin-shaped

7. _____ : Small circumscribed solid elevated skin lesion

8. _____ : Transient elevated patches (wheals)

9. _____ : Small pus-containing lesion

10. _____ : Mark remaining after wound healing

11. _____ : Any horny growth such as a wart or callosity

12. _____ : Bruise caused by bleeding under the skin

DEFINITIONS: SKIN TESTS

Describe the uses of the following skin tests:

1. Mantoux: _____

2. Dick: _____

3. Schick: _____

4. Allergy skin test: _____

5. Coccidioidin: _____

6. Histoplasmosis: _____

MATCHING: SKIN TERMS

Match the following terms to their definitions:

Terms	Definition
1. Ecchymosis	**a.** Scales or layers
2. Erosion	**b.** Scratching off (of skin)
3. Eruption	**c.** A rose-colored skin caused by disease or fever
4. Erythema	**d.** Narrow slit of the skin
5. Eschar	**e.** Redness
6. Exanthem	**f.** Breaking out
7. Excoriation	**g.** Itching
8. Exfoliation	**h.** A bruise
9. Fissure	**i.** Hard crust
10. Pruritus	**j.** Eating or gnawing

MATCHING: SKIN CONDITIONS

Match the terms on the left with their definitions on the right:

Term	Definition
1. Urticarial	**a.** Slit in the skin surface
2. Vesicle	**b.** Patch
3. Vitiligo	**c.** Yellow skin
4. Xanthoderma	**d.** Hives
5. Gangrene	**e.** Loss of pigment
6. Plaque	**f.** Dead skin
7. Superfluous	**g.** Small blister
8. Callus	**h.** A sac containing liquid
9. Cyst	**i.** Hyperplasia of the epidermis
10. Fissure	**j.** Excessive

COMPLETION: SKIN CONDITIONS

For each of the medical terms, list the common name:

Medical Term	Common Name
1. Verruca	**a.** _____
2. Miliaria	**b.** _____
3. Rubella	**c.** _____
4. Rubeola	**d.** _____
5. Varicella	**e.** _____
6. Erysipelas	**f.** _____
7. Urticaria	**g.** _____
8. Herpes zoster	**h.** _____
9. Tinea	**i.** _____
10. Pediculosis	**j.** _____

COMPLETION: SKIN INFECTIONS

For each skin infection, list the infectious agent as bacteria, virus, fungus, or parasite

Skin Infection	Infectious Agent
1. Acne vulgaris	**a.** _____
2. Tinea	**b.** _____
3. Herpes	**c.** _____
4. Impetigo	**d.** _____
5. Pediculosis	**e.** _____
6. Cellulitis	**f.** _____
7. Verruca	**g.** _____
8. Scabies	**h.** _____

IDENTIFYING WORD PARTS

For each of the medical terms, list the root word and the prefix and/or suffix:

Word	Root Word	Prefix	Suffix
1. Albinism	_____	_____	_____
2. Debridement	_____	_____	_____
3. Epidermis	_____	_____	_____
4. Escharotomy	_____	_____	_____
5. Excoriation	_____	_____	_____
6. Hemangioma	_____	_____	_____
7. Neurodermatitis	_____	_____	_____
8. Paronychia	_____	_____	_____
9. Pediculosis	_____	_____	_____
10. Subcutaneous	_____	_____	_____

CHAPTER

12

© teekid/iStock/Getty Images

Digestive System

OBJECTIVES

After completing this chapter and the exercises, the student should be able to:

1. Identify the organs of the digestive system.
2. Describe the location and label the structures of the digestive system.
3. List the function(s) of each organ and accessory organ in the digestive system.
4. Identify and define clinical disorders affecting the system.
5. Define and explain medical words pertaining to tests and procedures used in the diagnosis and treatment of digestive system disorders.

THE DIGESTIVE SYSTEM

The digestive system, also called the gastrointestinal (GI) system or alimentary tract, contains the organs involved in the ingestion and processing of food. Its general description is that of a long muscular tube extending from mouth to anus and the accessory organs, which includes the salivary glands, liver, gallbladder, and pancreas. The physician who specializes in diagnosis and treatment of disorders of the GI system is called a *gastroenterologist*. The *dentist* specializes in care of the teeth.

The primary function of the GI system is to provide the body with food, water, and electrolytes by digesting nutrients to prepare them for absorption. The following processes are involved in this function:

1. *Ingestion*: Taking food into the mouth
2. *Mastication*: Grinding or mincing food with the teeth and mixing with saliva from the salivary glands
3. *Deglutition*: Swallowing or movement of food from the mouth to the pharynx

ALLIED HEALTH PROFESSIONS

Dental Hygienists and Dental Assistants

Dental hygienists clean teeth and provide other preventive dental care; they also teach patients how to practice good oral hygiene. Hygienists examine patients' teeth and gums, recording the presence of diseases or abnormalities. They remove calculus, stains, and plaque from teeth; take and develop dental X-rays; and apply cavity preventive agents such as fluorides and pit and fissure sealants. In some states, hygienists administer local anesthetics and anesthetic gas; place and carve filling materials, temporary fillings, and periodontal dressings; remove sutures; and smooth and polish metal restorations.

Dental assistants perform a variety of patient care, office, and laboratory duties. They work at chairside as dentists examine and treat patients. They make patients as comfortable as possible in the dental chair, prepare them for treatment, and obtain dental records. Assistants hand instruments and materials to dentists and keep patients' mouths dry and clear by using suction or other devices. They also sterilize and disinfect instruments and equipment, prepare tray setups for dental procedures, and instruct patients on postoperative and general oral health care.

Some dental assistants prepare materials for making impressions and restorations, expose radiographs, and process dental X-ray film as directed by the dentist. State law determines which clinical tasks a dental assistant may perform, but in most states they may remove sutures, apply anesthetic and caries-preventive agents to the teeth and oral tissue, remove excess cement used in the filling process, and place rubber dams on the teeth to isolate them for individual treatment.

Those with laboratory duties make casts of the teeth and mouth from impressions taken by dentists, clean and polish removable appliances, and make temporary crowns. Dental assistants with office duties arrange and confirm appointments, receive patients, keep treatment records, send bills, receive payments, and order dental supplies and materials. Dental assistants should not be confused with dental hygienists, who are licensed to perform a wider variety of clinical tasks.

INQUIRY

Division of Education, American Dental Hygienists Association: www.adha.org
Dental Assisting National Board: www.danb.org
American Dental Assistants Association: www.dentalassistant.org
National Association of Dental Assistants: www.ndaonline.org

Data from Cross, Nanna and McWay, Dana. *Stanfield's Introduction to the Health Professions*, 7th ed. Burlington, MA: Jones & Bartlett Learning; 2017.

4. *Peristalsis*: Involuntary waves of smooth muscle contraction that move materials throughout the GI tract
5. *Digestion*: Chemical breakdown of large molecules into smaller ones so that absorption can occur
6. *Absorption*: The movement of end products of digestion from the lumen of the digestive tract into the blood and lymph circulation so that they can be used by body cells
7. *Egestion (defecation)*: Elimination of undigested wastes and bacteria from the tract as feces

The major and accessory organs are defined in Lesson One; the structures are seen throughout this chapter. **Figures 12-1** and **12-2** illustrate the positions of the various organs. A brief discussion of the function of the major parts and accessory organs follows.

The abdominal cavity and all its organs, including the organs of the GI system, are lined by a membrane called the *peritoneum*. The portion surrounding the abdominal organs is called the *visceral peritoneum* and that which lines the abdominal cavity is the *parietal peritoneum*. The peritoneum contains blood vessels, lymph vessels, and nerves (see Figure 12-1).

The upper digestive tract consists of the oral cavity, pharynx, esophagus, and stomach. The lower digestive tract is the small and large intestines. Accessory organs of the digestive system are the salivary glands, liver, pancreas, and gallbladder (see Figure 12-2).

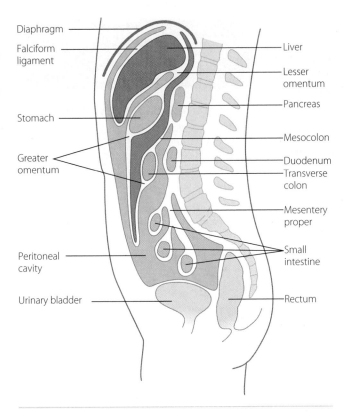

FIGURE 12-1 The peritoneal cavity.

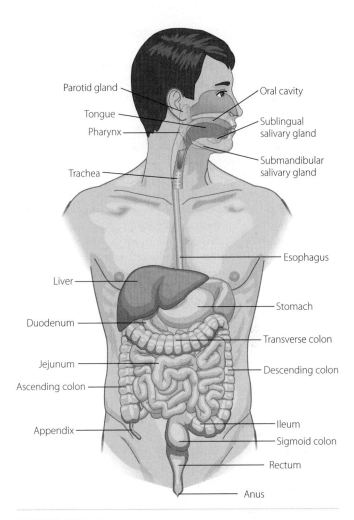

FIGURE 12-2 The digestive system.

The digestive tract begins with the oral cavity (also known as *buccal cavity*). The major parts of the cavity are the lips, cheeks, hard palate, soft palate, and tongue.

The lips surround the opening of the cavity, and the cheeks, which are continuous with the lips and lined with mucous membrane, form the walls of the oval-shaped cavity (**Figure 12-3**).

The hard palate forms the anterior portion of the roof of the mouth and the muscular soft palate lies posterior to it. The hard palate, or roof of the mouth, is supported by bone. It has irregular ridges in its mucous membrane lining called *rugae*. The soft palate is composed of skeletal muscle and connective tissue. The soft palate seals off the opening to the nose during swallowing. Hanging from the soft palate is a small soft tissue called a *uvula*. This structure aids in producing sound and speech (see Figure 12-3).

The tongue is a solid, strong, and flexible structure covered with mucous membrane. It extends across the floor of the oral cavity and strong, flexible, skeletal muscles attach it to the lower joint bone (*mandible*). It is the principal organ of taste and also assists in chewing by moving the food around (*mastication*) and swallowing (*deglutition*).

Across the surface of the tongue are small, rough elevations known as *papillae*. They contain taste buds that detect sweet, sour, salty, and bitter tastes of food (or liquid) as they move across the tongue (see Figure 12-3).

The tongue aids the digestive process by mixing food with saliva, shaping it into a small mass (called a *bolus*), and moving it toward the throat (*pharynx*) to be swallowed.

The release of saliva is triggered by the smell, taste, and sometimes even the thought of food.

Salivary glands are exocrine glands, of which there are three pairs—the *parotids*, *submandibulars*, and *sublinguals*—and they secrete most of the saliva produced each day. Saliva is a watery secretion released by the salivary glands containing some mucus and digestive enzymes.

The gums are made of fleshy tissue and surround the sockets of the teeth. Every individual has two sets of teeth during his or her lifetime. The first set, known as "baby teeth," are primary or *deciduous* teeth. There are 20 teeth in this set, 10 in each jawbone, and the baby will begin to cut them at about 6 months of age. The second set of teeth, the permanent teeth, begins to appear around age 6 years and replace the deciduous teeth. There are 32 permanent teeth, 16 in each jawbone. The last of these teeth, the third molars, or wisdom teeth, usually start erupting at about age 17 years.

The shape of the tooth determines its name. The incisors have a chisel shape with sharp edges for biting, canine or cuspid teeth have a single cusp (point) used for grasping and tearing, and the bicuspids or premolars and the molars have flat surfaces with multiple cusps for crushing and grinding (**Figure 12-3**).

The two main parts of the tooth are the crown which stands above the gum line and the root which is imbedded in *alveolar* bone below the gum line. The outer layer of the tooth consists of *enamel*, the hardest substance in the body. The second layer, *dentin*, is similar to the bone and surrounds the *pulp cavity* which contains connective tissue, nerves, and blood vessels. Blood vessels located in the pulp cavity transport nutrients to the tooth. The *periodontal* ligament is a connective tissue structure that surrounds the roots of the teeth and holds them in place in the dental alveoli. The *root canal* is the point at which the pulp cavity extends into the root of the tooth (**Figure 12-4**).

The digestive system begins with the throat and ends at the anus. This long tube has many parts and is connected to various accessory organs. Such parts and accessory organs are listed here (**Figure 12-5**):

1. *Esophagus*: Transports food from pharynx (throat) to *stomach* by peristalsis. Contains no digestive enzymes (see Figure 12-5).

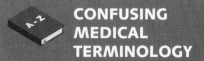

CONFUSING MEDICAL TERMINOLOGY

proct/o versus prostat/o

proct/o – anus and rectum, e.g., proctology (prok-<u>tol</u>-o-je) refers to a branch of medicine concerned with disorders of the rectum and anus

prostat/o – prostate, prostate gland, e.g., prostatorrhea (pros-tat-or-<u>re</u>-ah) refers to a discharge from the prostate

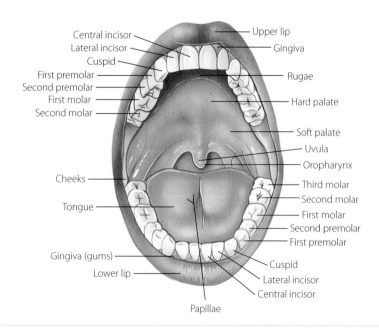

Central incisor
Lateral incisor
Cuspid
First premolar
Second premolar
First molar
Second molar
Cheeks
Tongue
Gingiva (gums)
Lower lip
Papillae
Upper lip
Gingiva
Rugae
Hard palate
Soft palate
Uvula
Oropharynx
Third molar
Second molar
First molar
Second premolar
First premolar
Cuspid
Lateral incisor
Central incisor

FIGURE 12-3 The oral cavity.

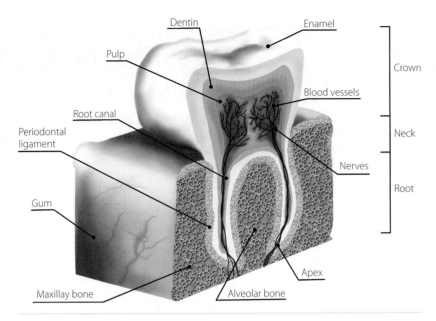

FIGURE 12-4 The parts of the tooth and supporting structures.
© Cessna152/Shutterstock.

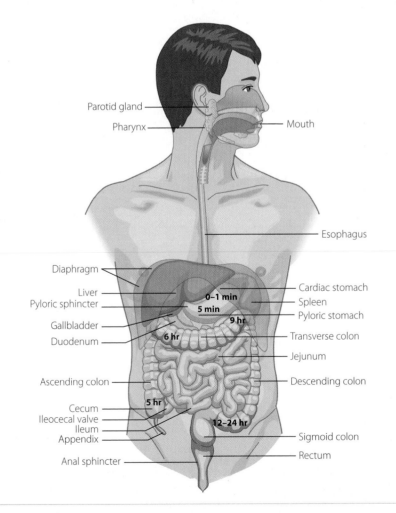

FIGURE 12-5 Human digestive tract; times indicated along the tract represent how long it takes food to pass through each area during the process of digestion.

2. *Stomach* (**Figure 12-6**): Primarily for food storage. Activity in the stomach results in formation of *chyme* and propels it into the *duodenum*. It secretes pepsin, hydrochloric acid, mucus, and intrinsic factor. The *gastric juices* initiate digestion of protein and fat.

3. *Small intestine*: Completes digestion that started in the mouth and stomach by its intestinal enzymes, pancreatic enzymes, and bile from the liver. Also absorbs products of digestion. Peristalsis moves undigested residue to the large intestine.

4. *Large intestine* (**Figure 12-7**): Performs the following functions:
   a. Absorbs 80–90 percent of water and electrolytes and reduces chyme to a semisolid mass
   b. Produces no digestive enzymes or hormones
   c. Bacteria present in the colon synthesize vitamin K, riboflavin, and thiamin
   d. Excretes waste and feces

5. *Pancreas* (**Figure 12-8**): This is the large, elongated gland located behind the greater curvature of the stomach. It contains both endocrine and exocrine glands. The endocrine cells, called islets of Langerhans, secrete the hormones insulin and glucagon. Exocrine glands secrete digestive enzymes, which allow them to digest protein, carbohydrate, and fat.

6. *Liver* (see Figure 12-8): Plays a major role in many body functions:
   a. Produces bile to emulsify fats
   b. Stores glycogen to maintain blood sugar levels
   c. Forms urea from excess amino acids and nitrogenous wastes
   d. Synthesizes fats from carbohydrate and protein
   e. Synthesizes cholesterol and lipoproteins from fats
   f. Synthesizes plasma proteins and blood clotting factors
   g. Stores minerals and fat-soluble vitamins
   h. Detoxifies drugs and toxins; inactivates hormones
   i. Produces heat
   j. Stores blood

7. *Gallbladder* (see Figure 12-8): Concentrates and stores bile used for digesting the fat in food

   Some common pathologies of the alimentary tract are shown in **Figure 12-9**.

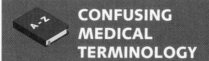

CONFUSING MEDICAL TERMINOLOGY

gastr/o versus abdomin/o, lapar/o, and celi/o

gastr/o – stomach, e.g., gastroenterologist (<u>gas</u>-troh-en-tuh-rol-uh-jist) refers to a physician who specializes in the study of the esophagus, stomach, and small and large intestines

abdomin/o, lapar/o, and celi/o – abdomen, belly; loin, flank, e.g., abdominocentesis (abdom-in-o-sen-<u>te</u>-sis) refers to surgical puncture of the abdomen; laparoscopy (<u>lap</u>-er-uh-skoh-pee) refers to use of a scope to penetrate the abdomen wall to study the abdominal cavity; celiotomy (se-li-<u>ot</u>-<u>ah</u>-me) refers to incision into the abdominal cavity

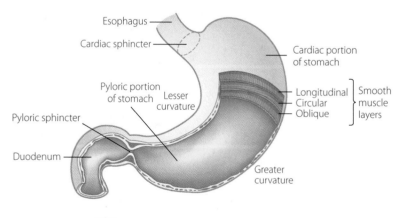

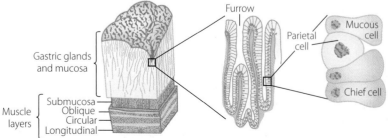

FIGURE 12-6 External and internal anatomy of the stomach.

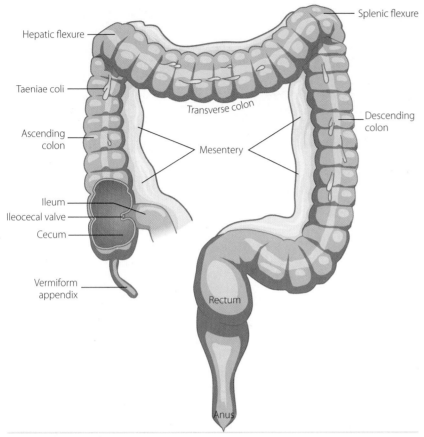

Splenic flexure

Hepatic flexure

Taeniae coli

Transverse colon

Ascending colon

Descending colon

Mesentery

Ileum

Ileocecal valve

Cecum

Vermiform appendix

Rectum

Anus

FIGURE 12-7 Large intestine; each segment is named according to the direction it travels or according to its shape.

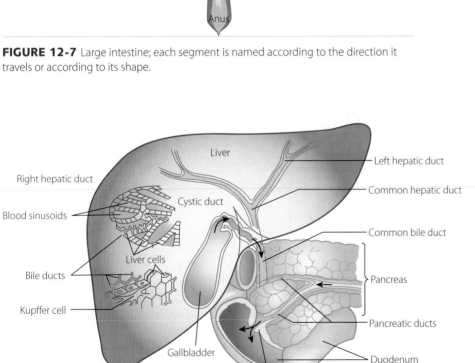

Liver

Left hepatic duct

Right hepatic duct

Common hepatic duct

Blood sinusoids

Cystic duct

Common bile duct

Liver cells

Pancreas

Bile ducts

Kupffer cell

Pancreatic ducts

Gallbladder

Duodenum

Ampulla of Vater

FIGURE 12-8 Liver and its interrelationship with the gallbladder, pancreas, and duodenum. A section has been removed from the liver and the area enlarged to show the arrangement of liver cells, bile ducts, Kupffer cells, and blood sinusoids to one another. Arrows indicate the direction of flow of bile from the gallbladder and liver and of digestive juices from the pancreas into the duodenum.

CONFUSING MEDICAL TERMINOLOGY

A-Z

hypo- versus hyper-

hypo- – under, decreased, deficient, below, e.g., hypoglossal (hi-po-<u>glos</u>-al) refers to under the tongue

hyper- – above, over, excess, increased, beyond, e.g., hyperbilirubinemia (hi-per-bil-i-<u>ru</u>-bin-e-me-ah) refers to excessive bilirubin (a chemical made by the liver) in blood as a result of obstruction of the biliary duct

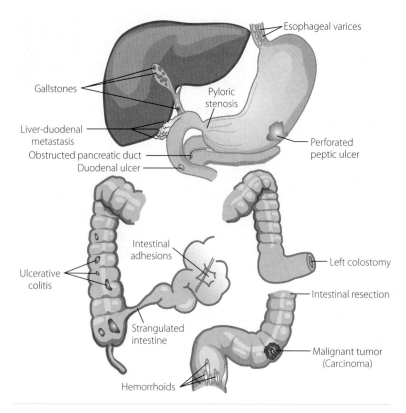

FIGURE 12-9 Pathologies of the alimentary tract.

LESSON ONE	Materials to Be Learned

The digestive system involves the processes of ingestion, digestion, absorption, and elimination of food and food products. The most essential medical terms related to this system are described in this lesson. Study them in conjunction with Figures 12-1 through 12-9.

The digestive system is a large organ system, which includes the accessory organs. It has myriad functions. In such a complex system, there will be many clinical disorders and diseases, some of which will require surgery. To properly diagnose and treat these conditions, specific medical tests are used. Great accuracy in pinpointing the exact location of the problem is essential (see Figure 12-9).

To provide a simple method of learning the major terms related to this system, this lesson is divided into four segments: the organ and accessory organs (and processes), selective clinical disorders, terms used in the diagnosis and treatment of the digestive system, and identification of divisions and quadrants of the abdomen.

MAJOR AND ACCESSORY ORGANS OF THE DIGESTIVE SYSTEM

Table 12-1 lists the major and accessory organs of the digestive system.

TABLE 12-1 Major and Accessory Organs of the Digestive System

Major and Accessory Organ	Pronunciation	Definition
Oral Cavity		
epiglottis	epi-glot-is	thin, leaf-shaped cartilage attached to the superior end of the larynx, protruding into the pharynx just behind the root of the tongue; covers the trachea during swallowing and opens during inhalation
gingiva (plural: Gingivae; [gums])	gin-gi-va	mucous membrane and supporting fibrous tissue that covers the aveolar jaw bone; separates the crown from the root of the tooth
palate	pal-ate	roof of the mouth which separates the mouth from the nose; *hard palate* is at the front and *soft palate* at the back of the mouth. The hard palate consists of bone covered with mucous membrane, while the soft palate consists of muscle and connective tissue
papillae	pah-pill-ay	small rough elevations on tongue and roof of the mouth; contain taste buds
salivary glands	sal-i-ver-e glands	three glands in the mouth that secrete saliva: the *parotid, submandibular*, and *sublingual* glands; saliva moistens food and starts carbohydrate digestion
tongue	tung	chief organ of taste; aids in mastication, swallowing, and speech
trachea	tray-kea	windpipe; wide, short tube that starts below the larynx and enters the thoracic cavity; passageway for air from the nose to the lungs
uvula	u-vu-la	small, fleshy mass of tissue that hangs from the soft palate at the roof of the mouth; aids in producing sound and speech
Teeth		
canine (cuspids)	key-nahyn (kuhs-pid)	fang-shaped teeth; function to grasp and tear food
deciduous	dih-sij-oo-uh s	baby teeth, milk teeth; primary teeth that erupt between 6 months and 4 years of age. Consists of a total of 20 teeth: incisors (8), canines (4), and molars (8)
incisor	in-sahy-zer	Chisel-shaped teeth located in the front of the mouth; function to slice or cut food
molar	moh-ler	largest and broadest teeth located in the back of the mouth; function to crush and grind food
permanent	per-ma-nent	push primary teeth out of their sockets between 6 and 25 years of age and add an additional 8 premolar and 4 molar teeth; consists of a total of 32 teeth
premolar (bicuspids)	pree-moh-ler (bahy-kuhs-pid)	teeth with a broad crown and cusp located between the canine and molars; function to crush and grind food

(continues)

TABLE **12-1** (*continued*)

Major and Accessory Organ	Pronunciation	Definition
Upper Alimentary Canal		
esophagus	e-<u>sof</u>-ah-gus	membranous passage extending from the pharynx to the stomach; moves food from the oral cavity to the stomach by *peristalsis* (alternating muscle contraction and relaxation)
lower esophageal sphincter (LES)	low-er e-soph-a-<u>ge</u>-al <u>sphinc</u>-ter	also, cardiac sphincter or gastroesophageal sphincter; ring of smooth muscle fibers at the junction of the esophagus and stomach that prevents backflow of stomach contents into the esophagus
pharynx	<u>far</u>-ingks	muscular cavity behind the nasal cavity, mouth, and larynx and anterior to the esophagus; allows passage of both air and food. Divided into three areas: the *nasopharynx* (top), *oropharynx* (center, behind the mouth), and *laryngopharynx* (bottom). The laryngopharynx also functions as a resonating organ in speech
pyloric sphincter	py-<u>lor</u>-ic <u>sphinc</u>-ter	circular muscle between the stomach and duodenum; controls the movement of the stomach contents into the duodenum
stomach	<u>stum</u>-ak	an expansion of the digestive tract between the esophagus and duodenum; allows for gradual movement of food into the small intestine for digestion. Gastric juice contains HCl, which activates pepsin to begin the digestion of dietary protein
Small Intestine		
duodenum	du-o-<u>de</u>-num	the first portion of the small intestine; as contents from the stomach (*chyme*) enter the duodenum, digestive enzymes are added from the pancreas for the digestion of carbohydrates and proteins, and bile is secreted from the liver to facilitate the digestion of dietary fat
jejunum	je-<u>joo</u>-num	part of the small intestine from the duodenum to the ileum; the majority of the digestion of food and nutrient absorption occurs here
ileum	<u>il</u>-e-um	last portion of the small intestine, from jejunum to cecum; two important functions of the ileum are absorption of vitamin B$_{12}$ and reabsorption of bile salts
ileocecal sphincter (valve)	il-eo-<u>ce</u>-cal <u>sphinc</u>-ter (valve)	circular muscle between the ileum and cecum (beginning of colon); controls the movement of contents from the ileum into the colon
peritoneum	per´-i´-to-<u>ne</u>-um	the peritoneal cavity; membrane lining abdominal walls and pelvis, body cavities, and surrounding the contained viscera (digestive organs)
Accessory Organs		
gallbladder	<u>gall</u>-blader	the pear-shaped organ behind the liver; stores and concentrates bile
liver	<u>liv</u>-er	the large, dark red gland in the right upper part of the abdomen just beneath the diaphragm; functions are storage and filtration of blood, secretion of bile, conversion of sugars into glycogen, and other metabolic activities
pancreas	<u>pan</u>-kre-as	a large, elongated gland situated transversely behind the stomach. Externally, it secretes digestive enzymes into the common duct; internally, its beta cells secrete insulin and glucagon

Major and Accessory Organ	Pronunciation	Definition
Large Intestine		
anus	<u>a</u>-nus	opening of the rectum on the body surface
appendix	ap-<u>pen</u>-dix	small tube at the junction of the small and large intestines on the right side of the body
ascending colon	a-<u>sen</u>-ding <u>ko</u>-lon	portion of the colon from the cecum to hepatic flexure; site for normal bacterial flora that break down dietary fiber and synthesize vitamin K, B_{12}, thiamin, and riboflavin
cecum	<u>se</u>-kum	the first part of the large intestine, a dilated pouch
descending colon	di-<u>send</u>-ing <u>ko</u>-lon	portion of the colon from the splenic flexure to the sigmoid colon; primary function is reabsorption of water and electrolytes
flexure	<u>flek</u>-sher	a bend or fold; as the hepatic flexure of the colon (near the liver)
rectum	<u>rek</u>-tum	the last portion of the large intestine; role is storage of undigested food, bacteria, and sloughed off cells (feces)
sigmoid colon	<u>sig</u>-moid <u>ko</u>-lon	portion of the large intestine between the descending colon and rectum; function is to store undigested food until evacuated through the rectum
transverse colon	trans-<u>vers</u> ko-lon	portion of the large intestine passing transversely across the upper part of the abdomen, between the hepatic and splenic flexure; primary function is reabsorption of water and electrolytes

CLINICAL DISORDERS

Table 12-2 lists common clinical disorders of the digestive system including dental conditions (see Figure 12-9)

TABLE **12-2** Clinical Disorders		
Clinical Disorder	**Pronunciation**	**Definition**
Oral Cavity		
abscessed tooth	<u>ab</u>-scessed	tooth infection with pus, pain, and inflammation; common causes are tooth fracture or decay
cleft lip/palate	cleft lip/<u>pal</u>-at	congenital fissure or split of the lip (cleft lip) or roof of the mouth (cleft palate)
dental caries	<u>den</u>-tal <u>cair</u>-eez	destruction of the tooth enamel by acids produced by bacterial plaque on dietary carbohydrates; caries can extend below the enamel
dental plaque	plak	bacterial plaque; result of action of bacteria on carbohydrates initially forming a sticky substance that hardens to tartar that adheres to the teeth
gingivitis (gum disease)	gin-gi-<u>vi</u>-tis	inflammation of the gums with irritation, redness, and swelling; most common cause is buildup of dental plaque and bacterial growth between the gums and teeth

(continues)

TABLE **12-2** (continued)

Clinical Disorder	Pronunciation	Definition
malocclusion	mal-oc-<u>clu</u>-sion	irregular bite, crossbite, or overbite; upper and lower teeth do not fit together during biting or chewing
oral leukoplakia	<u>or</u>-al loo-koh-<u>play</u>-kee-ah	precancerous lesion in the mouth
osteonecrosis of the jaw (ONJ)	os-te-o-<u>ne</u>-cro-sis	dead aveolar (jaw) bone after a tooth extraction; most common cause is history of treatment with bisphosphonates for osteoporosis
periodontitis	per-e-o-don-<u>ti</u>-tis	inflammatory disease of the periodontium; usually as a result of advanced stage of gingivitis; can cause loss of alveolar bone, the periodontal ligament, and tooth loss
pulpitis	pul-<u>pi</u>-tis	inflammation of the pulp; common cause is an infected tooth
sialolith	si-<u>al</u>-o-lith	salivary duct stone
temporomandibular joint syndrome (TMJ/TMD)	tem-po-ro-man-<u>dib</u>-u-lar	joint pain and headaches caused by clenching or grinding teeth, or joint injury
thrush	thrush	fungal infection of the mouth caused by *Candida albicans* resulting in painful, creamy white raised patches of the tongue and oral mucosa

Upper Alimentary Canal

achalasia	ak-al-<u>lay</u>-zee-ah	decreased motility of the lower two-thirds of the esophagus, along with constriction of the lower esophageal sphincter (LES); symptoms are vomiting and difficulty swallowing
esophageal atresia	e-sof´-ah-<u>je</u>-al ah-<u>tre</u>-zhe-ah	congenital absence of the opening between esophagus and stomach
esophageal varices	e-sof´-ah-<u>je</u>-al <u>var</u>-i-sez	enlarged, incompetent veins in the distal esophagus, usually caused by blocked ducts in the liver cirrhosis resulting in portal hypertension
esophagitis	e-sof´-ah-<u>ji</u>-tis	inflammation of the esophagus
gastric (peptic) ulcers	<u>gas</u>-trik (pep-tic) <u>ul</u>-serz	inflammation of the stomach or intestinal linings, with pain and sometimes bleeding from perforation
gastritis	gas-<u>tri</u>-tis	inflammation of the stomach lining
gastroesophageal reflux disease (GERD)	gas-tro-e-<u>soph</u>-a-<u>ge</u>-al re-<u>fluks</u> diz-<u>ez</u>	backflow of gastric acid contents into the esophagus causing heartburn and, if chronic, esophagitis (see Box 12-1)
Helicobacter pylori (*H. pylori*)	<u>Hel</u>-i-co-<u>bac</u>-ter py-<u>lor</u>-i	bacteria that causes gastritis and peptic ulcer disease of the stomach and duodenum
hiatal hernia	hi-<u>a</u>-tal	protrusion of the top of the stomach through the esophageal hiatus (opening) of the diaphragm
pyloric stenosis	pi-<u>lor</u>-ik ste-<u>no</u>-sis	an obstruction of the pyloric orifice of the stomach, congenital or acquired

Clinical Disorder	Pronunciation	Definition
Accessory Organs		
cholangitis	chol-an-gi-tis	inflammation of the bile ducts
cholecystitis	cho-le-cys-<u>ti</u>-tis	inflammation of the gall bladder, most commonly caused by gallstones or bacterial infection
cholelithiasis	ko´-le-li-<u>thi</u>-ah-sis	gallstones; hardened cholesterol stones formed from bile crystallization
cirrhosis	si-<u>ro</u>-sis	chronic inflammation of the liver and loss of normal architecture, with fibrosis and nodular regeneration; most common causes are chronic viral hepatitis or chronic alcoholism
hepatitis	hep´-ah-<u>ti</u>-tis	inflammation of the liver; caused by a virus, can be type A, B, or C; can also be caused by excessive alcohol use, e.g., alcoholic hepatitis
pancreatitis	pan´-kre-ah-<u>ti</u>-tis	inflammation of the pancreas; caused by activation of digestive enzymes within the pancreas causing severe pain; most common causes are gallstones and alcoholism
Small Intestine		
adhesion	ad-<u>he</u>-zhun	fibrous bands of scar tissue between internal organs and the intestinal tract or between different sites of the intestinal tract; abdominal surgery is the most common cause
celiac disease	<u>ce</u>-li-ac <u>diz</u>-ez	damage to the lining of the small intestine caused by the inability to digest wheat gluten, resulting in malabsorption of nutrients and malnutrition
fistula	<u>fis</u>-tu-la	permanent abnormal passageway at different sites of the intestinal tract, between the intestinal tract and other organs or between the intestinal tract and the exterior of the body
gastroenteritis	<u>gas</u>-tro-en´-ter-i-tis	inflammation of the stomach and intestine caused by ingested harmful bacterial toxin or a virus, with acute nausea and vomiting, cramps, and diarrhea
hernia	<u>her</u>-ni-a	a protrusion of an organ or part of the intestinal tract through connective tissue or through the abdominal wall
inflammatory bowel disease (IBD)	in-<u>flam</u>-uh-tawr-ee <u>bow</u>-el di-<u>zez</u>	autoimmune disorder with chronic inflammation of the gastrointestinal tract; *Crohn's disease* affects both the small and large intestine, while *ulcerative colitis* affects only the colon
intussusception	in´-tuh-suh-<u>sep</u>-shun	prolapse of a part of the intestine into the lumen of an immediately adjacent part; most common site is at the ileocecal junction and most common in newborn infants
lactose intolerance	<u>lac</u>-tose in-<u>tol</u>-erance	inability to digest lactose, sugar found in milk and dairy products; caused by a lack of the lactase enzyme in the small intestine
megacolon	meg-a-co-lon	dilation and hypertrophy of the colon; can be caused by chronic constipation, ulcerative colitis
volvulus	<u>vol</u>-vyoo-lus	loop of bowel twisting on itself resulting in bowel obstruction
Large Intestine		
appendicitis	ah-pen´-di-<u>si</u>-tis	inflammation of the appendix, which may rupture
diverticulitis	di´-ver-tik´-u-<u>li</u>-tis	inflammation of the *diverticula*, the pouches that form in the walls of the large intestine
hemorrhoids	hem-or-<u>rhoids</u>	engorged (varicose) veins under the rectal mucosa; caused by constipation, pregnancy, prolonged sitting, or infection of the anus

(continues)

TABLE 12-2 (*continued*)

Clinical Disorder	Pronunciation	Definition
Hirschsprung's disease	hirsh-sprungz diz-ez	congenital megacolon resulting from absence of autonomic ganglia in a segment of smooth muscle that normally stimulates peristalsis; usually requires surgery
inguinal hernia	ing-gwi-nal (pertaining to the groin)	hernia into the inguinal canal, the passage through the lower abdominal wall
irritable bowel syndrome (IBS) or spastic colon	eer-uh-tuh-bul bah-wul sin-drohm or spas-tic coh-lon	functional GI disorder that affects the large intestine; symptoms include abdominal pain or discomfort plus bowel movement patterns that vary between diarrhea and constipation
peritonitis	per´-i-to-ni-tis	inflammation of the peritoneal cavity; may be caused by chemical irritation or bacterial invasion
polyposis	pol´-i-po-sis	the formation of numerous polyps (growth hanging from a thin stalk); commonly found in the colon
rectocele	rek-to-sel	hernia of the rectum through the vaginal floor

TERMS USED IN THE DIAGNOSIS AND TREATMENT OF THE DIGESTIVE SYSTEM

Table 12-3 lists terms used to describe the symptoms, diagnosis and treatment of diseases of the digestive system.

TABLE 12-3 Terms Used in the Diagnosis and Treatment of the Digestive System

Clinical Disorder	Pronunciation	Definition
History and Physical Exam: Oral Cavity		
bruxism	brux-ism	chronic habit of clenching or grinding the teeth, commonly while sleeping
dysgeusia	dys-geu-si-a	distortion in the sense of taste
glossitis	glos-si-tis	inflammation of the tongue; caused by poorly fitting dentures, smoking, or systemic disease
hypogeusia	hypo-geu-si-a	decreased sense of taste
stomatitis	sto-ma-ti-tis	inflammation of the mucous membranes of all parts of the mouth
xerostomia	zeer-uh-stoh-mee-uh	dryness of the mouth caused by decreased secretion of saliva; caused by medications, disease, or aging

Clinical Disorder	Pronunciation	Definition
History and Physical Exam: Upper Alimentary Canal		
borborygmus	bor-boh-<u>rig</u>-mus	audible abdominal sound produced by hyperactive peristalsis of the small intestine; rumbling, gurgling, and tinkling noises can be heard with a stethoscope
dysphagia	dys-<u>pha</u>-gia	difficulty in swallowing
eructation (burping)	eh-ruk-<u>tay</u>-shun	belching; a unique sound resulting from the body attempting to bring air from the stomach through the mouth
emesis	<u>em</u>-eh-sis	material expelled from the stomach during vomiting; vomitus
fecal incontinence	<u>fe</u>-cal in-<u>con</u>-ti-nence	loss of bowel control from occasionally leaking a small amount of stool or passing gas, to not being able to control bowel movements; caused by muscle or nerve damage or physical inactivity
melena	<u>mell</u>-eh-nah	abnormal black, tarry stool containing digested blood
nausea and vomiting (N & V)	<u>naw</u>-ze-ah and <u>vom</u>-it-ing	nausea is an uneasiness of the stomach that often comes before vomiting; vomiting is the forcible involuntary emptying ("throwing up") of stomach contents through the mouth
odynophagia	o-dyn-<u>o</u>-pha-gia	painful swallowing due to a disorder of the esophagus
History and Physical Exam: Accessory Organs		
anorexia	an-o-<u>rex</u>-i-a	loss of appetite, especially if prolonged
ascites	as-<u>ci</u>-tes	abnormal accumulation of fluid in the spaces between tissues and organs in the cavity of the abdomen; complication of cirrhosis of the liver
jaundice	<u>jaun</u>-dice	yellowish pigmentation of the skin and eyes caused by the deposition of bile pigments; complication of obstructed bile duct found in diseases of the gallbladder, liver, or pancreas
History and Physical Exam: Small Intestine		
abdominal pain	ab-<u>dom</u>-i-nal	acute or chronic discomfort from mild to severe in the abdominal area; can be a symptom of an abnormal condition of any part of the GI tract, including the gallbladder, liver, or pancreas
diarrhea	di-ar-<u>rhe</u>-a	abnormally frequent intestinal evacuations with more or less fluid stools; can be watery diarrhea or bloody diarrhea
History and Physical Exam: Large Intestine		
constipation	con-sti-<u>pa</u>-tion	bowel movements that occur less often than usual or consist of hard, dry stools that are painful or difficult to pass; common causes are a diet low in fiber and certain medications

(continues)

TABLE **12-3** (*continued*)

Clinical Disorder	Pronunciation	Definition
flatulence	<u>flat</u>-u-lence	excessive passing of gas through the anus; certain foods increase gas production (e.g., beans, cabbage, fiber); also caused by bacterial action on undigested sugars (lactose), fiber, and polysaccharides in the colon
impaction (fecal)	im-<u>pak</u>-shun (<u>fek</u>-al)	hardened feces in the rectum or sigmoid colon; caused by constipation
tenesmus	te-<u>nes</u>-mus	sudden and constant feeling of a need to have a bowel movement; common symptom of ulcerative colitis
Diagnostic Tools		
biopsy	<u>bi</u>-op-se	removal of tissue for microscopic diagnosis
colonoscopy	ko-lon-<u>os</u>-ko-pe	endoscopic examination of the colon, either transabdominally during laparotomy or transanally by means of a colonoscope
digital examination	<u>dig</u>-i-tal eg-<u>zam</u>-i-na-shun	insertion of the gloved finger into the rectum
gastroscopy	gas-<u>tros</u>-ko-pe	inspection of the stomach's interior with a gastroscope
paracentesis	par-a-cen-<u>te</u>-sis	removal of fluid from the abdomen through a needle; used for diagnostic purposes or to remove fluid because of ascites
proctoscopy	prok-<u>tos</u>-ko-pe	inspection of the sigmoid colon and rectum with a proctoscope
Radiological Exams and Treatments		
barium swallow/upper GI series	<u>bah</u>-ree-um <u>swal</u>-o	the oral administration of a radiopaque contrast medium to view the esophagus by X-ray while swallowing
cholangiography	ko-lan´-je-<u>og</u>-rah-fe	X-ray examination of the bile ducts, using a radiopaque dye as a contrast medium
dental X-rays	den-tal ex-rays	X-ray of teeth, bones, and soft tissues; used to detect cavities, hidden dental structures (such as wisdom teeth), impacted teeth, abscesses, and bone loss
esophagogastroduodenoscopy (EGD)	e-sof´-ah-go-gas´-tro-du´-o-de-<u>nos</u>-ko-pe	using endoscopes to examine esophagus, stomach, and duodenum
extracorporeal shock wave lithotripsy (ESWL)	eks-trah-kor-<u>por</u>-ee-al shock wave <u>lith</u>-oh-trip-see	use of ultrasound to send shock waves to crush the gallstones, allowing contraction of the gallbladder to remove stone fragments
flat plate of abdomen	flat plate uv <u>ab</u>-do-men	an X-ray film of the abdomen
fluoroscopy	<u>floo</u>-or-<u>oh</u>-skop-ee	radiological technique to examine the function of an organ
magnetic resonance cholangiopancreatography (MRCP)	mag-<u>neh</u>-tic <u>rez</u>-oh-nans <u>chol</u>-an-gi-o-pan-<u>cre</u>-a-tog-ra-phy	use of magnetic resonance imaging; noninvasive alternative to an endoscopic procedure

Clinical Disorder	Pronunciation	Definition
percutaneous transhepatic cholangiography (PTC)	per-kyoo-<u>tay</u>-nee-us trans-heh-<u>pat</u>-ik koh-lan-jee-<u>og</u>-rah-fee	examination of the bile duct, using a needle to pass directly into the duct and to inject a contrast medium that can be seen by specialized equipment
scan	skan	an image produced using a sweeping beam of radiation, as in scintiscanning, B-mode ultrasonography, scanography, or CAT (computerized axial tomography)
ultrasonography	ul´-trah-son-<u>og</u>-rah-fe	using ultrasound to obtain a visual record of any organ
Laboratory Tests		
alkaline phosphatase (ALP)	<u>al</u>-ka-line <u>phos</u>-pha-tase	enzyme in liver cells and bile ducts; blood values are elevated with liver disease or a blocked bile duct
aspartate aminotransferase (AST)	as-<u>par</u>-tate a-mi-no-<u>trans</u>-fer-ase	enzyme in liver cells; high amounts in the blood indicate disease of liver cells
bilirubin	<u>bil</u>-i-<u>ru</u>-bin	pigment from breakdown of red blood cells; blood values are elevated in liver disease or obstruction of bile ducts in diseases of the gallbladder
lipase	<u>li</u>-pase	pancreatic enzyme that is elevated in the blood in acute and chronic pancreatitis
stool sample or specimen		a small stool sample for laboratory study, e.g., occult blood, parasites
Surgery for Diagnosis and Treatment of the Digestive Systsem: Oral Cavity		
cheiloplasty	<u>ki</u>-lo-plas´-te	surgical repair of a cleft lip
dental crown	den-tal crown	dental restoration which completely caps or encircles a tooth to restore strength; commonly done in teeth with a large cavity or after root canal therapy
dental filling	den-tal fill-ing	used to fill the space in a tooth because of a cavity or crack in the tooth
dental implant	den-tal im-plant	a post placed in the jawbone to substitute for the tooth root and provide a strong and sturdy foundation for a replacement tooth (crown)
endodontic/root canal therapy	en-doh-<u>don</u>-tik	treatment of inflamed or infected dental pulp, usually by removal of the nerve and other tissue of the pulp cavity and its replacement with suitable filling material
gingivectomy	gin-gi-<u>vek</u>-tuh-mee	surgical removal of diseased gum tissue and the bacteria that can cause periodontitis
gingivoplasty	gin-gi-<u>vo</u>-plas-ty	surgical reshaping of the gum tissue after removal of the gum because of gingivitis
tooth extraction	tooth ex-<u>trac</u>-tion	removal of a tooth because of infection, decay, or impaction

(continues)

TABLE **12-3** (continued)

Clinical Disorder	Pronunciation	Definition
Surgery for Diagnosis and Treatment of the Digestive Systsem: Upper and Lower Gastrointestinal Tract and Accessory Organs		
anastomosis	ah-nas´-to-<u>mo</u>-sis	surgical formation of a connection between two parts; ileorectal anastomosis connects the ileum and rectum after removal of the colon
appendectomy	ap´-en-<u>dek</u>-to-me	excision of the appendix
bypass	<u>bi</u>-pas	a shunt, e.g., a surgically created pathway
cholecystectomy	ko´-le-sis-<u>tek</u>-to-me	excision of the gallbladder
colectomy	kuh-<u>lek</u>-tuh-mee	surgical removal of all or part of the large intestine because of cancer or ulcerative colitis
colostomy	ko-<u>los</u>-to-me	surgical creation of an opening (stoma) between the colon and the body surface; often done at the same time as a colectomy
esophageal manometry	e-soph-a-<u>ge</u>-al ma-<u>nom</u>-et-ry	measurement of coordination and force of muscles, including the lower esophageal sphincter
gastrectomy	gas-<u>trek</u>-to-me	excision of the stomach, may be partial or subtotal
herniorrhaphy	her´-ne-<u>or</u>-ah-fe	surgical repair of a hernia
ileostomy	il´-e-<u>os</u>-to-me	surgical creation of an opening into the ileum with a stoma on the abdominal wall
laparotomy	lap´-ah-<u>rot</u>-o-me	incision through any part of the abdominal wall
portacaval shunt	por´-tah-<u>ka</u>-val shunt	connecting the portal vein and inferior vena cava to bypass a cirrhotic liver
stoma	<u>sto</u>-mah	"mouth"; an artificially created opening (e.g., in ileostomy) on the surface of the abdomen

DIGESTION AND NUTRITION TERMS

These terms are used to describe the processes of digestion and metabolism, nutrition assessment, and intervention (see **Table 12-4**).

TABLE **12-4** Digestion and Nutrition Terms

Term	Pronunciation	Definition
anabolism	a-<u>nab</u>-o-lizm	building up, using nutrients (proteins) for growth and development
absorption	ab-<u>sorp</u>-shun	uptake from intestinal cells—fluids, solutes, proteins, fats, and other nutrients—into the blood and lymph systems
BMI	body mass index	estimate of body fat based on weight in relation to height

Term	Pronunciation	Definition
cachexia	kah-<u>kek</u>-se-ah	severe malnutrition and wasting, emaciation
catabolism	kah-<u>tab</u>-o-lizm	burning nutrients; breakdown in the presence of oxygen
deglutition	de´-glu-<u>ti</u>-shun	the act of swallowing
digestion	di-<u>jes</u>-chun	the act of converting food and fluids into chemical substances that can be absorbed and assimilated
elimination	e-lim-i-<u>na</u>-shun	excreting solid waste (feces)
emaciation	ee-may-she-<u>ay</u>-shun	excessive leanness caused by disease or lack of nutrition
excretion	ek-<u>skre</u>-shun	excreting body solid and liquid waste (feces and urine)
hyperalimentation	hi´-per-al´-i-men-<u>ta</u>-shun	an intravenous feeding program similar to total parenteral nutrition
mastication	mas-ti-<u>kay</u>-shun	chewing
nasogastric (NG)	na´-zo-<u>gas</u>-trik	a soft flexible tube introduced through the nose into the stomach for gavage, lavage, or suction
NPO (nothing per os)		no food or fluid by mouth or other body orifice (*os* means any body orifice)
obesity	o-<u>bes</u>-i-te	body mass index (BMI) of ≥ 30 using the formula: weight (kg) ÷ height squared (m²)
peristalsis	peri-<u>stal</u>-sis	muscular movement of food and liquid through the GI tract
total parenteral nutrition (TPN)	pah-<u>ren</u>-ter-al nu-<u>trish</u>-un	intensive intravenous feeding most often introduced through a subclavian vein; alternate route for providing nutrition

BOX 12-1 provides an overview of gastroesophageal reflux disease (GERD).

Box 12-1 Gastroesophageal Reflux Disease (GERD)

Gastroesophageal reflux (GER) is a common condition found in people of all ages. GER occurs when the stomach contents back up into the esophagus because of relaxation of the lower esophageal sphincter (LES) or muscle; when acid touches the lining of the esophagus, the most common symptom is pain in the chest called heartburn. Chronic acid reflux causes an inflammatory condition of the esophagus, esophagitis.

About 50 percent of infants "spit up" after feeding because the LES has not completely developed. This condition is usually painless and by 1–1½ years of age, the majority of babies no longer spit up after eating or drinking. If the child has other symptoms, including abdominal pain, heartburn, poor weight gain, or breathing problems, then the condition is considered the chronic disease— gastroesophageal reflux disease (GERD).

About 20 percent of adults also have GERD. Those more likely to have the disease are pregnant women, those who are overweight or obese, and smokers. Additional symptoms of chronic disease are coughing, asthma, and laryngitis. Treatment involves lifestyle changes to promote weight loss and elimination of medications and foods that relax the LES plus the use of acid-inhibiting medications.

ABDOMINAL REFERENCE TERMS

These terms are used to describe the location of symptoms during a physical exam and documentation in the medical record Refer to **Table 12-5** and **Figure 12-10**.

TABLE **12-5** Abdominal Reference Terms			
Area	**Right**	**Middle**	**Left**
quadrant (<u>kwod</u>-rant) (see Figure 12-10)	right upper quadrant (RUQ) and right lower quadrant (RLQ)		left upper quadrant (LUQ) and left lower quadrant (LLQ)
divisions (nine)	right hypochondrium (hi´-po-<u>kon</u>-dre-um) (RH)	epigastric (ep´-i-<u>gas</u>-trik) (E)	left hypochondrium (LH)
	right lumbar (<u>lum</u>-bar) (RL)	umbilical (um-<u>bil</u>-i-kal) (U)	left lumbar (LL)
	right inguinal (<u>ing</u>-gwi-nal) or iliac (<u>il</u>-e-ak) (RI)	suprapubic (<u>soo</u>-prah-pu-bik) (S) or hypogastrium (hy-po-<u>gas</u>-tri-um) (H)	left inguinal or iliac (LI)

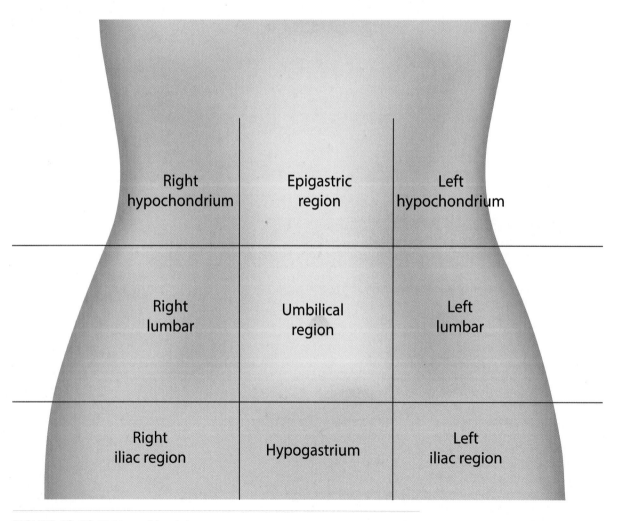

FIGURE 12-10 Divisions of the abdomen.
© joshya/Shutterstock.

THE ORIGIN OF MEDICAL TERMS

Table 12-6 explains the origin of several terms used in this chapter.

TABLE **12-6** The Origin of Medical Terms		
Word	**Pronunciation**	**Origin and Definition**
appendectomy	ap-en-<u>dek</u>-to-me	Latin, *appendere*, to cause to hang + Greek, *ektomia*, cutting out of
bruxism	<u>brux</u>-ism	Greek, *bryyx(is)*, gnashing of teeth
epiglottis	epi-<u>glot</u>-is	Greek, *epi*, near to + Greek, *glotta*, tongue
malocclusion	mal-oc-<u>clu</u>-sion	Latin, *malus*, bad + Latin, *occludere*, close up
osteonecrosis	os-te-o-<u>ne</u>-cro-sis	Greek, *osteon*, bone + Greek, *nekrosis*, death
peritoneum	per-ĭ-to-<u>ne</u>-um	Greek, *peri*, around, surrounding + Greek, *teinein*, to stretch
pharynx	<u>far</u>-ingks	Greek, *pharynx*, throat
sigmoid	<u>sig</u>-moid	Greek, *sigmoeides*, shaped like a sigma
volvulus	<u>vol</u>-vyoo-lus	Latin, *volv*, to turn, twist + Latin, *ule*, small, little
xerostomia	<u>zeer</u>-uh-<u>stoh</u>-mee-uh	Greek, *xeros*, dry + Greek, *stoma*, mouth

ABBREVIATIONS

These abbreviations listed in **Table 12-7** are frequently used to describe the digestive system, including clinical disorders and diagnostic tools.

TABLE **12-7** Abbreviations			
Abbreviation	**Definition**	**Abbreviation**	**Definition**
ALP	alkaline phosphatase	GI	gastrointestinal
AST	aspartate aminotransferase	IBD	inflammatory bowel disease
BMI	body mass index	IBS	irritable bowel syndrome
E	epigastric	LES	lower esophageal sphincter
EGD	esophagogastro-duodenoscopy	LLQ	left lower quadrant
ESWL	extracorporeal shock wave lithotripsy	LL	left lumbar
GERD	gastroesophageal reflux disease	MRCP	magnet resonance cholangiopancreatography

(continues)

TABLE **12-7** (continued)			
Abbreviation	**Definition**	**Abbreviation**	**Definition**
N & V	nausea and vomiting	RH	right hypochondrium
NG	nasogastric	S	suprapubic
NPO	nothing per os	TMJ/TMD	temporomandibular joint syndrome/disease
ONJ	osteonecrosis of the jaw	TPN	total parenteral nutrition
PTC	percutaneous transhepatic cholangiography	U	umbilical

The following box describes common drugs used to treat diseases of the digestive system.

PHARMACOLOGY AND MEDICAL TERMINOLOGY

Drug Classification	antidiarrheal (an-tih-dye-ah-<u>ree</u>-ul)	antiemetic (an-tih-ee-<u>met</u>-ik)	proton pump inhibitors (in-hib-i-tors) (PPIs)
Function	treats diarrhea	relieves nausea and vomiting	treats gastric acid hypersecretion
Word Parts	**anti-** = against; **diarrheal** = pertaining to diarrhea	**anti-** = against; **emetic** = pertaining to "vomiting"	**inhibit** = prevent ; **acid** = pertaining to ulcers (e.g., stomach or espophageal)
Active Ingredients (examples)	diphenoxylate-atropine sulfate (Lomotil); loperamide hydrochloride (Imodium)	meclizine (Antivert); metoclopramide (Reglan); ondansetron (Zofran)	esomeprazole (Nexium); lansoprazole (Prevacid); pantoprazole (Protonix)

CLINICAL *Note*

Dental Office Visit Note

EXAM: A 22-year-old female presents today for routine cleaning and checkup. Routine removal of **calculus**, **plaque**, and stains performed prior to examination. Hygienist exam reports no obvious abnormalities. Gums appear pink and healthy with no bleeding or evidence of **gingivitis**. Of interest was slight swelling of tissue around the third lower left molar indicating possible early **abscess**.

X-RAY: Dental radiology shows **dental caries** of the third left lower molar.

DIAGNOSIS: Mild abscess of third lower left **molar**.

PLAN: Amoxicillin 500mg po **TID** × 10 days. Recheck tooth at that time. Drill and fill tooth as needed.

Direction: For the portions of the clinical note shown by a colored font, provide the definition and/or words for abbreviation.

LESSON TWO	Progress Check

LIST: DIGESTIVE PROCESSES

List terms used to describe the seven major digestive processes:

1. _____

2. _____

3. _____

4. _____

5. _____

6. _____

7. _____

MATCHING: ORAL CAVITY TERMS

Match the parts of the oral cavity listed on the left with their respective functions listed on the right:

Terms	**Definition**
1. Tongue	**a.** Roof of the mouth
2. Pharynx	**b.** Windpipe
3. Parotid, submaxillary, sublingual	**c.** Covers trachea during swallowing
4. Trachea	**d.** Produce saliva
5. Palate	**e.** Swallowing takes place here
6. Epiglottis	**f.** Primary or baby teeth
7. Gingiva	**g.** Broad tooth used for crushing and grinding
8. Deciduous	**h.** Chisel-shaped tooth used for cutting food
9. Molar	**i.** Separates crown from root of the tooth
10. Incisor	**j.** Moves food to facilitate chewing

COMPLETION: CLINICAL CONDITIONS OF THE ORAL CAVITY

Write the medical terms for the following descriptions of clinical conditions:

1. _____: Builds up on the teeth from the action of bacteria on carbohydrates

2. _____: Congenital fissure of the roof of the mouth

3. _____: Infected tooth with pus and inflammation

4. _____: Inflammation, redness, and swelling of the gums

5. _____: Salivary duct stone

6. _____: Joint pain from chronic grinding of the teeth

7. _____: Inflammatory disease of the jaw bone

8. _____: Destruction of tooth enamel by acids produced by bacteria

9. _____: Upper and lower teeth do not fit together during biting or chewing

10. _____: Precancerous lesion in the mouth

WORD POOL: ORAL CAVITY

Select appropriate terms from the word pool below to complete these sentences:

1. _____: Removal of a tooth

2. _____: Removal of infected dental pulp

3. _____: Surgical correction of a cleft lip

4. _____: Surgical removal of diseased gum

5. _____: Post in the jawbone for a replacement tooth

6. _____: Surgical reshaping of gum tissue

7. _____: Treating space in a tooth because of a cavity

8. _____: Capping a tooth after a root canal

Word pool: Cheiloplasty, crown, extraction, filling, gingivectomy, gingivoplasty, implant, root canal

MATCHING: DIGESTIVE TRACT TERMS

Match the parts of the digestive tract listed on the left with their respective functions listed on the right:

Terms	Function
1. Stomach	**a.** Peristalsis moves food into the stomach
2. Lower esophageal sphincter	**b.** Digests food and absorbs nutrients
3. Rectum	**c.** Removes water before excretion
4. Esophagus	**d.** Prevents backflow of stomach contents into the esophagus
5. Gallbladder	**e.** Function is storage of feces
6. Liver	**f.** Stores fat-soluble vitamins; manufactures bile
7. Pancreas	**g.** Secretes acid for digestion of protein
8. Ileum	**h.** Stores bile
9. Gastric mucosa	**i.** Releases enzymes to aid in digestion
10. Colon	**j.** Function is to store food

COMPLETION: CLINICAL CONDITIONS OF THE GI TRACT

Write in the medical terms for the following descriptions of clinical conditions:

1. _____: Abnormal constriction of the lower esophageal sphincter

2. _____: Stones in the gallbladder

3. _____: Autoimmune disorder of the small intestine or colon

4. _____: Abnormal backflow of gastric acid into the esophagus

5. _____: Acute inflammation of the liver

6. _____: Obstruction of the pyloric sphincter

7. _____: Chronic inflammation of the liver

8. _____: Inability to digest and absorb wheat gluten

9. _____: Fibrous bands of scar tissue between different sites of the intestinal tract

10. _____: Varicose veins of the rectum

11. _____: Inability to digest lactose (milk sugar)

12. _____: Inflammation of the appendix

13. _____: Congenital megacolon

14. _____: Bowel loop twisting on itself

15. _____: Abnormal passageway between the colon and abdominal wall

16. _____: Protrusion of part of the intestinal tract through the abdominal wall

17. _____: Numerous polyps in the colon

18. _____: Functional GI disorder with abdominal discomfort and changes in bowel movement patterns

19. _____: Inflammation of the peritoneal membrane

20. _____: Abnormal out pouches of the colon

WORD POOL: DIGESTIVE TRACT

Select appropriate terms from the word pool below to complete these sentences:

1. _____: The first part of the digestive system

2. _____: The chief organ of digestion

3. _____: The first part of the large intestine

4. _____: Three accessory organs

5. _____: The lower part of the large intestine

6. _____: The last part of the alimentary canal

7. _____: The three divisions of the small intestine

8. _____: Contains bacteria that produces vitamin K

Word pool: Cecum, duodenum, gallbladder, ileum, jejunum, liver, mouth or oral cavity, pancreas, sigmoid colon, rectum, small intestine, large intestine

MATCHING: DIAGNOSTIC AND SURGICAL PROCEDURES FOR TREATING DISEASES OF THE GI TRACT

Match the term on the left with the description of the procedure on the right:

Terms	Description
1. Barium swallow	**a.** Incision through the abdominal wall
2. Extracorporeal shock wave lithotripsy (ESWL)	**b.** Removal of excess abdominal fluid with a needle
3. Laparotomy	**c.** Used to evaluate for obstruction in the gallbladder or liver
4. Colostomy	**d.** Use of radiopaque contrast to view the esophagus by X-ray
5. Paracentesis	**e.** Used to diagnose pancreatitis
6. Bilirubin	**f.** Use of ultrasound to crush gallstones
7. Proctoscopy	**g.** Elevated in liver disease
8. Lipase	**h.** Analyzed for blood and parasites
9. Aspartate aminotransferase (AST)	**i.** Examination of the sigmoid colon and rectum
10. Stool sample	**j.** Creation of a stoma between the colon and abdominal wall

IDENTIFYING WORD PARTS

For each of the medical terms, list the root word and the prefix and/or suffix:

Word	Root Word	Prefix	Suffix
1. Achalasia	_____	_____	_____
2. Antiemetic	_____	_____	_____
3. Endodontic	_____	_____	_____
4. Epigastric	_____	_____	_____
5. Gingivitis	_____	_____	_____
6. Hypochondrium	_____	_____	_____
7. Hyperalimentation	_____	_____	_____
8. Parenteral	_____	_____	_____
9. Paracentesis	_____	_____	_____
10. Polyposis	_____	_____	_____

Design Credits: Confusing Medical Terminology Icon: Icon made by Treepik from www.flaticon.com; Allied Health Professions Icon: Icon made by Pixel Buddha from www.flaticon.com

CHAPTER

13

© teekid/iStock/Getty Images

Respiratory System

OBJECTIVES

After completing this chapter and the exercises, the student should be able to:

1. Identify the organs of the respiratory system.
2. Describe the location and label the structures of the respiratory system.
3. List the functions of the respiratory system.
4. Identify and define clinical disorders affecting the respiratory system.
5. List and explain diagnostic tools and medical procedures used to treat disorders of the respiratory system.

THE RESPIRATORY SYSTEM

The respiratory system consists of a series of tubes that transport air into and out of the lungs. Its function is to supply O_2 to the body cells and to transport CO_2 produced by the body cells into the atmosphere. The respiratory organs also have important functions for normal speech, acid–base balance, hormonal regulation of blood pressure, and defense against foreign material. The respiratory system also allows humans to perceive odors and to filter and moisten air.

Respiration involves the following processes:

1. Pulmonary ventilation (breathing)
2. External respiration (diffusion of O_2 and CO_2 between air in the lungs and the capillaries)
3. Internal respiration (diffusion of CO_2 and O_2 between blood and tissue cells)
4. Cellular respiration (use of O_2 by the body cells in production of energy and release of CO_2 and H_2O)

177

ALLIED HEALTH PROFESSIONS

Respiratory Therapists and Respiratory Therapy Technicians

The term *respiratory therapist* used here includes both respiratory therapists and respiratory therapy technicians. Respiratory care therapists work to evaluate, treat, and care for patients with breathing disorders. They work under the direction of a physician.

Most respiratory therapists work with hospital patients in three distinct phases of care: diagnosis, treatment, and patient management. In the area of diagnosis, therapists test the capacity of the lungs and analyze the oxygen (O_2) and carbon dioxide (CO_2) concentrations and potential of hydrogen (blood pH), a measure of the acidity or alkalinity of the blood. To measure lung capacity, the therapist has the patient breathe into a tube connected to an instrument that measures the volume and flow of air during inhalation and exhalation. By comparing the reading with the norm for the patient's age, height, weight, and sex, the therapist can determine whether lung deficiencies exist.

To analyze O_2, CO_2, and pH levels, therapists need an arterial blood sample, for which they generally draw arterial blood. This procedure requires greater skill than is the case for routine tests, for which blood is drawn from a vein. Inserting a needle into a patient's artery and drawing blood must be done with great care; any slip can damage the artery and interrupt the flow of oxygen-rich blood to the tissues. Once the sample is drawn, it is placed in a gas analyzer, and the results are relayed to the physician.

INQUIRY

American Association for Respiratory Care: www.aarc.org
National Board for Respiratory Care: www.nbrc.org

Data from Cross, Nanna, and McWay, Dana. *Stanfield's Introduction to the Health Professions*, 7th ed., Burlington, MA: Jones & Bartlett Learning; 2017.

The respiratory tract is divided into the upper respiratory tract, consisting of the *nose*, *pharynx*, and *larynx*, and the lower respiratory tract, the *trachea*, *bronchi*, and *lungs*. These structures are defined and illustrated in Lesson One (**Figure 13-1**). A brief discussion of their respective functions is:

1. **Nose (nostrils or nares)**: The external portion of the respiratory tract that filters small particles, warms and humidifies incoming air, and receives odors. It is the primary organ for the sense of smell.
2. **Pharynx (throat)**: A five-inch muscular tube that extends from the base of the skull to the esophagus. It is the airway that connects the mouth and nose to the larynx. Although it is a single organ, it is divided into three sections—the *nasopharynx*, *oropharynx*, and *laryngopharynx*. The nasopharynx is behind the nose and serves to equalize pressure on both sides of the tympanic membrane (eardrum). The oropharynx, behind the mouth, is a muscular soft palate containing the uvula and palatine tonsils. The laryngopharynx surrounds the opening of the esophagus, which is the gateway to the rest of the respiratory system. The pharynx is the common passageway for both air and food. To prevent food from entering the respiratory tract, a small flap called the *epiglottis* covers the opening of the larynx during the act of swallowing.
3. **Larynx (voice box)**: This connects the pharynx with the trachea. It is a short tube shaped like a triangular box and is supported by nine cartilages, three paired and three unpaired. It contains the vocal cords and supporting tissue that make vocal sounds possible.
4. **Trachea (windpipe)**: A four-inch-long tube, the trachea extends into the chest and serves as a passageway for air into the bronchi. It lies in front of the esophagus. It is kept permanently open by 16–20 C-shaped cartilaginous rings.
5. **Bronchi**: The trachea branches into two tubes called the bronchi (the bronchial tree). Each bronchus enters a lung. The right primary (main) bronchus is shorter

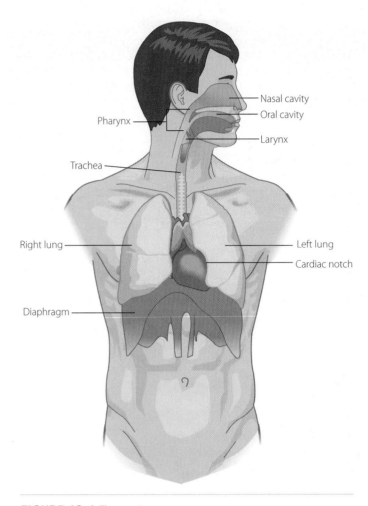

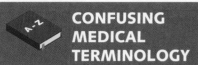

CONFUSING MEDICAL TERMINOLOGY

ox/i versus oxy-

ox/i – oxygen, e.g., oximetry (<u>ok</u>-sim-i-tree) refers to the measuring of oxygen saturation of the blood by means of an oximeter

oxy- – sharp, quick, sour, rapid, e.g., oxyblepsia (ok-si-<u>blef</u>-see-uh) refers to the unusual acuity of vision

FIGURE 13-1 The respiratory system.

than the left because the arch of the aorta displaces the lower trachea to the right. Foreign objects falling into the trachea are more likely to lodge in the right bronchus. Each bronchus subdivides into progressively smaller branches called *bronchioles*, which terminate in the *alveoli* (air space).

6. *Lungs*: They are pyramid-shaped, spongy, air-filled organs that are molded into the thoracic cavity that contains them. The right lung has three lobes, the left has two. In the lungs, alveoli are surrounded by a network of tiny blood vessels called *capillaries*: O_2 from the lungs passes into these capillaries for distribution to the cells and CO_2 from the blood cells passes into the lungs for removal (by exhalation). When O_2 is absorbed into the blood it attaches to *hemoglobin* and is released as needed.

The pleura are the serous membrane coverings that enclose each lung. The *parietal* pleura lines the *thoracic* (chest) cavity (rib cage, diaphragm, and mediastinum). The *visceral* pleura covers the lung and is continuous at the root of the lung, where it joins with the parietal pleura. The parietal and visceral pleura lie close together; between them is a thin film of lubricating fluid that prevents friction when the two slide against each other during respiration.

Pulmonologists are physicians who specialize in the diagnosis and treatment of diseases of the respiratory system, including infectious diseases, cancer, and chronic diseases of the lungs, as described in this chapter.

The overview described the structure, function, and supporting systems of the respiratory system. The respiratory system involves the exchange of O_2 and CO_2. We inhale O_2 and exhale CO_2. This process is also known as *respiration* (inspiration and expiration). To facilitate the learning of myriad medical terms within the respiratory system, the terms are divided into tables. Table 13-1 in Lesson One describes components and processes of the respiratory system and Table 13-2 names and defines common respiratory diseases and disorders. Table 13-3 provides terms pertaining to diagnostic tools and aspects of treatment as well as terminology needed for an understanding of the respiratory system. Refer to **Figures 13-2** through **13-5** as needed.

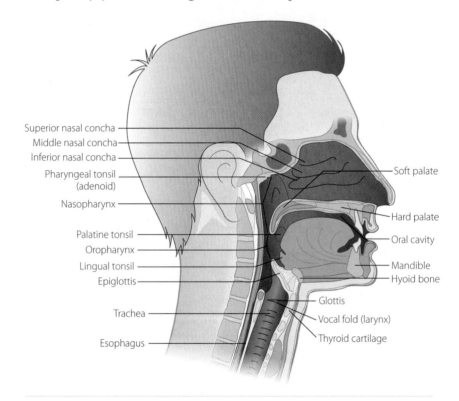

FIGURE 13-2 Sagittal section of the head and neck, showing the respiratory passage down to the bifurcation of the trachea.

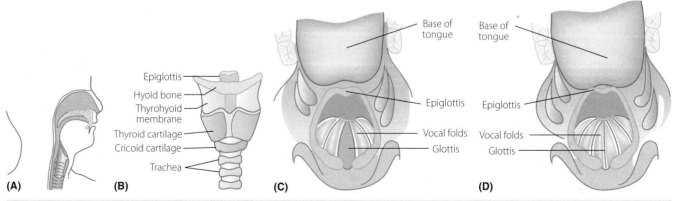

FIGURE 13-3 Larynx. **(A)** In relation to the head and neck. **(B)** Anterior aspect. **(C)** Superior aspect with vocal folds open. **(D)** Superior aspect with vocal folds closed.

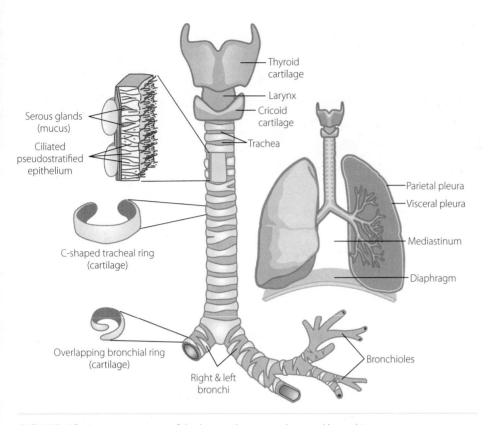

FIGURE 13-4 Anterior aspect of the human larynx, trachea, and bronchi.

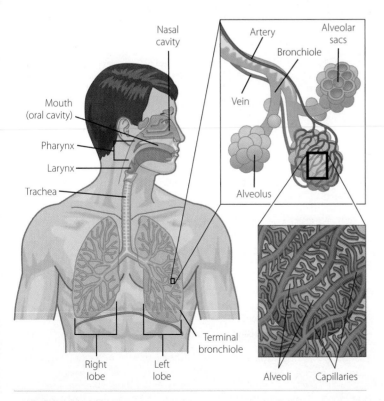

FIGURE 13-5 Internal structure of the lungs.

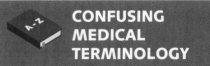

CONFUSING MEDICAL TERMINOLOGY

germ versus germ

germ – sprout, seed, fetus, e.g., wheat germ

germ – pathogenic microorganism, e.g., germ warfare

TERMS THAT DESCRIBE THE COMPONENTS AND FUNCTIONS OF THE RESPIRATORY SYSTEM

Table 13-1 lists terms that describe structure and functions of the respiratory tract.

TABLE **13-1** Terms that Describe the Components and Functions of the Respiratory System		
Component/ Function	**Pronunciation**	**Definition**
alveolus (plural: alveoli)	al-<u>ve</u>-o-lus (al-<u>ve</u>-ol-i)	a small saclike dilation (outpocketing) of the alveolar ducts
bifurcation	bi´-fer-<u>ka</u>-shun	a division into two branches, e.g., bronchi
bronchus (plural: bronchi)	<u>brong</u>-kus (<u>brong</u>-ki)	one of the larger passages conveying air to (right or left principal lobe) and within the lungs
bronchioles	<u>brong</u>-ke-olz	one of the subdivisions of the branched bronchial tree
capillaries (pulmonary)	<u>cap</u>-il-lar-y	smallest arteries in the lung located next to the alveoli; functions are to pick up O_2 from inhaled air and return CO_2 to be exhaled (see Figure 13-5)
diaphragm	<u>dye</u>-ah-fram	muscular partition that separates the thoracic cavity from the abdominal cavity and aids in the process of breathing
expiration/exhalation	ex-pi-<u>ra</u>-tion/ex-ha-<u>la</u>-tion	act of breathing out; CO_2 moves out of the body in this order: lungs, bronchi, trachea, larynx, pharynx, nose (mouth)
hilus	<u>hi</u>-lus	part of lung where vessels, nerves, and bronchi enter
inspiration/inhalation	in-spi-<u>ra</u>-tion/in-ha-<u>la</u>-tion	act of breathing in; O_2 enters the body in this order: nose (mouth), pharynx, larynx, trachea, bronchi, lungs
larynx	<u>lar</u>-inks	voice organ, containing the vocal cords
lung	lung	two cone-shaped spongy organs consisting of alveoli, blood vessels, nerves, and elastic tissue; each is enveloped in a double-folded membrane called the pleura
nasal cavity	<u>na</u>-zal <u>kav</u>-i-te	nose, nares, cavity separated by septum
parenchyma (lung)	pah-<u>reng</u>-ki-mah	the essential elements or "working parts" of an organ, e.g., alveoli in the lung
parietal pleura	par-ry-<u>e</u>-tal <u>ploo</u>-rah	the serous membrane that lines the thoracic (chest) cavity
perfusion	per-<u>fu</u>-zhun	the passage of blood through capillaries in the lung where O_2 and CO_2 are exchanged
pharynx	<u>far</u>-ingks	throat, cavity behind the nasal cavities, and mouth
respiration/ventilation	res-pi-<u>ra</u>-tion/ven-til-<u>a</u>-tion	act of breathing air into the lungs (inhaling) and removing CO_2 out of the lungs (exhaling)
sputum	<u>spu</u>-tum	matter ejected from the trachea, bronchi, and lungs through the mouth
surfactant	sur-<u>fac</u>-tant	lipoprotein mixture that coats and prevents collapse of the alveoli by reducing surface tension of pulmonary fluids
trachea/windpipe	<u>tra</u>-ke-ah/wind-pipe	air passageway from the throat to the lungs that carries air in and out of the lungs
visceral pleura	<u>viss</u>-or-al <u>ploo</u>-rah	membrane that covers the lungs; this membrane and the parietal membrane are close together; between them is a thin film of lubricating fluid that prevents friction when they slide against each other

COMMON DISORDERS OF THE RESPIRATORY SYSTEM

Table 13-2 describes common disorders of the respiratory system.

Condition	Pronunciation	Definition
acute respiratory distress syndrome (ARDS)	a-<u>cute</u> <u>res</u>-pi-ra-to-ry di-<u>stress</u> <u>syn</u>-drome	infection, injury, or other conditions cause fluid build-up in the alveoli preventing the lungs from filling with air
anthracosis/black lung disease	an-thrah-<u>koh</u>-sis	accumulation of carbon deposits in the lung due to breathing smoke or coal dust
asbestosis	as-bes-<u>to</u>-sis	lung disease caused by inhaling asbestos particles; associated with development of mesothelioma, a type of lung cancer
asphyxia	as-<u>fik</u>-se-<u>a</u>	suffocation from lack of O_2
asthma	<u>az</u>-mah	inflammation and swelling of bronchial tubes and bronchial spasms causing a narrowing of bronchi, bronchial airway obstruction, and mucus production. Triggers in those with a genetic predisposition are irritants which include respiratory infections, pollutants, and exposure to allergens
atelectasis	at'-e-<u>lek</u>-tah-sis	incomplete expansion of the lungs at birth or collapse of the adult lung
bronchiectasis	<u>brong</u>-ke-ek-tah-sis	chronic dilation of one or more bronchi
bronchitis	brong-<u>ki</u>-tis	inflammation of one or more bronchi; in chronic bronchitis, the lining of the airways are constantly irritated, inflamed and swollen, and forms lots of thick mucus; low blood O_2 causes cyanosis, right heart failure, and edema (blue bloaters)
bronchospasm	<u>brong</u>-ko-spazm	spasmodic contraction of bronchi muscles, as in asthma
byssinosis/brown lung disease	bis-ih-<u>noh</u>-sis	lung disease resulting from inhaling dust from cotton, flax, or hemp
coccidioidomycosis/valley fever	kok-<u>sid</u>-e-oi-do-mi-<u>ko</u>-sis	respiratory infection caused by inhaling fungal spores of *Coccidioides immitis*, fungus found in the soil in Southwestern United States and Washington state, parts of Mexico, Central and South America; symptoms vary in severity from that of a common cold to those resembling influenza
chronic obstructive pulmonary disease (COPD)	<u>chron</u>-ic ob-<u>struc</u>-tive <u>pul</u>mo-nar-y dis-<u>ease</u>	chronic progressive lung disease: emphysema or chronic bronchitis; poor airflow in the lungs; symptoms are wheezing, shortness of breath with difficulty exhaling, and cough
cor pulmonale	kor <u>pul</u>-mo-nay-lee	heart failure from pulmonary disease
coryza/common cold	ko-ri-<u>zah</u>/com-mon cold	acute inflammation of the mucous membrane of the nose, with mucus discharge
croup	kroop	viral upper airway infection in children; symptoms include a barking cough, difficulty (suffocative) breathing, stridor, and spasm of the larynx
cystic fibrosis (CF)	sis-<u>tik</u> fi-<u>bro</u>-sis	hereditary disease of mucus and sweat glands; chronic disease present at birth affects the lungs, pancreas, liver, intestines, sinuses, and sex organs. Thick and sticky mucus clogs the lungs and blocks the release of pancreatic enzymes

(continues)

TABLE 13-2 (*continued*)

Condition	Pronunciation	Definition
deviated septum	de-<u>vi</u>-ated <u>sep</u>-tum	defect in the wall between the nostrils that can cause partial or complete obstruction
diphtheria	<u>dif</u>-the-re-ah	an acute upper respiratory infection caused by the *Corynebacterium diphtheriae* bacterium primarily affecting the membranes of the nose, throat, or larynx accompanied by fever and pain; the bacteria produces a toxin which destroys healthy tissues in the respiratory system; the disease is prevented by childhood immunization
effusion	e-fu-<u>zhun</u>	escape of a fluid; exudation or transudation (from the lungs)
emphysema	em-fi-<u>se</u>-mah	walls between the aveoli are permanently damaged causing aveoli to lose shape, resulting in an abnormal accumulation of air in the lungs and retention of CO_2; patients often use forceful exhalation to remove excess air (pink puffers); nearly always caused by smoking
fibrosis	fi-<u>bro</u>-sis	formation of fibrous or scar tissue (in lungs), usually caused by previous infections
"flu"	floo	popular name for influenza
hay fever/allergic rhinitis	hay <u>fe</u>-ver/al-<u>ler</u>-gic rhi-<u>ni</u>-tis	a hypersensitive state, e.g., allergy to pollen; symptoms are similar to the common cold
hemothorax	he-mo-<u>tho</u>-raks	blood in the pleural thoracic cavity
histoplasmosis	his-to-<u>plaz</u>-mo-sis	fungal infection of the lungs caused by *Histoplasma* fungus. The fungus lives in soil that contains large amounts of bird or bat droppings; may be symptomatic or asymptomatic, resembling tuberculosis
influenza	in-floo-<u>en</u>-zah	an acute viral infection of the respiratory tract; serious for the very young and old
laryngitis	lar-in-<u>ji</u>-tis	inflammation of the larynx
laryngotracheo-bronchitis	la-<u>rin</u>-go-<u>tra</u>-ke-o-brong-<u>ki</u>-tis	inflammation of the larynx, trachea, and bronchi
lobar pneumonia	<u>lo</u>-bar pneu-<u>mo</u>-ni-ae	acute inflammation of lobes of the lungs, most often caused by *Streptococcus pneumoniae*, but can be caused by viral or fungal infections; consolidation of the lungs when alveoli fill up with fluid or pus; serious complications can be prevented with Pneumococcal pneumonia vaccine
lung abscess	lung <u>ab</u>-sess	pus formed by the destruction of lung tissue and microorganisms by white blood cells that have gone to a localized area to fight infection
lung cancer/carcinoma	lung <u>can</u>-ser/car-sih-<u>noh</u>-muh	leading cause of death from cancer in the United States; most cases of lung cancer are caused by smoking; two main types are non-small cell lung cancer and small cell lung cancer
pertussis/whooping cough	per-<u>tus</u>-is/hoop-ing kof	acute upper respiratory infectious disease caused by bacterium *Bordetella pertussis*; marked by peculiar paroxysms of cough, ending in a prolonged crowing or whooping respiration; can be prevented by childhood immunization

Condition	Pronunciation	Definition
pharyngitis	far-in-ji-tis	inflammation of the pharynx
pleural effusion	ploo-ral eh-fyoo-shun	accumulation of fluid in the pleural space, which compresses the underlying portion of the lung, resulting in dyspnea
pleurisy	ploor-i-se	inflammation of the pleura
pneumococcal disease	pneu-mo-coc-cal di-sease	infection caused by bacteria (*Streptococcus pneumoniae*), most often of the lungs, but can also infect the meninges causing meningitis
pneumoconiosis	nu-mo-ko-ne-o-sis	any lung disease, e.g., anthracosis, silicosis, caused by permanent deposition of substantial amounts of particulate matter in the lungs
pneumothorax	nu-moh-thor-acks	a collection of gas or air in the pleural cavity, resulting from a perforation through the chest wall or the visceral pleura; caused by pneumonia or trauma
pulmonary embolism (PE)	pul-mo-nar-y em-bo-lism	blood clot of pulmonary arteries, most frequently by detached fragments of thrombus from a leg or pelvic vein; risk factors are recent surgery or hospitalization
pulmonary fibrosis	pul-mo-nar-y fi-bro-sis	formation of scar tissue (in lungs); most common type is idiopathic pulmonary fibrosis and the cause is unknown, although one cause is sarcoidosis, an inflammatory disease primarily of the lungs
respiratory distress syndrome (RDS)	res-pi-ra-to-ry di-stress syn-drome	disease of newborns, born premature (<37 weeks gestation); deficiency of surfactant, fluid secreted by alveolar cells that reduces surface tension of pulmonary fluids which prevents aveoli from collapsing
rhinitis rhinorrhea	ri-ni-tis ri-nor-re-ah	inflammation and discharge from the nasal membrane; "runny nose"
sudden infant death syndrome (SIDS)	sud-den in-fant death syn-drom (sidz)	crib death; cause unknown; associated failure of synapse of nerves to activate the diaphragm
silicosis	sill-ih-koh-sis	a lung disorder caused by inhalation of silica (quartz) dust, resulting in the formation of small nodules in the lung
sinusitis	si-nu-si-tis	inflammation of the sinuses; caused by bacteria, viruses, or allergens
sleep apnea	sleep ap-ne-a	pauses in breathing lasting from seconds to minutes, 30 or more times an hour; two main types: obstructive (blocking of the airway) or central (brain does not send proper signals to muscles that control breathing)
streptococcal throat/strep throat	strep-to-kok-al/strep throat	sore throat caused by the spore bacteria group A *Streptococcus*; a complication is acute rheumatic heart disease
tonsillitis	ton-si-li-tis	inflammation of the tonsils, especially the palatine tonsils
tuberculosis (TB)	too-ber-ku-lo-sis	an infectious disease caused by bacteria, *Mycobacterium tuberculosis*; marked by tubercles and caseous necrosis in tissues of the lung; can be latent and develop into active disease if untreated (see Box 13-1 later in this chapter)
upper respiratory tract infection (URI)	up-per res-pi-ra-to-ry tract in-fec-tion	general term for colds; can be a viral or bacterial infection that affects the throat (pharyngitis), nasopharynx (nasopharyngitis), sinuses (sinusitis), larynx (laryngitis), trachea (tracheitis), or bronchi (bronchitis).

Signs and Symptoms of Respiratory Diseases

The signs and symptoms of respiratory diseases are unique to the system. They provide doctors, nurses, and patients with clues in terms of sight and sound, for example, wheezing (sound), a certain color of sputum (sight), coughing (sound), sneezing (sight and sound), and so forth. These manifestations are all helpful in making a diagnosis. The medical terminology included in Table 13-3 on diagnostics should become part of your vocabulary.

TERMS USED IN THE DIAGNOSIS AND TREATMENT OF RESPIRATORY DISORDERS

Table 13-3 explains terms documented by the health practitioner when conducting a history and physical exam, the tools for making a diagnosis and forms of treatment for respiratory disorders.

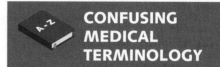

CONFUSING MEDICAL TERMINOLOGY

bronch/o versus brachi/o

bronch/o (or bronchi/o) – bronchus (one of two branches leading from the trachea); e.g., bronchitis (brong-<u>kahy</u>-tis) refers to inflammation (-itis) or infection of the bronchus; bronchiectasis (brong-<u>keee</u>ek-tuh-sis) refers to a condition of dilation (-ectasis) of the bronchus

brachi/o (brachio-, brachi-) – arm, e.g., brachialis (brey-kee-uhl-<u>al</u>-is) refers to a muscle of the upper arm

TABLE 13-3 Terms Used in the Diagnosis and Treatment of Respiratory Disorders

Term	Pronunciation	Definition
History and Physical Exam		
anoxia	an-<u>ok</u>-se-ah	without O_2
apnea	<u>ap</u>-ne-ah	temporary cessation of breathing; asphyxia
bradypnea	brad-ip-<u>nee</u>-ah	abnormally slow breathing
Cheyne-Stokes breathing	<u>chan</u>-stokes breath-ing	waxing and waning of the depth of respiration: the patient breathes deeply a short time and then breathes slightly or stops altogether; the cycle repeats
consolidation	kon-sol´-i-<u>da</u>-shun	solidification of lung tissue because aveola are filled with fluid, as in pneumonia
cough	koff	inhalation and forceful expiration; usually caused by irritation of the airways from dust, smoke, infection, or mucus; can be described as croupy, rasping, harsh, hollow, loose, dry, productive, brassy, bubbly, or wracking
cyanosis	si-ah-<u>no</u>-sis	a bluish discoloration of skin and mucous membranes caused by insufficient O_2 in the blood
dysphonia	dis-<u>fo</u>-ne-ah	voice impairment; difficulty in speaking; complication of laryngitis
dyspnea	<u>disp</u>-ne-ah	labored or difficult breathing
epistaxis	ep-ih-<u>staks</u>-is	hemorrhage from the nose; nosebleed
expectoration	ex-pek-toh-<u>ray</u>-shun	the act of coughing up and spitting out mucus from the lungs, bronchi, and trachea
flail chest	flal chest	chest wall moves paradoxically with respiration as a result of multiple fractures of the ribs

Term	Pronunciation	Definition
hemoptysis	he-<u>mop</u>-ti-sis	the spitting of blood or of blood-stained sputum (from the lungs)
hiccup	hik-<u>up</u>	sharp respiratory sound with spasm of the glottis and diaphragm
hypercapnia	hi´-per-<u>kap</u>-ne-ah	an excess of CO_2 in the blood
hyperventilation	hi´-per-ven´-ti-<u>la</u>-shun	increased rate and/or depth of respiration, e.g., from anxiety
hypoxia	hi-<u>pok</u>-see-ah	insufficient O_2
Kussmaul breathing	<u>koos</u>-mowl breath-ing	gasping, labored breathing; also called air hunger
orthopnea	or´-thop-<u>ne</u>-ah	difficult breathing, except in the upright position
palpation	<u>pal</u>-pay-shun	application of hands and fingers to external surfaces to detect abnormalities
percussion and auscultation (P & A)	per-<u>kush</u>-un and aw´-skul-<u>ta</u>-shun	striking the chest with short, sharp blows of the fingers and listening through a stethoscope for the sounds produced
productive cough	pro-<u>duk</u>-tiv kof	cough with spitting of mucus or phlegm from the bronchi
rales, rhonchi	rahlz, <u>rong</u>-ki	an abnormal respiratory sound (crackling) heard on auscultation, indicating some pathologic condition
shortness of breath (SOB)	short-ness of breath	difficult or labored breathing; symptom of lung disease
sneeze	sneeze	spasmodic contraction of muscles causing air to be expelled forcefully through the nose and mouth
tachypnea	tak´-ip-<u>ne</u>-ah	very rapid respiration
wheeze	hweez	breathing with a raspy or whistling sound; common symptom of asthma

Diagnostic Tools: Laboratory Tests

arterial blood gases	ar-<u>ter</u>-i-al blud <u>gas</u>-iz	O_2, CO_2, and other gases in the arterial blood
complete blood count (CBC)	com-plete blood count	measurement of red blood cells, white blood cells, and platelets to determine the presence of infection
enzyme immunoassay (EIA)	<u>en</u>-zyme im-mu-no-a-<u>ssay</u>	test for diagnosing either histoplasmosis or coccidioidomycosis
immunoreactive trypsinogen (IRT)	im-mu-no-<u>re</u>-ac-tive tryp-<u>sin</u>-o-gen	newborn screening test for cystic fibrosis
pleural fluid culture	<u>pleu</u>-r-al <u>flu</u>-id <u>cul</u>-ture	culture of fluid sample taken from the pleural space to determine presence of bacteria-causing infection
rapid strep test	<u>ra</u>-pid strep test	throat swab to collect mucus from the back of the throat to test for strep throat
sputum culture	<u>spu</u>-tum <u>cul</u>-ture	sputum collected after a deep cough; spitting phlegm from the lungs into a special container which is cultured to determine if bacteria or other disease-causing germs grow

(continues)

TABLE 13-3 (*continued*)

Term	Pronunciation	Definition
Diagnostic Tools: Skin Tests		
Mantoux (test)	man-<u>too</u>	tuberculosis skin test
purified protein derivative (PPD)	<u>pu</u>-ri-fied <u>pro</u>-tein di-<u>riv</u>-a-tiv	tuberculin protein used in skin tests (as the Mantoux test) to detect tubercle bacillus infection
sweat test	sweat test	sweat is collected and tested for salt; used as a diagnostic test for cystic fibrosis in infants at 2 weeks of age
tine test	tīn test	skin test for tuberculosis
Diagnostic Tools: Lung Function Tests		
forced vital capacity (FVC)	forced <u>vi</u>-tal kah-<u>pas</u>-i-te	amount of air that can be expelled from the lungs after deep inspiration (pulmonary function test)
peak expiratory flow rate (PEFR)	pek ex-pi-<u>ra</u>-tory <u>flo</u> rat	measurement of how fast a person can exhale using a small handheld device to monitor treatment in asthma or COPD
pulmonary function tests (PFTs)	<u>pul</u>-mo-ner´-e <u>fungk</u>-shun tests	tests to assess ventilatory status
pulse oximetry	pulse ox-<u>im</u>-e-try	measurement of the O_2 saturation of arterial by blood pulse oximeters, a photoelectric device with a probe that is taped to a finger
residual volume (RV)	re-<u>zed</u>-u-al vol-ume	air remaining in the lungs after complete expiration
spirometer (spirometry)	spi-<u>rom</u>-e-ter (spi-<u>rom</u>-e-tre)	an instrument for measuring air taken into and expelled from the lungs; spirometry is the measurement of lung capacity
total lung capacity (TLC)	to-tal lung ca-pac-i-ty	volume of air in the lungs after maximum inhalation
Other Diagnostic Tools		
bronchoscope	<u>brong</u>-ko-skop	an instrument for inspecting the bronchi
bronchoscopy	brong-<u>kos</u>-ko-pe	lung examination using a bronchoscope
computed tomography scan (CT)	com-<u>put</u>-ed <u>to</u>-mog-ra-phy	imaging that uses special X-ray equipment to make cross-sectional pictures of the lungs and inside the chest; CT angiography combines a CT scan with the injection of dye
laryngoscopy	lar´-ing-<u>gos</u>-ko-pe	visual examination of the interior larynx with an instrument called a laryngoscope
scan (lung, pleura)	skan	an image or a "picture" produced using radioactive isotopes, e.g., B-mode ultrasonography
X-ray examination	X-ray ex-am-i-na-tion	visual record made using X-rays for diagnostic examination of the chest; may be AP (anteroposterior) or Lat (side) views
Treatment Including Surgery		
aerosol	<u>a</u>-er-o-sol´	a medication sprayed from a pressurized container to relieve bronchial distress, especially asthma

Term	Pronunciation	Definition
bronchodilator	brong´-ko-di-<u>la</u>-tor	an agent capable of dilating the bronchi
cardiopulmonary resuscitation (CPR)	car-di-o-<u>pul</u>-mo-nar-y re-<u>sus</u>-ci-ta-tion	artificial means of providing circulation and breathing during cardiac and respiratory arrest; e.g., mouth-to-mouth resuscitation and external chest compression
continuous positive airway pressure (CPAP)	con-<u>tin</u>-u-ous <u>pos</u>-i-tive <u>air</u>-way <u>pres</u>-sure	mild air pressure used to keep breathing airways open; includes a mask and tube that connects to a machine's motor that blows air into the tube; used to treat sleep apnea
endotracheal (ET) tube	en´-do-<u>tra</u>-ke-al	catheter inserted in the trachea during surgery and for a temporary airway to provide O_2 in emergency situations
expectorant	ek-<u>spek</u>-to-rant	an agent that promotes expectoration (loosening of secretions)
hyposensitization	hi´-po-sen´-si-ti-<u>za</u>-shun	used to reduce the symptoms of allergies by exposing a patient to an offending substance to reduce sensitivity to the substance
laryngectomy	lah-rin-<u>jek</u>-to-me	excision of the larynx, e.g., because of cancer
lavage of sinuses	lah-<u>vahzh</u> of si-<u>nus</u>-es	the irrigation or washing out of sinuses; used to treat acute or chronic sinus infection
lobectomy	lo-<u>bek</u>-to-me	excision of a lobe of the lung, e.g., to remove lung tissue damaged by disease
nebulizer	<u>neb</u>-u-liz-er	device for converting a drug from liquid to mist, which is inhaled through a mask to deliver medication to the deep part of the respiratory tract
oxygen therapy	<u>ox</u>-y-gen <u>ther</u>-a-py	supplemental O_2 provided when lung disease prevents adequate oxygenation of body tissues; the patient wears a nasal cannula which is attached to an O_2 delivery system
pneumococcal vaccine	pneu-mo-<u>coc</u>-cal vac-<u>cine</u>	used to prevent infection by *Streptococcus pneumoniae*; recommended for those over 65 years of age or for those with chronic disease
postural drainage	<u>pos</u>-chur-al <u>dran</u>-ij	treatment for mucus congestion in the lungs; the patient's head is placed downward so that the trachea will be inclined below the lungs and the secretions mobilized
respirator (ventilator)	<u>res</u>-pi-ra´-tor (ven´-ti-<u>la</u>-tor)	a device for giving artificial respiration or to assist in pulmonary ventilation
rhinoplasty	<u>ri</u>-no-plas´-te	plastic surgery of the nose; may be done to correct deformities that prevent normal breathing
submucous resection (SMR)	sub-mu-<u>co</u>-sal re-<u>sec</u>-tion	excision of a portion of the submucous membrane of the nose to correct a deviated septum
thoracentesis	thor´-rah-sen-<u>te</u>-sis	surgical puncture of the chest wall into the parietal cavity to remove fluid
tracheostomy	tra´-ke-<u>os</u>-to-me	creation of an opening into the trachea through the neck, e.g., insertion of a tube to facilitate ventilation
tracheotomy	tra´-ke-<u>ot</u>-o-me	incision of the trachea through the skin and muscles of the neck
ventilator	ven´-ti-<u>la</u>-tor	an apparatus to assist in pulmonary ventilation; see also *respirator*

BOX 13-1 explains the importance of a TB test before beginning work at a hospital.

Box 13-1 Why Do I Need a TB Test Before I Begin Working in the Hospital?

Tuberculosis (TB) is primarily a disease of the lungs and can be spread to others through the air when an infected person sneezes, sings, speaks, or coughs. Not everyone who is exposed to the bacteria, *Mycobacterium tuberculosis*, develops active TB. Instead, a person can have inactive or latent TB for many years. Those with latent TB will have no symptoms and cannot spread the disease to others, but are at risk for active TB when their immune system becomes suppressed, e.g., during chemotherapy for cancer.

A person with latent TB will test positive when TB skin tests are administered and will need treatment to prevent developing active TB in the future. Public health officials recommend that groups at risk for developing active TB receive treatment to prevent the development of active TB. High-risk groups include residents and employees of correctional facilities, nursing homes, homeless shelters, hospitals, and other health-care facilities.

Treatment for those with latent TB is a combination of two drugs—rifapentine and isoniazid—taken once a week for 12 weeks. Those with active TB are treated with a combination of medications for 6–9 months and can continue to expose others to the disease for the first 2–3 weeks of drug treatment.

Since the development of antibiotics and other medications, TB is no longer the dreaded disease that it was in the early 1900s when it was the leading cause of death in the United States. However, all health-care workers can expect to be asked to have a TB skin test as a measure to prevent the spread of TB.

Source: Centers for Disease Control and Prevention. *Tuberculosis (TB)*. Internet: https://www.cdc.gov/tb/default.htm

THE ORIGIN OF MEDICAL TERMS

Table 13-4 explains the origin of terms used to describe the respiratory system.

TABLE 13-4 The Origin of Medical Terms		
Word	**Pronunciation**	**Origin and Definition**
asbestosis	as-bes-<u>to</u>-sis	Greek, *asbestos*, inextinguishable + Greek, *osis*, condition
atelectasis	at´-e-<u>lek</u>-tah-sis	Greek, *atelēs*, incomplete + Greek, *ektasis*, extension
coccidioidomycosis	coc-<u>cid</u>-i-oi-do-my-<u>co</u>-sis	Greek, *kokkos*, berry + Greek, *eidos*, form + Greek, *mykes*, fungus + Greek, *osis*, condition
diphtheria	<u>diph</u>-the-ri-a	Greek, *diphthera*, leather membrane
effusion	ef-fu-<u>sion</u>	Latin, *effusio*, a pouring out
hemoptysis	he-<u>mop</u>-ty-sis	Latin, *hemo*, blood + Greek, *ptyeine*, to spit
pneumothorax	pneu-mo-<u>thor</u>-ax	Greek, *pneuma*, air, + Greek, *thorax*, the chest
rhinorrhea	<u>rhi</u>-nor-rhe-a	Greek, *rhis*, nose

Word	Pronunciation	Origin and Definition
thoracentesis	tho-ra-cen-<u>te</u>-sis	Greek, *thorax*, the chest + Greek, *kentēsis*, puncture
tracheotomy	tra-che-<u>ot</u>-o-my	Greek, *tracheia*, rough artery + Greek, *tomē*, incision

ABBREVIATIONS

The abbreviations listed in **Table 13-5** are used frequently in respiratory care, including diagnosis and treatment.

TABLE **13-5** Abbreviations Used Frequently in Respiratory Care

Abbreviation	Definition	Abbreviation	Definition
ARDS	acute respiratory distress syndrome	O_2	oxygen
CBC	complete blood count	PEFR	peak expiratory flow rate
CF	cystic fibrosis	PPD	purified protein derivative
CO_2	carbon dioxide	RDS	respiratory distress syndrome
COPD	chronic obstructive pulmonary disease	RV	residual volume
CPAP	continuous positive airway pressure	SIDS	sudden infant death syndrome
CPR	cardiopulmonary resuscitation	SMR	submucosa resection
CT	computed tomography	SOB	shortness of breath
EIA	enzyme immunoassay	TB	tuberculosis
ET	endotracheal tube	TLC	total lung capacity
FVC	forced vital capacity	VQ	ventilation perfusion
IRT	immunoreactive trypsinogen		

The following box describes common drugs used to treat respiratory diseases.

PHARMACOLOGY AND MEDICAL TERMINOLOGY

Drug Classification	antitussive (an-tih-<u>tuss</u>-iv)	bronchodilator (brong-koh-<u>dye</u>-lay-tor)
Function	to reduce cough from various causes	expands the bronchial tubes by relaxing the bronchial muscles
Word Parts	**anti-** = against; **tussive** = pertaining to a cough	**bronch**/o = airway; **dilator** = pertaining to dilate or become wider
Active Ingredients (examples)	dextromethorphan hydrobromide (Benylin DM, Robitussin Pediatric, Vick's Formula 44); pseudoephedrine hydrochloride and guaifenesin (Mucinex D, Robitussin PE)	theophylline (Quibron-TSR, Theo-Dur, Theo-24, Theochron); aminophylline (Norphl, Phyllocontin, Quibron-T)

Pulmonologist Consult Note

I have been requested by pediatric specialist, Dr. Jones, to evaluate a 7-year-old African American male, admitted last night through the ER for **Status Asthmaticus**. See attending physician **H&P** for detailed review of systems. Patient currently displays **anoxic** symptoms with severe **dyspnea** and both **inspiratory** and **expiratory wheezing**. **Pulse oximeter** shows O_2 levels in mid-80s. This patient is currently experiencing moderate respiratory distress after a full 12 hours of continuous respiratory treatment with I.V. steroids and **bronchodilators**. Plan at this time is to increase IV hydration, add theophylline and beta-agonist to the pulmonary treatment. O_2 saturation will be continuously monitored with doctor being notified of decreasing levels.

PLAN: Add meds as instructed, continue monitoring, and reevaluate in a.m.

Direction: For the portions of the clinical note shown by a colored font, provide the definition and/or words for abbreviation.

LESSON TWO   Progress Check

LISTS: PARTS OF THE RESPIRATORY SYSTEM

List the anatomical parts of the upper respiratory tract:

1. _____

2. _____

3. _____

List the anatomical parts of the lower respiratory tract:

4. _____

5. _____

6. _____

MATCHING: SYMPTOMS RELATED TO DISORDERS OF THE RESPIRATORY SYSTEM

Match the terms on the left column to their definitions on the right:

Terms	Definition
1. Apnea	**a.** Incomplete expansion or collapse of the lung
2. Dyspnea	**b.** Bloody nose
3. Bradypnea	**c.** Voice impairment
4. Tachypnea	**d.** Difficult breathing
5. Atelectasis	**e.** Abnormally slow breathing
6. Bronchiectasis	**f.** Runny nose
7. Hemoptysis	**g.** Very rapid breathing
8. Rhinorrhea	**h.** Chronic dilation of one or more bronchi
9. Dysphonia	**i.** Temporary cessation of breathing
10. Epistaxis	**j.** Spitting up of blood-tinged sputum

CLINICAL *Note*

MULTIPLE CHOICE: TERMS THAT DESCRIBE SYMPTOMS, DIAGNOSTIC TOOLS, AND DISORDERS OF THE RESPIRATORY SYSTEM

Circle the letter of the correct answer:

1. The pulmonary function test is used to:
   a. diagnose abnormal lung tissue
   b. demonstrate abnormal pulmonary blood flow
   c. evaluate how a patient breathes
   d. measure obstructions to pulmonary function

2. When the chest wall is punctured with a needle to obtain fluid for diagnosis, the procedure is known as:
   a. thoracentesis
   b. bronchoscopy
   c. pleural biopsy
   d. pulmonary angiogram

3. Coccidioidomycosis is:
   a. a malignant lung tumor
   b. a disease caused by a fungus
   c. coughing up of blood
   d. a collection of fluid in the pleural cavity

4. Which of the following statements describes eupnea?
   a. Shortness of breath
   b. Lack of oxygen
   c. Difficult breathing
   d. Normal breathing

5. Heart failure caused by pulmonary disease is called:
   a. coryza
   b. cor pulmonale
   c. COPD
   d. carcinoma

6. A deviated septum is a:
   a. malfunctioning alveoli
   b. defect in the wall between nostrils
   c. broken nose
   d. pulmonary obstruction

7. Which of the following terms describes the coughing up of blood?
   a. Expectorate
   b. Hypoxia
   c. Hemoptysis
   d. Sputum

8. A hemothorax is a:
   a. blood in the pleural thoracic cavity
   b. collapsed lung
   c. creation of a new opening into the chest
   d. nosebleed

9. The common name for pertussis is:
   a. measles
   b. hay fever
   c. hiccups
   d. whooping cough

10. A respiratory condition with a collection of air in the pleural cavity is:
    a. hemothorax
    b. effusion
    c. pleurisy
    d. pneumothorax

MATCHING: DISORDERS OF THE RESPIRATORY SYSTEM

Match the terms in the disorder on the left column to their definitions on the right:

Disorder
1. Silicosis
2. Pulmonary embolism
3. Byssinosis
4. Croup
5. Diphtheria
6. Anthracosis
7. Asthma
8. Emphysema
9. Respiratory distress syndrome
10. Histoplasmosis

Definition
a. Brown lung disease
b. Viral upper respiratory infection in children
c. Lung infection caused by fungal spores in soil with bird or bat droppings
d. Damage to alveoli with retention of CO_2
e. Inflammation and swelling of bronchial tubes caused by allergies
f. Lung disorder caused by inhalation of silica or quartz dust
g. Blood clot in the lungs
h. Lung disease of infants born prematurely
i. Black lung disease
j. Acute bacterial respiratory infection that destroys membranes of the respiratory tract

ABBREVIATIONS: TERMS USED TO DESCRIBE DISORDERS, DIAGNOSIS, OR TREATMENT OF DISEASES OF THE RESPIRATORY SYSTEM

Define the following abbreviations:

1. URI: _____

2. PEFR: _____

3. ARDS: _____

4. CF: _____

5. CPAP: _____

6. COPD: _____

7. TB: _____

8. SIDS: _____

9. ET tube: _____

10. VQ: _____

IDENTIFYING WORD PARTS

For each of the medical terms, list the root word and the prefix and/or suffix:

Word	Root Word	Prefix	Suffix
1. Anthracosis	_____	_____	_____
2. Asphyxia	_____	_____	_____
3. Dysphonia	_____	_____	_____
4. Emphysema	_____	_____	_____
5. Epistaxis	_____	_____	_____
6. Hypercapnia	_____	_____	_____
7. Pertussis	_____	_____	_____
8. Pneumonia	_____	_____	_____
9. Sinusitis	_____	_____	_____
10. Tuberculosis	_____	_____	_____

© teekid/iStock/Getty Images

Cardiovascular System

OBJECTIVES

After completing this chapter and the exercises, the student should be able to:

1. Identify the organs of the cardiovascular system.
2. Describe the location and functions of the structures of the heart.
3. List the functions of the cardiovascular system.
4. Identify the structure and functions of the lymphatic system.
5. Name blood components of the cardiovascular and lymphatic systems.
6. Identify and describe the types and functions of the blood vessels.
7. Identify and define medical words pertaining to tests and procedures used in the diagnosis and treatment of selected clinical disorders affecting the cardiovascular and lymphatic systems.
8. Correctly spell and pronounce new medical terms.

The cardiovascular system is a subset of the circulatory system. It consists of the heart, blood vessels, and blood. The lymphatic system is also a part of the circulatory system, consisting of lymph vessels and lymph nodes within the larger vessels. Associated with the circulatory system are the blood-forming organs, that is, the spleen, liver, bone marrow, thymus gland, and lymph tissue (**Figures 14-1** through **14-3**).

The heart is a four-chambered hollow organ that lies between the lungs in the middle of the *thoracic* cavity. Two-thirds of the heart lies left of the *midsternum*. It is about the size of the owner's fist. It is cone shaped, the base directed toward the right shoulder and the apex pointed toward the left hip.

The heart is covered with a double-walled sac called the *pericardium* that encloses the heart and great blood vessels. It is attached to the *diaphragm*, the *sternum*, and the lung pleura. The tough outer layer of the pericardium protects the heart. The inner *serous* layer contains the visceral membrane (*epicardium*) that covers the heart surface and the parietal membrane that lines the inside of the pericardium. There is fluid in the space between these layers that lubricates the membrane and prevents friction.

ALLIED HEALTH PROFESSIONS

Diagnostic Medical Sonographers, Cardiovascular Technologists and Technicians, Nuclear Medicine Technologists, and Surgical Technologists

Diagnostic medical sonographers use special equipment to direct sound waves into areas of the patient's body. Sonographers operate the equipment, which collects reflected echoes and forms an image that may be videotaped, transmitted, or photographed for interpretation and diagnosis by a physician. Before the exam, the sonographers usually spread a special gel on the skin to aid in the transmission of sound waves, and during the exam, use a transducer which transmits sound waves in a cone or rectangle-shaped beam. Sonographers select images for storage, take measurements, calculate values, and analyze results in preliminary findings for the physician.

Cardiovascular technologists and technicians assist physicians in diagnosing and treating cardiac (heart) and peripheral vascular (blood vessel) ailments. They schedule appointments, perform ultrasound or cardiovascular procedures, review doctors' interpretations and patient files, and monitor patients' heart rates. They also operate and maintain testing equipment, explain test procedures, and compare test results to a standard to identify problems. Other day-to-day activities vary significantly between specialties.

Surgical technologists, also called scrubs and surgical or operating room technicians, assist in surgical operations under the supervision of surgeons, registered nurses, or other surgical personnel. Surgical technologists are members of operating room teams, which most commonly include surgeons, anesthesiologists, and circulating nurses.

Before an operation, surgical technologists help prepare the operating room by setting up surgical instruments and equipment, sterile drapes, and sterile solutions. They assemble both sterile and nonsterile equipment, as well as check and adjust it to ensure that it is working properly. Technologists also prepare patients for surgery by washing, shaving, and disinfecting incision sites. They transport patients to the operating room, help position them on the operating table, and cover them with sterile surgical drapes. Technologists also observe patients' vital signs, check charts, and help the surgical team put on sterile gowns and gloves.

Nuclear medicine technologists operate cameras that detect and map the radioactive drug in a patient's body to create diagnostic images. After explaining test procedures to patients, technologists prepare a dosage of the radiopharmaceutical and administer it by mouth, injection, inhalation, or other means. They position patients and start a gamma scintillation camera or "scanner," which creates images of the distribution of a radiopharmaceutical as it localizes in, and emits signals from, the patient's body. The images are produced on a computer screen or on film for a physician to interpret.

INQUIRY

Alliance of Cardiovascular Professionals: www.acp-online.org
Association of Surgical Technologists: www.ast.org
Society of Diagnostic Medical Sonography: www.sdms.org
Society of Nuclear Medicine Technologists: www.snm.org

Data from Cross, Nanna, and McWay, Dana. *Stanfield's Introduction to the Health Professions*, 7th ed. Burlington, MA: Jones & Bartlett Learning; 2017.

There are four heart chambers: upper right and left *atria* and lower right and left *ventricles*. The ventricles are separated by the *interventricular* septum. The *tricuspid* valve lies between the right atrium and right ventricle. Blood flows forward through the valve in one chamber, backward in another. It regulates blood pressure in the heart, sending blood into the right ventricle when the pressure is greater in the right atrium and preventing backflow of blood into the right atrium.

The blood vessels are a series of closed tubes that carry blood from the heart to the tissue and back to the heart. The three major types of vessels are *arteries*, *capillaries*, and *veins*.

Arteries carry blood from the heart. Elastic arteries are the largest arteries from the heart. Muscular arteries branch into medium-sized and small arteries that contain both muscular and elastic tissue. The smallest, the *arterioles*, deliver blood to capillary beds in the tissues.

Veins carry blood back to the atria of the heart. The venous system holds 75 percent of total blood volume and returns blood under low pressure. The venous system begins at the *capillary* beds and flows into larger *venules*, and then into small, medium, and large veins. The *vena cava*, the largest vein in the body, returns deoxygenated blood to the right atrium of the heart.

The major arteries of systemic circulation are the *aorta*, the largest vessel in diameter in the body, and the branches from the aorta leading toward the head and neck and descending into the trunk and lower extremities (see Figures 14-1 through 14-3 for complete details).

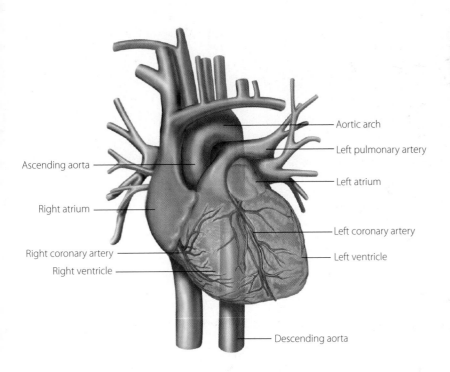

- Aortic arch
- Left pulmonary artery
- Left atrium
- Left coronary artery
- Left ventricle

Ascending aorta

Right atrium

Right coronary artery

Right ventricle

Descending aorta

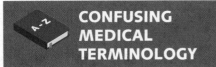

CONFUSING MEDICAL TERMINOLOGY

hemostasis versus **homeostasis**

hemostasis – control of blood flow
(hee-<u>muh</u>-stey-sis)

homeostasis – a steady state
(<u>hoh</u>-mee-uh-stey-sis)

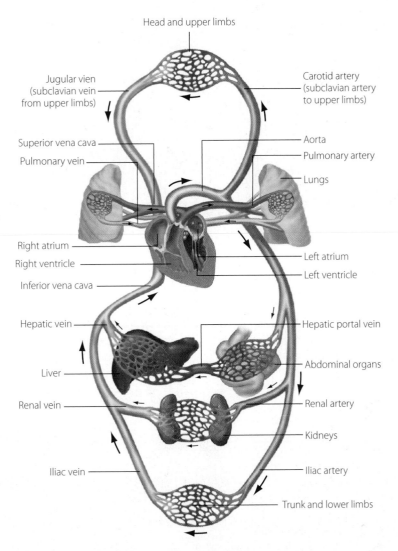

Head and upper limbs

Jugular vien
(subclavian vein
from upper limbs)

Carotid artery
(subclavian artery
to upper limbs)

Superior vena cava

Pulmonary vein

Aorta

Pulmonary artery

Lungs

Right atrium

Right ventricle

Inferior vena cava

Left atrium

Left ventricle

Hepatic vein

Hepatic portal vein

Liver

Abdominal organs

Renal vein

Renal artery

Kidneys

Iliac vein

Iliac artery

Trunk and lower limbs

FIGURE 14-1 The heart and blood circuits.

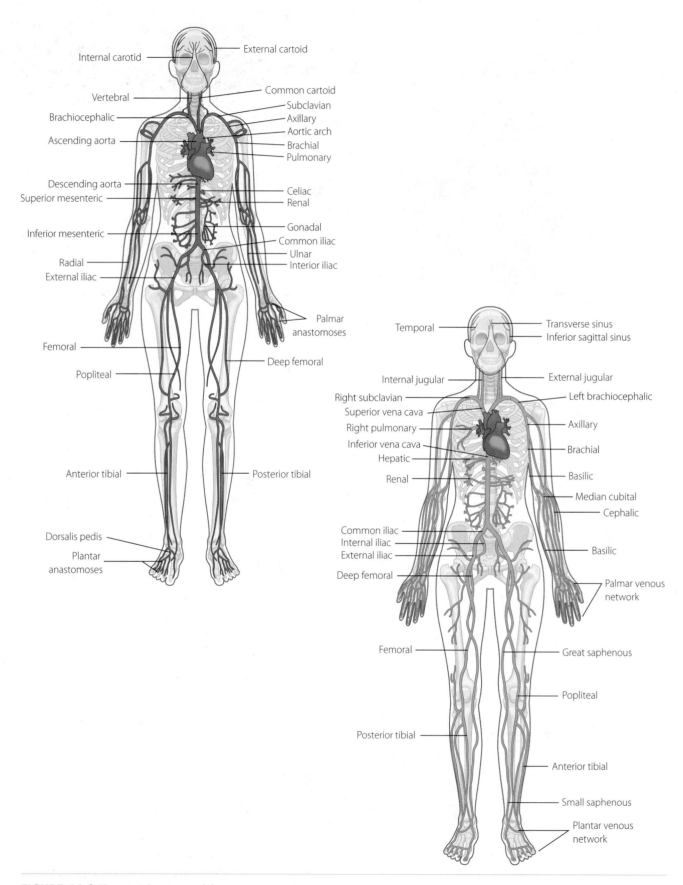

FIGURE 14-2 The arterial system and the venous system.

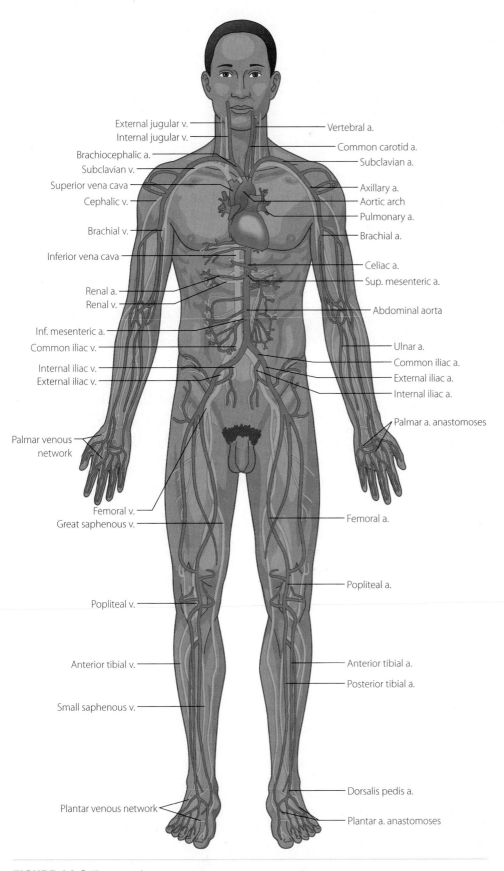

FIGURE 14-3 The arterial–venous system.

The circulatory system can be divided into three types of circulation: pulmonary (lung), systemic (whole body), and portal (intestine, liver, and spleen). Functions of the circulatory system are:

1. *Transport*: Gases, hormones, minerals, enzymes, and other vital substances are carried in the blood to every cell in the body; all waste materials are carried by the blood to the lungs, skin, or kidneys for elimination from the body (*pulmonary circulation*).
2. *Body temperature*: The blood vessels maintain body temperature by dilating at the skin surface to dissipate heat or by constricting to retain heat.
3. *Protection*: The blood and lymphatic systems protect the body against injury and foreign invasion through the immune system; blood clotting mechanisms protect against blood loss.
4. *Buffering*: Blood proteins provide an acid–base buffer system to maintain optimum pH of the blood.

Parts of the heart are defined and illustrated in Lesson One of this chapter.

LESSON ONE Materials to Be Learned

The human circulatory system consists of a pump (the heart) and a network of vessels that transport blood throughout the body. The workhorse of the circulatory system is the heart, propelling blood through approximately 60 miles of blood vessels in the body.

Lesson One explains the parts and functions of the heart and blood vessels and the terminology related to them. It also describes disorders/diseases affecting the system and some means of diagnosis and treatment. Blood pressure terminology, blood types, blood components, and other general and related terms are included. The lymphatic system, which is an integral part of the circulatory system, is discussed in Lesson Two.

THE CARDIOVASCULAR SYSTEM

This information should be studied in conjunction with Figures 14-4 through 14-10.

The Heart

The heart is a muscular, cone-shaped organ (about the size of a clenched fist) that pumps blood throughout the body and beats normally about 70 times per minute by coordinated nerve impulses and muscular contractions. *Pulmonary circulation* provides for oxygenation of blood and *systemic circulation* is responsible for transportation of blood to and from body cells. The heart is enclosed in a fibroserous sac and is divided into four chambers.

The Circulatory System

The circulatory system in the body transports oxygen and nutrients *to* and carbon dioxide and wastes *away from* the cells. The receiving chambers of the heart are the atria while the pumping chambers of the heart are the ventricles. The top two heart chambers (the atria) receive blood while the bottom two chambers (the ventricles) pump blood out of the heart. The right side of the heart receives blood that is low in oxygen from the large vein, the vena cava, while the left side of the heart receives oxygenated blood from the left pulmonary veins coming from the lungs. The right ventricle pumps blood to the lungs to drop off carbon dioxide and collect oxygen. The left ventricle pumps oxygenated blood out of the heart to all parts of the body to supply tissues with oxygen. This information should be studied in conjunction with **Figures 14-4** through **14-8**.

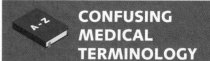

CONFUSING MEDICAL TERMINOLOGY

aort/o versus atri/o versus arteri/o versus arteriol/o

aort/o – aorta, e.g., aortostenosis (a-or-to-steh-no-sis) refers to narrowing of the aorta (a-or-toh)

atri/o – atrium, e.g., atrium (a-tre-um) refers to each of the two (left and right) upper chambers of the heart

arteri/o – artery, e.g., arteriosclerosis (ar-te-re-o-skleh-ro-sis) refers to hardening of an artery

arteriol/o – arteriole, e.g., arteriolitis (ar-ter-i-o-li-tis) refers to inflammation of an arteriole

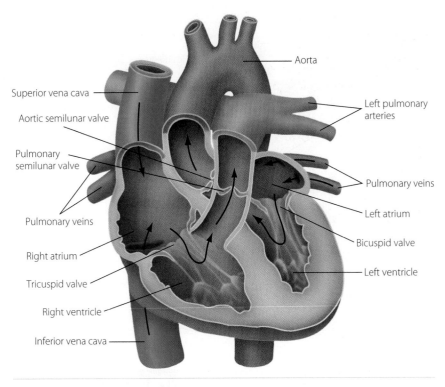

Aorta

Superior vena cava

Aortic semilunar valve

Pulmonary
semilunar valve

Pulmonary veins

Right atrium

Tricuspid valve

Right ventricle

Inferior vena cava

Left pulmonary
arteries

Pulmonary veins

Left atrium

Bicuspid valve

Left ventricle

FIGURE 14-4 Diagram of the heart; arrows indicate direction of blood flow.

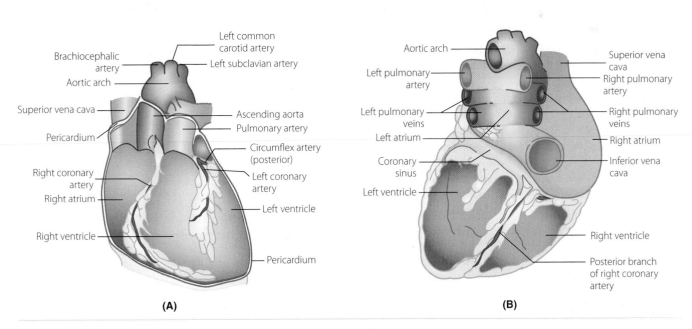

Brachiocephalic
artery

Aortic arch

Superior vena cava

Pericardium

Right coronary
artery

Right atrium

Right ventricle

Left common
carotid artery

Left subclavian artery

Ascending aorta

Pulmonary artery

Circumflex artery
(posterior)

Left coronary
artery

Left ventricle

Pericardium

(A)

Aortic arch

Left pulmonary
artery

Left pulmonary
veins

Left atrium

Coronary
sinus

Left ventricle

Superior vena
cava

Right pulmonary
artery

Right pulmonary
veins

Right atrium

Inferior vena
cava

Right ventricle

Posterior branch
of right coronary
artery

(B)

FIGURE 14-5 (A) Anterior structure of the heart. **(B)** Posterior structure of the heart.

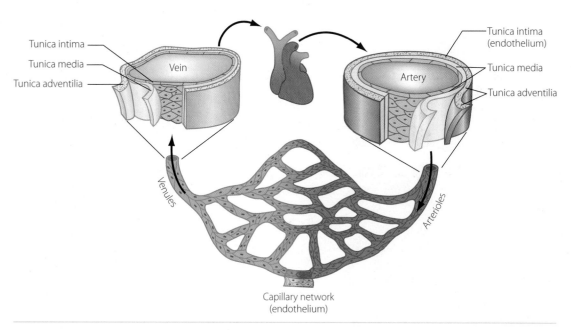

FIGURE 14-6 Blood vessels, showing the single-cell endothelium of all the vessels and the layered muscular coats of arteries and veins.

The Cardiac Conduction System

The *cardiac conduction system* or the electrical system controls how the heart pumps blood. The electrocardiogram (EKG) is a graphical picture of the conduction system of the heart. The heart's electrical system is made up of three main parts:

1. Sinoatrial (SA) node, located in the right atrium
2. Atrioventricular (AV) node, located on the atrial septum
3. His-Purkinje system, located along the walls of the ventricles

A heartbeat is a single cycle in which the heart chambers relax and contract to pump blood. This cycle includes the opening and closing of the valves of the right and left ventricles of the heart.

Each heartbeat has two basic parts: diastole and systole. During diastole, the atria and ventricles of the heart relax and begin to fill with blood. At the end of diastole, the atria contract (atrial systole) and pump blood into the ventricles. The atria then begin to relax. The ventricles then contract (ventricular systole), pumping blood out of the heart.

Each heart beat is set in motion by an electrical signal from within the heart muscle. In a normal, healthy heart, each beat begins with a signal from the *SA node*. The heart rate or pulse is the number of signals the SA node produces per minute. The electrical signal is generated as the vena cava fills the right atrium with blood from other parts of the body. The signal spreads across the cells of the right and left atria. This signal causes the atria to contract to push blood through the open valves from the atria into both ventricles.

The signal arrives at the AV node near the ventricles. It slows for an instant to allow the right and left ventricles to fill with blood. The signal is released and moves along a pathway called the *bundle of His*, which is located in the walls of the ventricles. From the bundle of His, the signal fibers divide into left and right bundle branches through the *Purkinje fibers*. The signal spreads across the cells of the ventricle walls, and both ventricles contract. However, this does not happen at exactly the same moment. The left ventricle contracts an instant before the right ventricle. This pushes blood through the aortic valve (for the left ventricle) to the rest of the body and through the pulmonary valve (for the right ventricle) to the lungs. As the signal passes, the walls of the ventricles relax and await the next signal.

This process continues over and over as the atria refill with blood and more electrical signals come from the SA node.

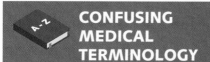

CONFUSING MEDICAL TERMINOLOGY

apheresis versus -poiesis

apheresis – removal of blood, e.g., therapeutic apheresis (ah-fer-ee-cis) refers to the removal of a component of the blood that contributes to a disease state

-poiesis – formation, e.g., hematopoiesis (hi-mat-oh-poi-ee-sis) refers to formation of blood

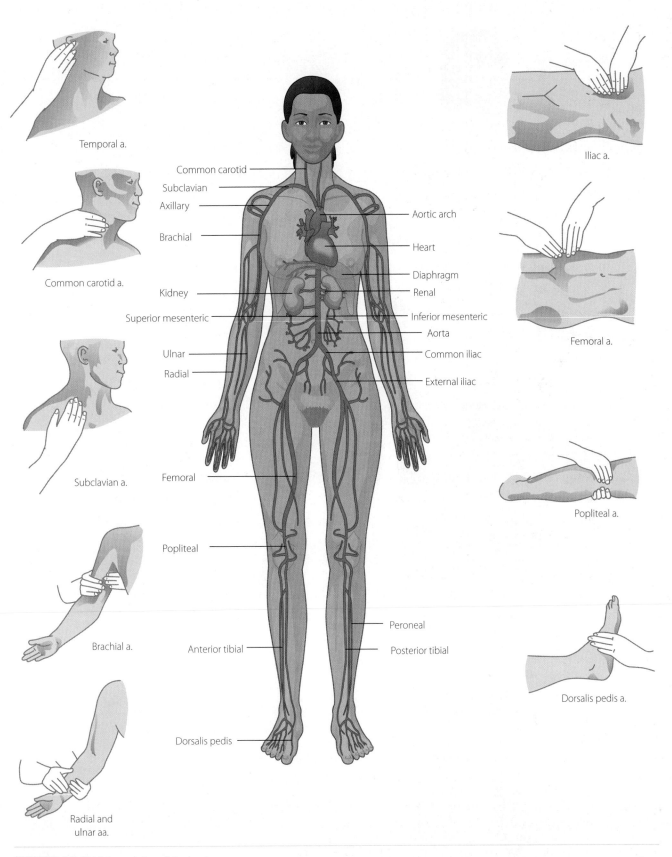

Temporal a.

Common carotid a.

Subclavian a.

Brachial a.

Radial and
ulnar aa.

Common carotid
Subclavian
Axillary
Brachial
Kidney
Superior mesenteric
Ulnar
Radial
Femoral
Popliteal
Anterior tibial
Dorsalis pedis

Aortic arch
Heart
Diaphragm
Renal
Inferior mesenteric
Aorta
Common iliac
External iliac
Peroneal
Posterior tibial

Iliac a.

Femoral a.

Popliteal a.

Dorsalis pedis a.

FIGURE 14-7 Major arteries of the body.

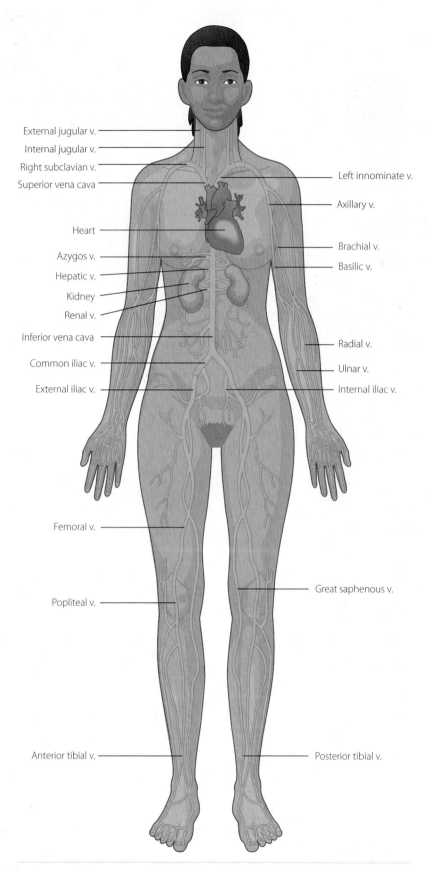

External jugular v.
Internal jugular v.
Right subclavian v.
Superior vena cava

Heart
Azygos v.
Hepatic v.
Kidney
Renal v.
Inferior vena cava
Common iliac v.
External iliac v.

Left innominate v.
Axillary v.
Brachial v.
Basilic v.
Radial v.
Ulnar v.
Internal iliac v.

Femoral v.

Popliteal v.

Great saphenous v.

Anterior tibial v.

Posterior tibial v.

FIGURE 14-8 Major veins of the body.

PARTS OF THE HEART

Table 14-1 lists major and minor parts of the heart and cardiac conduction system.

TABLE **14-1** Parts of the Heart		
Parts of the Heart	**Pronunciation**	**Definition**
apex	<u>a</u>-peks	the pointed end (of the heart)
atrium (plural: atria)	<u>a</u>-tre-um (<u>a</u>-tre-uh)	one of the two (left and right) upper chambers of the heart; these upper chambers receive blood
septum	<u>sep</u>-tum	a dividing wall between the right and left sides of the heart
ventricle	<u>ven</u>-tri-kul	one of the two (left and right) lower chambers of the heart; they pump blood out of the heart
valves	valvz	a membrane in a passage to prevent backward flow of blood
aortic	a-<u>or</u>-tic	located between the left ventricle and the aorta
mitral	<u>mi</u>-tral	shaped like a miter, also called bicuspid valve; situated between the left atrium and the left ventricle
pulmonary semilunar	<u>pul</u>-mon-ner´-e sem´-i-<u>lu</u>-nar	pertaining to the lung and resembling a crescent valve; located between the right ventricle and the pulmonary artery
tricuspid	tri-<u>kus</u>-pid	having three points or cusps, situated between the right atrium and the right ventricle
membranes	<u>mem</u>-brânz	
endocardium	en´-do-<u>kar</u>-de-um	inner lining membrane of the four heart chambers and heart valves
epicardium	ep´-i-<u>kar</u>-de-um	the outer layer of the heart wall; the visceral pericardium; protects the heart by reducing friction between the layers of the heart
myocardium	mi´-o-<u>kar</u>-de-um	middle, thickest layer of the heart wall, made of cardiac muscle; the layer between the epicardium and endocardium layers
pericardium	per´-i-<u>kar</u>-de-um	the fibroserous sac enclosing the heart; the sac contains fluid that reduces friction between the pericardium and other heart layers (epicardium, myocardium, and endocardium)
The Cardiac Conduction System		
atrioventricular (AV) node	a´-tre-o-ven-<u>trik</u>-u-lar nod	specialized cardiac tissue located beneath the endocardium of the septum of the right atrium; provides a normal conduction pathway between the right atrium and right ventricle
bundle of His (A-V bundle)	<u>bun</u>-d´-l of his	electrical conduction passes from the cardiac fibers at the A-V node to the atria and ventricles of the heart; this bundle splits into right and left bundle branches that travel between the right and left ventricles
purkinje fibers	per-kin-<u>jee</u>	specialized cardiac muscle fibers that conduct impulses from the atrioventricular node down the outside of the right and left ventricles; stimulates the ventricles to contract and force blood into the aorta and pulmonary trunk
sinoatrial node (SA) node (pacemaker)	si´-no-<u>a</u>-tre-al nod (<u>pace</u>-mak-er)	atypical cardiac muscle fibers at the junction of the superior vena cava and right atrium; originates the cardiac rhythm, and is therefore called the pacemaker of the heart
sinus rhythm	<u>si</u>-nus <u>rith</u>-uh-m	the normal heart rhythm originating in the sinoatrial (SA) node

TERMS USED TO DESCRIBE BLOOD CIRCULATION

Table 14-2 defines terms used to describe the circulation of blood in the heart and blood vessels.

TABLE **14-2** Terms Used to Describe the Circulation of Blood		
Circulation	**Pronunciation**	**Definition**
circulation	ser´-ku-<u>la</u>-shun	movement in circuitous course; as the movement of blood through the heart and blood vessels
collateral	ko-<u>lat</u>-er-al	circulation by secondary channels that develop after obstruction because of atherosclerosis, e.g., in the coronary arteries
coronary	<u>kor</u>-o-ner-e	circulation of blood in the coronary arteries that supply blood and oxygen to the heart tissues
portal	<u>por</u>-tal	circulation of blood from the gastrointestinal tract and spleen through the portal vein to the liver
pulmonary	<u>pul</u>-mo-ner´-e	movement of blood through the lungs and the pulmonary artery
systemic	sis-<u>tem</u>-ic	pertaining to movement of blood to the body as a whole

TYPES OF BLOOD VESSELS

Three types of vessels carry blood throughout the body. Each has a unique structure and function. **Table 14-3** describes different types of blood vessels.

TABLE **14-3** Types of Blood Vessels		
Blood Vessels	**Pronunciation**	**Definition**
artery	<u>ar</u>-ter-e	a vessel in which blood flows away from the heart, carrying oxygenated blood
aorta	a-<u>or</u>-tah	the great artery arising from the left ventricle; largest artery
arterioles	ar-<u>ter</u>-ri-oles	the smallest arteries in which blood flows into capillaries where blood is exchanged with venules
coronary arteries	<u>kor</u>-o-ner´-e <u>ar</u>-ter-es	arteries from the base of the aorta that supply the heart muscle with blood
vein	vân	a vessel in which blood flows toward the heart, carrying blood with little oxygen
vena cava	<u>ve</u>-nah <u>ca</u>-vah	largest vein. *Inferior:* The venous trunk for the lower viscera. *Superior:* The venous trunk draining blood from head, neck, upper limbs, and thorax
venules	<u>ve</u>-nules	the smallest veins in which blood flows into capillaries where blood is exchanged with arterioles
capillary	<u>kap</u>-i-ler´-e	a minute, hair-like vessel connecting arterioles and venules

BLOOD COMPONENTS

Table 14-4 describes components of the blood that support many body functions.

TABLE **14-4** Blood Components

Component	Pronunciation	Definition
red blood cells/ erythrocytes (RBCs)	red blud/ e-<u>ryth</u>-ro-cyte	red corpuscles; one of the formed elements in peripheral blood. They contain hemoglobin and transport oxygen
reticulocytes	re-<u>tik</u>-u-lo´-sitz	immature red blood cells, produced by the bone marrow
white blood cells/ leukocytes (WBCs)	wahyt blud	colorless blood corpuscles capable of ameboid movement; protect the body against pathogenic microorganisms
agranulocytes	ah-<u>gran</u>-u-lo-sitz´	nongranular leukocytes, produced by the spleen and lymph nodes
basophils	<u>ba</u>-so-filz	any structure cells staining readily with basic dyes; functions unknown
eosinophils	e´-o-<u>sin</u>-o-filz	having a nucleus with two lobes and cytoplasm containing coarse, round granules. May be associated with allergy
granulocytes	<u>gran</u>-u-lo-sitz´	any cells containing granules, especially a granular leukocyte; formed in the bone marrow. There are three types: neutrophils, eosinophils, and basophils
neutrophils	<u>nu</u>-tro-filz	having a nucleus with three to five lobes and cytoplasm containing very fine granules. Neutrophils defend the body by ingesting invaders
lymphocytes	<u>lim</u>-fo-sitz	white blood cell with immune functions; made in the bone marrow and found in blood and lymph tissue. Two main types: B lymphocytes make antibodies and T lymphocytes help kill tumor cells and help control immune responses
monocytes	<u>mon</u>-o-sitz	destroy foreign invaders in the body
Clotting Factors		
fibrinogen	fi-<u>brin</u>-o-jen	promotes blood clotting
platelet/thrombocyte	<u>plât</u>-let/ <u>throm</u>-bo-cyte	a disk-shaped structure in the blood, for blood coagulation
Liquid Components		
plasma	<u>plas</u>-mah	the fluid portion of the blood or lymph, without the cells, amber colored; when whole blood is undisturbed in a tube, clotting cells settle in the bottom and the clear plasma is on top
serum	<u>se</u>-rum	the clear portion of the blood separated from solid elements; plasma minus fibrinogen
Terms Used in Blood Banking		
landsteiner types	<u>land</u>-sti-ner	refers to the type of red blood cell: A, B, AB, and O
Rh factors		a genetically determined antigen, present on the surface of erythrocytes. One Rh factor present in blood means it is Rh positive; if no factor is found, the blood is Rh negative
type and crossmatch (x match)		determination of the compatibility of the blood of a donor and that of a recipient before transfusion; donor's cells are placed in the recipient's serum and recipient's cells are placed in the donor's serum; absence of agglutination, hemolysis, and cytotoxicity indicates compatibility
universal donor	<u>do</u>-ner	a person with group O blood; frequently used in emergency transfusion
universal recipient	re-<u>sip</u>-e-ent	able to receive blood of any type; group AB

TERMS USED TO DESCRIBE BLOOD PRESSURE

Table 14-5 describes common terms used to describe blood pressure.

TABLE **14-5** Terms Used to Describe Blood Pressure		
Term	**Pronunciation**	**Definition**
diastolic pressure	di-ah-<u>stol</u>-ic <u>presh</u>-ur	the bottom number of a blood pressure reading; taken during the dilation of the heart, especially of the ventricles
normal blood pressure (BP)		an acceptable range for systolic pressure is <120 and for diastolic < 80; usually recorded as $^{80}/_{120}$
hypertension	hi´-per-<u>ten</u>-shun	persistently high arterial blood pressure with diastolic pressures > 90 and systolic pressure > 140
systolic pressure	sis-<u>tol</u>-ic <u>presh</u>-ur	the top number in a blood pressure reading; reflects pressure during the contraction of the heart, especially of the ventricles

CLINICAL DISORDERS OF THE CARDIOVASCULAR SYSTEM

Table 14-6 describes clinical disorders of the cardiovascular system.

TABLE **14-6** Clinical Disorders of the Cardiovascular System		
Condition	**Pronunciation**	**Definition**
aortic stenosis (AS)	a-<u>or</u>-tic ste-<u>no</u>-sis	narrowing or stricture of the aortic valve which obstructs the flow of blood from the left ventricle into the aorta, causing decreased cardiac output; may lead to congestive heart failure
anemia	ah-<u>ne</u>-me-ah	reduction below normal of red blood cells, hemoglobin, or the volume of packed red cells in the blood; a symptom of various disorders. Severe anemia increases the work load of the heart
aneurysm	<u>an</u>-u-rizm	a sac formed by localized dilation of an artery or vein
angina pectoris	an-<u>ji</u>-nah <u>pek</u>-to-ris	chest pain caused by decreased supply of oxygen to the heart muscle; precipitated by increased activity or stress. Symptom of coronary heart disease
arteriosclerosis	ar-te´re-o-skle-<u>ro</u>-sis	thickening and loss of elasticity of the arterial walls, slowing the flow of blood; causes hypertension
atherosclerosis	ath´-er-o-skle-<u>ro</u>-sis	cholesterol plaque buildup causing arteries to narrow and become stiff; increases risk for hypertension, heart attack, and stroke
cardiomyopathy	car-di-o-my-<u>op</u>-a-thy	disease of the heart muscle causing weak contractions that prevent movement of blood out of the heart; results in inadequate oxygen levels in body tissues
congestive heart failure (CHF)	kon-<u>jes</u>-tiv hart <u>fâl</u>-yer	defective blood-pumping system, marked by shortness of breath and abnormal retention of sodium and water or edema (**Figure 14-9**)
coronary artery disease/ coronary heart disease (CAD/CHD)	<u>cor</u>-o-nar-y	atherosclerosis of the coronary arteries; cholesterol plaque inside coronary arteries; the plaque can break off and block the blood and oxygen supply to the heart muscles, resulting in a heart attack

Condition	Pronunciation	Definition
dyscrasia	dis-<u>kra</u>-ze-ah	any abnormal condition of the blood components, e.g., the number or shape of red blood cells, white blood cells, or clotting factors
embolism	<u>em</u>-bo-lizm	the sudden blocking of an artery by an embolus
embolus	<u>em</u>-bo-lus	a foreign object (i.e., air, fat, tissue, or blood) brought by the blood and forced into a smaller vessel, thus obstructing the circulation
infective endocarditis (IE)	en´-do-kar-<u>di</u>-tis	inflammation of the endocardium, usually caused by a bacterial infection in those with a heart defect
ischemia	is-<u>ke</u>-me-ah	reduced blood flow and oxygen to an organ; usually caused by a constricted or blocked artery
mitral valve prolapse (MVP)	<u>mi</u>-tral valve pro-<u>lapse</u>	condition in which the flaps of the mitral valve do not close tightly; this condition may cause blood to leak from the ventricle back into the atrium. Symptoms are chest pain, shortness of breath, and palpitations
myocarditis	mi´-o-kar-<u>di</u>-tis	inflammation of the myocardium; usually caused by a viral infection
pericarditis	per´-i-kar-<u>di</u>-tis	inflammation of the pericardium; symptom is a "creaking" heart sound from the heart rubbing against the pericardial sac
peripheral artery disease (PAD)/peripheral vascular disease (PVD)	pe-<u>riph</u>-er-al <u>ar</u>-ter-y dis-<u>ease</u>/<u>vas</u>-cu-lar	atherosclerosis of the arteries in the legs, preventing adequate blood flow; causes leg cramps and pain when walking (claudication)
rheumatic heart disease (RHD)	roo-<u>mat</u>-ik	complication of rheumatic fever with scaring and malfunction of valves of the heart
stroke (cerebrovascular accident [CVA])	strôk	a sudden and acute vascular lesion of the brain caused by hemorrhage, embolism, thrombosis, or rupturing blood vessels
transient ischemic attack (TIA)	<u>tran</u>-s-hən is-<u>kem</u>-ik ah-<u>tak</u>	brief interruption of circulation to a portion of the brain owing to vascular spasm, causing temporary loss of function; a precursor to CVA

Terms Related to the Conduction System

arrhythmia	ah-<u>rith</u>-me-ah	variation from the normal rhythm of the heartbeat
asystole	a-<u>sis</u>-to-le	cardiac standstill; no heartbeat
fibrillation	fi´-bri-<u>la</u>-shun	irregular contractions of the muscle fibers of the heart resulting in a lack of synchronism between heartbeat and pulse
heart block	hart blok	type of arrhythmia; often applied specifically to arterioventricular heart block
premature contractions (PACs/PVCs)	pre-ma-<u>ture</u> con-<u>trac</u>-tions	early beat of the upper chamber of the heart (premature atrial contractions [PACs]) or lower chamber of the heart (premature ventricular contractions [PVCs]); palpitations or "skipped beat"
congenital defects	kon-<u>jen</u>-i-tal <u>de</u>-fekts	defects present at birth (see Box 14-1)
coarctation of the aorta	ko´-ark-<u>ta</u>-shun a-or-ta	narrowing of the aorta, the largest artery that branches off the heart and delivers oxygen-rich blood throughout the body; increases the work load of the heart
hemophilia	he´-mo-<u>fil</u>-e-ah	a hereditary hemorrhagic condition caused by lack of one or more clotting factors

(continues)

TABLE 14-6 *(continued)*

Condition	Pronunciation	Definition
patent ductus arteriosus (PDA)	pa-tent duk-tus ar-te-re-o-sus	birth defect; duct with an abnormal opening in the ductus arteriosus, the artery that connects the two main arteries that carry blood out of the heart (aorta and pulmonary arteries); results in abnormal blood mixing of oxygenated and deoxygenated blood
septal defect	sep-tal de-fect	abnormal hole in the septum that separates the left and right sides of the heart; the hole can be between the upper chambers (*atrial septal defect [ASD]*) or between the lower chambers (*ventricular septal defect [VSD]*); if the hole is large, it allows oxygenated and deoxygenated blood to mix and would require surgery
sickle cell anemia/sickle cell disease (SCD)	sick-el cell ah-ne-me-ah	genetic blood disorder with sickle- or crescent-shaped red blood cells; the abnormal shape impairs blood flow and causes blockage. Those with the disease are at risk of heart attack or stroke
Heart Attack		
cardiac arrest	kar-de-ak ah-rest	cessation of heart function; heart attack
coronary thrombosis	kor-o-ner-e throm-bo-sis	thrombosis of a coronary artery, often leading to myocardial infarction
infarction	in-fark-shun	a localized area of ischemic necrosis owing to occlusion of the arterial supply
myocardial infarction (MI)	mi-o-kar´-de-al in-fark-shun	gross necrosis of the myocardium, caused by decreased blood supply to the area
occlusion	o-kloo-zhun	obstruction, a closing off of the coronary arteries, leading to a heart attack
plaque	plak	a deposit of fatty material in the artery (atherosclerosis)
Vein Disorders		
thrombophlebitis	throm´-bo-fle-bi-tis	inflammation of a vein associated with thrombus formation
varicose veins	var-i-kos vânz	a dilated, tortuous vein, usually in the leg, caused by a defective venous valve
venous thromboembolism (VTE)	ve-nous throm-bo-em-bo-lism	blood clots that occur in the veins; two types: pulmonary embolism (PE) and deep vein thrombosis (DVT)

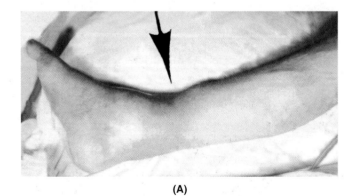

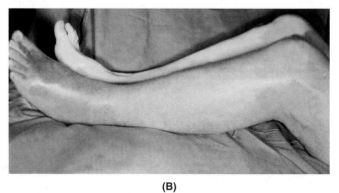

(A)   (B)

FIGURE 14-9 (A) Marked pitting edema of leg as a result of chronic heart failure. **(B)** Localized edema of left leg caused by venous obstruction; right leg appears normal.

Courtesy of Leonard V. Crowley, MD, Century College.

TERMS USED IN DIAGNOSIS AND TREATMENT OF CARDIOVASCULAR DISEASES

Table 14-7 describes terms used in the diagnosis and treatment of cardiovascular diseases.

Term	Pronunciation	Definition
TABLE 14-7 Terms Used in the Diagnosis and Treatment of Diseases of the Cardiovascular System		
History and Physical Exam		
auscultation	aws´-kul-ta-shun	the act of listening for sounds within the body, chiefly to ascertain the condition of the thoracic or abdominal viscera; may be performed with an unaided ear or with a stethoscope
bradycardia	brad´-e-kar-de-ah	slowness of the heartbeat, as evidenced by a pulse rate of < 60
cyanosis	sigh´-ah-no-sis	dark, slightly bluish discoloration of the skin, lips, and fingernails; occurs because the oxygen level of blood leaving the heart is below normal
dyspnea on exertion (DOE)	dysp-ne-a on ex-er-tion	shortness of breath, present in congestive heart failure and brought on by physical activity
edema	e-de-ma	abnormally large fluid volume in tissues between the body's cells; can be caused by congestive heart failure. Symptoms are swelling in the ankles or legs
extrasystole	ex-tra-sys-to-le	a premature contraction of the heart, resulting in momentary interruption of the normal heartbeat
heart murmur	hart mer-mer	auscultatory sound (soft, blowing); a periodic sound of short duration of cardiac origin; may be the result of an incompetent heart valve
orthopnea	or´-thop-ne-ah	shortness of breath when lying flat; symptom of congestive heart failure
tachycardia	tak´-e-kar-de-ah	abnormally rapid heart rate; pulse rate of 100 beats per minute
Laboratory Tests		
arterial blood gases	ar-ter-i-al	measures O_2, CO_2, and pH to evaluate heart function, especially in heart failure
B-type natriuretic peptide (BNP)	na-tri-ur-et-ic pep-tide	cardiac neurohormone secreted by the left ventricle in response to elevated blood volume and pressure; used to diagnose congestive heart failure
cardiac enzyme test	kar-de-ak en-zym test	blood enzymes measured to determine if there is damage to the myocardial muscle; injury of heart muscle releases enzymes into the bloodstream. Enzymes measured are creatine kinase and troponin
hemoglobin (Hg/Hb)	he´-mo-glo-bin	measured to evaluate for anemia; the oxygen-carrying pigment of the red blood cells
prothrombin time (PT)	pro-throm-bin	blood test to measure how long it takes blood to clot; used to check whether anticoagulant medicine to prevent blood clots is working
serum lipid test	see-rum lip-id test	determination of triglycerides, cholesterol, and lipoproteins (low density lipoprotein [LDL] and high density lipoprotein [HDL]); high levels of serum lipids are a risk for heart attack and stroke

(continues)

TABLE 14-7 *(continued)*

Term	Pronunciation	Definition
Diagnostic Tools		
exercise stress test		assessment of cardiac function by subjecting the patient to controlled amounts of physical stress, such as the treadmill or pedaling a stationary bike while monitoring heart function
holter monitor	<u>hol</u>-tur	a portable device for monitoring blood pressure or heart/respiratory rate, e.g., ECG; usually worn for a 24-hour period
phlebotomy	fle-<u>bot</u>-o-me	incision of a vein to draw blood for lab analysis
sphygmomanometer	sfig´-mo-mah-<u>nom</u>-e-ter	an instrument for measuring arterial blood pressure
venipuncture	ven´-i-<u>pungk</u>-chur	puncture of a vein with a needle to withdraw blood or infuse fluid
Radiological Exams		
angiography	an´-je-<u>og</u>-rah-fe	X-ray technique using an injected contrast medium to visualize the heart and blood vessels
cardiac catheterization	<u>kar</u>-de-ak kath´-e-ter-i-<u>za</u>-tion	evaluation of heart function, including valves and coronary arteries; a long, fine catheter is navigated through a peripheral blood vessel into the chambers of the heart using X-ray visualization as a guide
computed axial tomography (CAT scan or CT scan)	kuh-m-<u>pyoot</u>-ed <u>ak</u>-see-al toh-<u>mog</u>-rah-fee	diagnostic X-ray technique that uses ionizing radiation to produce cross-sectional images; used to examine the heart, coronary arteries, and brain
echocardiography	ek-oh-car-dee-<u>og</u>-rah-fee	diagnostic procedure using ultrasound waves to study the structure and motion of the heart and to detect changes in some heart disorders
electrocardiogram (ECG/EKG)	e-lek´-tro-<u>kar</u>-de-o-gram´	record produced by electrocardiography to evaluate electrical activity of the heart; used to evaluate for an irregular heartbeat and the strength and timing of electrical impulses
doppler	<u>dop</u>-ler	a device for measuring blood flow to evaluate for atherosclerosis of carotid arteries and peripheral arteries; transmits and reflects sound waves
magnetic resonance imaging (MRI)	mag-<u>neh</u>-tic rehz-oh-nans <u>im</u>-uh-jing	noninvasive procedure that uses strong magnetic fields and radiofrequency waves to produce images of the heart, blood vessels, and brain; it can also show the heartbeat and blood flow
positron emission tomography (PET)	<u>pawz</u>-ih-tron ee-mish-<u>un</u> toh-<u>mog</u>-rah-fee	computerized X-ray technique using radioactive substances, which are given by injection, to measure blood flow and metabolic activity of the heart and blood vessels; the radiation emitted is measured by the PET camera
thallium stress test	thal-<u>ee</u>-um stress test	thallium injections are given intravenously in conjunction with the stress test to determine whether there are changes in coronary blood flow during exercise; changes may be indicative of ischemia, severe coronary narrowing, or infarction
Treatments		
cardiopulmonary resuscitation (CPR)	car-di-o-<u>pul</u>-mo-nar-y re-<u>sus</u>-ci-ta-tion	emergency procedure that involves providing mouth-to-mouth resuscitation and applying external chest compression to restore heart function in someone who has had a heart attack

Term	Pronunciation	Definition
Dietary Approaches to Stop Hypertension (DASH)		consists of low fat meats and dairy products, whole grains, nuts, legumes, fruits, and vegetables; limits added salt, saturated fat and sugar; diet to lower blood pressure, and LDL cholesterol while maintaining normal body weight
low-salt diet		diet low in sodium content to reduce body water level; recommended for preventing hypertension and for treating congestive heart failure
pacemaker	pâs-mâk-er	electrical device for stimulating the heartbeat or reestablishing normal heart rhythm; used to treat arrhythmias

Medications

Term	Pronunciation	Definition
anticoagulant	an´-ti-ko-ag-u-lant	any substance that removes or prevents blood clotting
antihypertensive drug	an´-ti-hi´-per-ten-siv	a drug that reduces or eliminates high blood pressure; includes diuretics, beta blockers, and calcium channel blockers
digitalis	dij´-i-tal-is	drug used to maintain optimal heart contraction; used to treat congestive heart failure and heart arrhythmias
diuretic	di´-u-ret-ik	drug used to remove excess interstitial fluid that results in increased urine excretion; used to treat hypertension or congestive heart failure
heparin	hep-ah-rin	a substance that counteracts blood clotting, existing both as a natural substance in the blood and as a drug
statins	stat-ins	class of drugs that lower serum cholesterol by reducing production of cholesterol by the liver
thrombolytic ("clot buster")	throm-bo-lyt-ic	drug injected to dissolve a blood clot and restore blood flow in the coronary artery during a heart attack or in ischemic stroke
vasodilator	vas´-o-di-la-tor	drugs that dilate blood vessels; used to treat hypertension
vasopressor	vas´-o-pres-or	an agent that constricts blood vessels; used to treat hypotension, usually in a medical emergency

Surgery

Term	Pronunciation	Definition
angioplasty	an-je-o-plas´-te	surgical or percutaneous reconstruction of blood vessels
commissurotomy	kom´-i-shur-ot-o-me	surgical incision of a defective heart valve to increase the size of the orifice; commonly done to separate adherent, thickened leaflets of a stenotic mitral valve
coronary artery bypass graft (CABG)	kor-o-ner-e ar-ter-e bi-pas	use of a leg vein or synthetic material to substitute for an occluded artery in the heart
endarterectomy	en´-dar-ter-ek-to-me	excision of thickened areas of the innermost coat of an artery to increase blood flow
percutaneous transluminal coronary angioplasty (PTCA)	per´-ku-ta-ne-us trans-lum-i-nul kor-o-ner-e an-je-o-plas´-te	dilation of a blood vessel by means of a balloon catheter inserted through the skin and into the chosen vessel, and then passed through the lumen of the vessel to the site of the lesion, where the balloon is inflated to flatten plaque against the artery wall

BOX 14-1 describes common forms of congenital heart disease in newborns.

Box 14-1 Why do Some Babies have Congenital Heart Disease?

Congenital heart disease (CHD) is the most common birth defect in infants in the United States. One in four newborns have heart defects that affect the structure and function of the heart. Examples are a septal defect or hole between the right and left side of the heart or an abnormal opening in the ductus arteriosus, the artery that connects the two main arteries: the aorta and the pulmonary artery. Both of these defects result in a mixing of oxygenated and deoxygenated blood. "Blue babies" or cyanosis is a symptom of a lack of oxygen in body tissues. Other symptoms are excessive sleeping and poor feeding. A diagnosis can be made during pregnancy or in early infancy with the use of an echocardiogram that shows ultrasound pictures of the heart. Treatment can include medications and surgery.

Can CHD Be Prevented?
Although some CHDs are likely to be caused by defective genes, other preventable factors are also important. These factors are the mother's diet and her overall health condition. Women who are obese, have poorly controlled diabetes, or smoke, are more likely to deliver babies with heart defects. Heart defects in infants can be prevented when women achieve a healthy weight and desirable blood glucose levels, take a daily folic acid supplement, and stop smoking.

Congenital Heart Defects (CHDs). Division of Birth Defects and Developmental Disabilities, Centers for Disease Control and Prevention. https://www.cdc.gov/ncbddd/heartdefects/facts.html

LESSON TWO   **Materials to Be Learned**

THE LYMPHATIC SYSTEM

The lymphatic system is an accessory component of the circulatory system. It consists of *lymphocytes* (produced in the bone marrow) and *lymph fluid* (derived from tissue fluid). Lymph vessels return lymph fluid to the circulation via two collecting ducts: the right lymphatic duct and the left thoracic duct. The *right lymphatic duct* receives lymph from the right side of the head and neck, right upper arm, and right thorax. It empties into the right subclavian vein near the right jugular vein. The *left thoracic duct* receives lymph from the legs, abdominal regions, left arm, and left side of the head, neck, and thorax. It empties into the left subclavian vein near the left jugular vein. Lymph then moves from the two collecting ducts into the venous system, becoming part of the plasma (see Figures 14-2 and 14-8 in Lesson One and **Figure 14-10** in this lesson).

Functions of the lymphatic system are:

1. Returns excess tissue fluid that has leaked from the capillaries. If not removed, this fluid collects in spaces between the cells and results in *edema.*
2. Returns plasma proteins that have leaked out of the capillaries into the circulation. If not returned, these proteins would accumulate, increase the osmotic pressure in the tissue fluid, and upset capillary function.
3. Transports absorbed nutrients. Specialized lymph vessels transport nutrients, especially fats, from the digestive system to the blood.

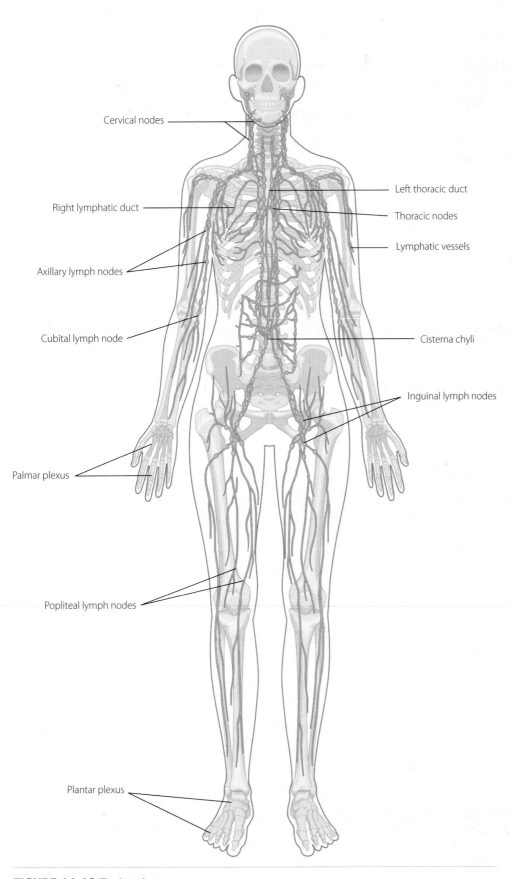

Cervical nodes

Right lymphatic duct

Axillary lymph nodes

Cubital lymph node

Palmar plexus

Popliteal lymph nodes

Plantar plexus

Left thoracic duct

Thoracic nodes

Lymphatic vessels

Cisterna chyli

Inguinal lymph nodes

FIGURE 14-10 The lymphatic system.

4. Removes toxic substances and other cellular debris from circulation in tissues after infection or tissue damage.

5. Controls quality of tissue fluid by filtering it through lymph nodes before returning it to the circulation.

PARTS AND FUNCTIONS OF THE LYMPHATIC SYSTEM

Components of the lymphatic system include lymph fluid, lymph vessels, lymph nodes, and lymphocytes. The functions of this system are:

1. Transporting fluid from the tissues back to the bloodstream.
2. Assisting in controlling infection caused by microorganisms.
3. Transporting fats away from the digestive organs.

Table 14-8 describes the parts and functions of the lymphatic system.

TABLE **14-8** Parts and Functions of the Lymphatic System

Term	Pronunciation	Definition
Lymphoid Tissues and Cells		
adenoids	add-<u>eh</u>-noyds	mass of lymphoid tissue located at the back of the nose in the upper part of the throat; normally present only in children
antibodies	an-tih-<u>bod</u>-eez	substances produced by the body in response to foreign organisms
capillaries	cap-<u>ih</u>-lair-eez	smallest of the lymph vessels, they transport interstitial fluid back to the blood via large lymph vessels
ducts	ducts	the largest of the lymph vessels, point of entry to blood circulation; *right lymphatic duct* and *left thoracic duct* (see Figure 14-10)
lymphocytes	lim-<u>foh</u>-sights	leukocytes originating from stem cells, developing in the bone marrow, and carried by both the blood and lymph systems
macrophage	<u>mack</u>-roh-fayj	large cell involved in defending against infection; found in lymph nodes, liver, spleen, lungs, brain, and spinal cord
nodes	nodes	collections of lymphatic tissue; located in several parts of the body (see Figure 14-10)
phagocytes	<u>fag</u>-oh-sights	cells that engulf and destroy bacteria
spleen	spleen	large organ located behind the stomach that filters blood to remove pathogens and serves as a blood reservoir
T cells	t sels	important part of the immune response; provide defense against disease by attacking foreign and abnormal cells
thymus gland	<u>thigh</u>-mus	endocrine gland that stimulates red bone marrow to produce T lymphocytes (T cells)
tonsils	<u>ton</u>-sills	two oval-shaped tissues at the back of the throat that lie between the mouth and the pharynx; prevent infections of the breathing passages but often become infected themselves

PATHOLOGICAL CONDITIONS OF THE LYMPHATIC SYSTEM

Table 14-9 describes pathological conditions of the lymphatic system.

TABLE 14-9 Pathological Conditions of the Lymphatic System

Term	Pronunciation	Definition
carinii pneumonia	kah-rye-nee-eye noo-mon-ia	pneumonia caused by a common worldwide parasite to which most people have a natural immunity
dyscrasia	dis-kra-ze-ah	any abnormal condition of the blood components, e.g., the number or shape of red blood cells, white blood cells, or clotting factors
hypersplenism	high´-per-splen-izm	enlargement of the spleen; splenomegaly
lymphadenopathy	lim-fad-en-noh-pa-thee	chronic or excessive lymph node enlargement
lymphedema/lymphatic edema	lim-fuh-dee-muh/ lim-fat-ik e-de-ma	localized fluid retention and tissue swelling caused by obstruction in the lymphatic system; interstitial fluid is normally reabsorbed by the lymph system and recirculated in the bloodstream
mononucleosis	moh-oh-noo-klee-oh-sis	benign self-limiting acute infection of B lymphocytes, usually caused by Epstein-Barr virus
pneumonocystic pneumonia	noo-moh´-noh-sis-tik noo-mon-ia	a rare form of pneumonia in AIDS patients
sarcoidosis	sar-koyd-oh-sis	a systemic inflammatory disease characterized by small rounded lesions forming on the spleen, lymph nodes, and other organs

THE ORIGIN OF MEDICAL TERMS

Table 14-10 explains the origin of several terms used in this chapter.

TABLE 14-10 The Origin of Medical Terms

Word	Pronunciation	Origin and Definition
auscultation	aws-kul-ta-shun	Latin, *auscultare*, to listen to
lymphadenopathy	lim-fad-en-noh-pa-thee	Latin, *lympha*, lymph fluid + Greek, *adenos*, a gland + Greek, *pathos*, suffering
fibrinogen	fi-brin-o-jen	Latin, *fibra*, fiber; + Greek, *genes*, born, produced
ischemia	is-ke-me-ah	Greek, *ischaimos*, from *ischein*, to restrain + Greek, *haima*, blood
orthopnea	or-thop-ne-a	Greek, *orthos*, straight + Greek, *pnoia*, breathing
lymphocytes	lim-foh-sights	Latin, *lympha*, lymph fluid + Greek, *kytos*, cell

(continues)

TABLE **14-10** (continued)

Word	Pronunciation	Origin and Definition
myocardium	mi-o-<u>kar</u>-de-um	Latin, *myo*, muscle + Greek, *kardia*, heart
resuscitate	re-<u>sus</u>-ci-tate	Latin, *resuocitat*, raised again, from *re*, back + Latin, *suscitare*, raise
thrombocyte	<u>throm</u>-bo-cyte	Greek, *thrombos*, "clot of blood" + Greek, *kutos*, container, hollow vessel
varicose	<u>var</u>-i-kos	Latin, *varicōsus*, from *varix*, *varic*, swollen vein

ABBREVIATIONS

Abbreviations in **Table 14-11** are frequently used when diagnosing and/or charting cardiovascular disorders.

TABLE **14-11** Abbreviations

Abbreviation	Definition	Abbreviation	Definition
ASD	arterial septal defect	DVT	deep vein thrombosis
ASHD	arteriosclerotic heart disease	ECG/EKG	electrocardiogram
AS	aortic stenosis	ECHO	echocardiogram
AV	atrioventricular	Hg/Hb	hemoglobin
BNP	B-type natriuretic peptide	HDL	high-density lipoprotein
BP	blood pressure	LDL	low-density lipoprotein
CABG	coronary artery bypass graft	Mono	mononucleosis
CBC	complete blood count	MRI	magnetic resonance imaging
CCU	coronary care unit	MVP	mitral valve prolapse
CHF	congestive heart failure	O_2	oxygen
CO_2	carbon dioxide	PAD/PVD	peripheral artery disease/ peripheral vascular disease
CPR	cardiopulmonary resuscitation	PET	positron emission tomography
CVA	cerebrovascular accident	PT	prothrombin time
DASH	Dietary Approaches to Stop Hypertension	PTCA	percutaneous transluminal coronary angioplasty
DOE	dyspnea on exertion	PVC	premature ventricular contractions

Abbreviation	Definition	Abbreviation	Definition
RBC	red blood cell, red blood (cell) count	TIA	transient ischemic attack
SA	sinoatrial	VSD	ventricular septal defect
SCD	sickle cell disease/anemia		

The following box describes common drugs used to treat cardiovascular disease.

PHARMACOLOGY AND MEDICAL TERMINOLOGY

Drug Classification	antiarrhythmic (an-tee-ah-rith-mik)	anticoagulant (an-tih-koh-ag-yoo-lant)	antihypertensive (an-tih-high-per-ten-siv)
Function	corrects cardiac arrhythmias (irregular beats)	prevents clot continuation and formation	opposes high pressure (blood)
Word Parts	**anti-** = against; **arrhythm/o** = rhythm; **-ic** = pertaining to	**anti-** = against; **coagul/o** = clotting	**anti-** = against; **hyper-** = excess; **tensive** = pertaining to tension or pressure
Active Ingredients (examples)	digoxin (Lanoxin); propranalol hydrochloride (Inderal)	heparin calcium (Calcilean); warfarin sodium (Coumadin)	nadolol (Corgard); furosemide (Lasix); diltiazem hydrochloride (Cardizem, Cardizem CD)

CLINICAL *Note*

ED Note

Patient is a 55-year-old Caucasian female with complaint of midsternal pressure with pain from the left jaw, extending down the left arm. Patient thought she had indigestion and self-medicated with 6 OTC chewable Tums. When pain began to radiate to neck, jaw, and arm, patient chewed a 325 mg **ASA** tablet and asked her husband to transport her to the ED. Upon arrival, patient was clearly in distress with anxiety, profuse sweating, **SOB**, and **cyanosis**. EKG showed active **MI** with anterior ST segment elevation, indicating an **anterior STEMI**. Suspect **acute thrombotic occlusion** of the left anterior descending coronary artery. Patient was put on O_2 at 4 L via nasal cannula, given **sublingual** nitroglycerin. Patient remained unstable and was transported to the cath lab for immediate cardiac cath with possible stent placement. Surgical team and OR on standby for possible **CABG**.

Direction: For the portions of the clinical note shown by a colored font, provide the definition and/or words for abbreviation.

LESSON THREE	Progress Check

LIST: FUNCTIONS OF THE CIRCULATORY AND LYMPHATIC SYSTEMS

List the functions of the circulatory system:

1. _____

2. _____

3. _____

4. _____

List the functions of the lymphatic system:

5. _____

6. _____

7. _____

8. _____

9. _____

COMPLETION: CARDIOVASCULAR SYSTEM

Name the structure or fluid from the cardiovascular system for the definitions given below:

1. _____: One of two lower chambers of the heart that pump blood out of the heart

2. _____: Upper chambers of the heart that receive blood from other parts of the body

3. _____: Largest vein where blood from the body is returned to the heart

4. _____: Heart chamber that pumps oxygenated blood out of the heart to all parts of the body

5. _____: Largest artery that carries oxygenated blood out of the heart

6. _____: The sac that contains fluid and surrounds the heart

7. _____: Cardiac muscle fibers that conduct electrical impulses from the A-V node along the outside of the ventricles

8. _____: Carry blood away from the heart while _____ carry blood to the heart

9. _____: Measurement of heartbeat when heart muscles are relaxed

10. _____: Normal blood pressure numbers

11. _____: Prevent backflow of blood between chambers of the heart

12. _____: Liquid part of the blood after red blood cells and clotting factors have been removed

13. _____: Blood type O

14. _____: Blood components that promote blood clotting

COMPLETION: LYMPHATIC SYSTEM

Name the structure or fluid from the lymphatic system for the definitions given below:

1. _____ : Large lymph vessel in the chest that drains the lymph from the upper right part of the body

2. _____ : Masses of lymph tissue in the nasopharynx

3. _____ : Organ in the mediastinum that produces T-cell lymphocytes and helps in the immune response

4. _____ : Tiniest lymph vessels

5. _____ : Stationary lymph tissue along the path of lymph vessels all over the body

6. _____ : Large lymph vessel in the chest that drains lymph from the lower part and left side of the body above the diaphragm

7. _____ : Fluid that lies between cells and becomes lymph as it enters lymph capillaries

8. _____ : Organ near the stomach that produces, stores, and eliminates blood cells

9. _____ : Cells that engulf and destroy bacteria

10. _____ : Substances produced by the body in response to foreign organisms or substances

MATCHING: DIAGNOSTIC TOOLS—CARDIOVASCULAR SYSTEM

Match the following diagnostic procedures to their function:

Terms	**Definition**
1. Echocardiogram	**a.** Complete blood count
2. Holter monitor	**b.** Measurement of O_2, CO_2, pH
3. Exercise stress test	**c.** Reflected sound waves from the heart
4. Angiography	**d.** X-ray record of heart and blood vessels
5. Arterial blood gases	**e.** X-ray record of an artery
6. CBC	**f.** Blood coagulation test
7. Cholesterol	**g.** Recording device for ECG/EKG activity
8. ECG/EKG	**h.** Electrical recording of heart activity
9. Prothrombin time	**i.** A fatlike substance found in vessel walls
10. Angiocardiography	**j.** Evaluation of heart function while exercising

MATCHING: CLINICAL DISORDERS

Match the definition with the following clinical conditions:

Clinical Condition	**Definition**
1. Angina pectoris	**a.** Low volume of red blood cells
2. Congestive heart failure	**b.** A sac formed by a localized dilation of an artery or vein
3. Mitral valve prolapse	**c.** Chest pain caused by lack of oxygen to heart muscle
4. Coronary heart disease	**d.** Scarring of heart valves; complication of rheumatic fever
5. Hemophilia	**e.** Irregular contractions of the heart
6. Cerebrovascular accident	**f.** Defective blood pumping system, causing shortness of breath and edema
7. Venous thromboembolism	**g.** Localized fluid retention and swelling caused by obstruction in the lymphatic system
8. Myocardial infarction	**h.** Congenital lack of clotting factors
9. Rheumatic heart disease	**i.** Viral infection of the B lymphocytes
10. Fibrillation	**j.** Blood pressure above 80/120
11. Mononucleosis	**k.** Stroke
12. Lymphedema	**l.** Cholesterol buildup and blockage of blood flow
13. Hypertension	**m.** Necrosis of the blood supply with lack of oxygen
14. Anemia	**n.** Blood clot in a vein
15. Aneurysm	**o.** Valves fail to close tight resulting in backflow of blood

ABBREVIATIONS: CARDIOVASCULAR SYSTEM

Define the following commonly used abbreviations:

1. ASD: _____

2. BP: _____

3. CBC: _____

4. CCU: _____

5. CHF: _____

6. CO_2: _____

7. CPR: _____

8. CVA: _____

9. ECG, EKG: _____

10. MI: _____

11. O_2: _____

12. PVC: _____

13. RBC: _____

14. TIA: _____

15. WBC: _____

IDENTIFYING WORD PARTS

For each of the medical terms, list the root word and the prefix and/or suffix.

Word	Root Word	Prefix	Suffix
1. Anticoagulant	_____	_____	_____
2. Arrhythmia	_____	_____	_____
3. Cardiogram	_____	_____	_____
4. Cyanosis	_____	_____	_____
5. Dyspnea	_____	_____	_____
6. Endocarditis	_____	_____	_____
7. Hypertension	_____	_____	_____
8. Natriuretic	_____	_____	_____
9. Phagocyte	_____	_____	_____
10. Sarcoidosis	_____	_____	_____

CHAPTER

15

© teekid/iStock/Getty Images

Nervous System

OBJECTIVES

After completing this chapter and the exercises, the student should be able to:

1. Identify the organs of the nervous system.
2. List the functions of the nervous system.
3. Identify and define clinical disorders affecting the nervous system.
4. List and explain medical and surgical procedures used in diagnosing and treating nervous system disorders.
5. List and define psychiatric clinical disorders.
6. Create new medical terms using combining forms and give their meanings.
7. Correctly spell and pronounce new medical terms.

THE NERVOUS SYSTEM

The human nervous system (NS) provides functions not seen in other animal species, for instance, the formation of ideas. We are able to think and reason, that is, judge right from wrong, separate logical from illogical, and plan for the future. Our NS is the center of all mental activity, including thought, learning, and memory. It is no wonder then that any abnormal condition that affects the NS affects the entire body.

This chapter briefly describes the anatomy and physiology of the NS and its disorders. The study of the NS is called *neurology*. There are two physician specialties for the treatment of NS conditions: the *neurologist* diagnoses and treats diseases and disorders, while a *neurosurgeon* specializes in surgery involving the brain, spinal cord, or peripheral nerves. In addition, the *psychiatrist* is the physician who specializes in the diagnosis and treatment of diseases of the brain that affect behavior, thoughts and feelings. When studying materials in this chapter, refer to Figures 15-1 through 15-7.

ALLIED HEALTH PROFESSIONS

Physical Therapists and Physical Therapist Assistants and Aides

Physical therapists provide services that help restore function, improve mobility, relieve pain, and prevent or limit permanent physical disabilities. They restore, maintain, and promote overall fitness and health. Their patients include accident victims and individuals with disabling conditions such as low-back pain, arthritis, heart disease, fractures, head injuries, and cerebral palsy.

Therapists examine patients' medical histories and then test and measure the patients' strength, range of motion, balance and coordination, posture, muscle performance, respiration, and motor function. Next, physical therapists develop plans describing a treatment strategy and its anticipated outcome.

Physical therapist assistants and aides help physical therapists to provide treatment that improves patient mobility, relieves pain, and prevents or lessens physical disabilities of patients. A physical therapist might ask an assistant to help patients exercise or learn to use crutches, for example, or an aide to gather and prepare therapy equipment. Patients include accident victims and individuals with disabling conditions such as low-back pain, arthritis, heart disease, fractures, head injuries, and cerebral palsy.

Physical therapist assistants perform a variety of tasks. Under the direction and supervision of physical therapists, they provide part of a patient's treatment. This might involve exercises, massages, electrical stimulation, paraffin baths, hot and cold packs, traction, and ultrasound. Physical therapist assistants record the patient's responses to treatment and report the outcome of each treatment to the physical therapist.

Physical therapist aides help make therapy sessions productive, under the direct supervision of a physical therapist or physical therapist assistant. They usually are responsible for keeping the treatment area clean and organized and for preparing for each patient's therapy. When patients need assistance moving to or from a treatment area, aides push them in a wheelchair or provide them with a shoulder to lean on. Physical therapist aides are not licensed and do not perform the clinical tasks of a physical therapist assistant in states where licensure is required.

The duties of aides include some clerical tasks, such as ordering depleted supplies, answering the phone, and filling out insurance forms and other paperwork. The extent to which an aide or an assistant performs clerical tasks depends on the size and location of the facility.

INQUIRY

American Physical Therapy Association: www.apta.org

Data from Cross, Nanna, and McWay, Dana. *Stanfield's Introduction to the Health Professions,* 7th ed. Burlington, MA: Jones & Bartlett Learning; 2017.

The NS consists of two main anatomic subdivisions: the *central nervous system* (CNS) and the *peripheral nervous system* (PNS). The three main components of the NS are the brain, spinal cord and nerves (**Figure 15-1**). The brain and spinal cord constitute the CNS and are housed in the skull and vertebral canal, respectively. The brain and spinal cord receive, store, and process all sensory and motor data and control consciousness. The PNS transmits sensory and motor information back and forth between the CNS and the rest of the body. There are 12 pairs of cranial nerves and 31 pairs of spinal nerves in the PNS (see Table 15-2 and Figures 15-6 and 15-7).

The Central Nervous System

The human brain (**Figure 15-2**) comprises 2 percent of the body's total weight, consumes 25 percent of its oxygen, and receives 15 percent of its cardiac output (see Figure 15-1). The protective outer coverings of the brain are the bony skull and the *meninges*, the three connective tissue layers. The innermost covering, called the *pia mater*, is thin and delicate and closely adheres to the brain. The *arachnoid* is the middle layer and is separated from the pia mater by *subarachnoid* space. It contains cerebrospinal fluid, blood vessels, and web-like tissue that secure it to the pia mater. The *dura mater* is the thick outermost layer that adheres to the inner surface of the skull (**Figure 15-3**).

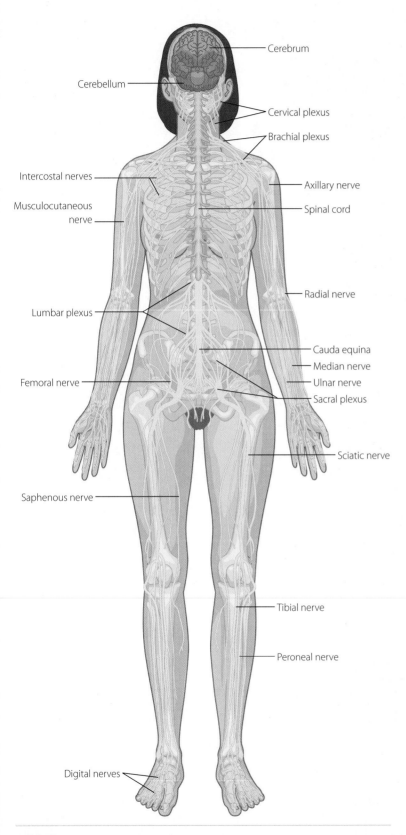

Cerebrum

Cerebellum

Cervical plexus

Brachial plexus

Intercostal nerves

Axillary nerve

Musculocutaneous nerve

Spinal cord

Radial nerve

Lumbar plexus

Cauda equina

Median nerve

Ulnar nerve

Femoral nerve

Sacral plexus

Sciatic nerve

Saphenous nerve

Tibial nerve

Peroneal nerve

Digital nerves

FIGURE 15-1 The nervous system.

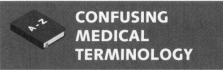

CONFUSING MEDICAL TERMINOLOGY

MS versus MS versus MS

MS – musculoskeletal system

MS – mitral stenosis

MS – multiple sclerosis

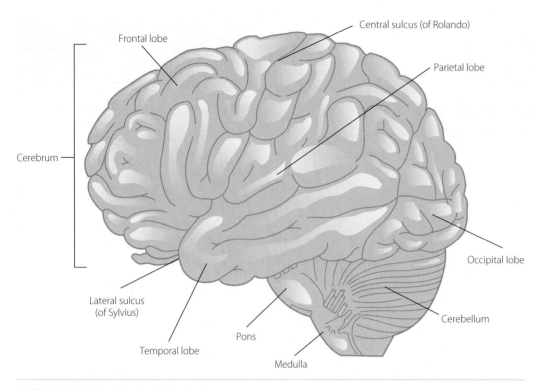

FIGURE 15-2 Surface view of the brain.

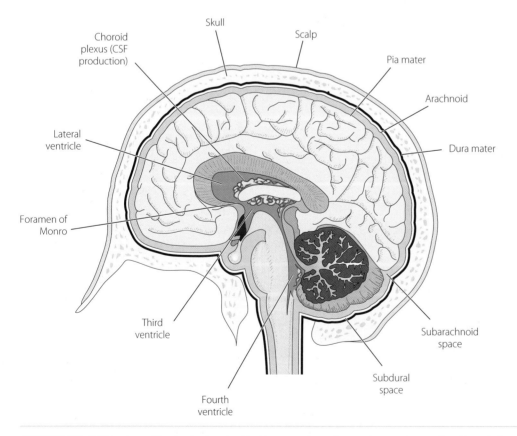

FIGURE 15-3 Side view of the brain showing the three meninges layers, dura mater, arachnoid, and pia mater.

Cerebrospinal fluid surrounds the *subarachnoid* spaces around the brain and spinal cord and fills the ventricles within the brain. White and gray matter is contained in the brain and spinal cord.

The *cerebrum* is the largest part of the brain. It has two hemispheres: the left and right hemispheres. The functional areas of the *cerebral cortex* include primary motor areas, primary sensory areas, and secondary areas that function at a higher level than the primary areas.

The *hypothalamus* lies inferior to the thalamus and forms the floor and lower part of the side walls of the third *ventricle*. It plays an important role in the regulation of appetite, heart rate, body temperature, water balance, digestion, and sexual activity.

The *cerebellum* lies inferior to the *pons* and is the second largest area of the brain. A cross section of the cerebellum looks like a tree and is often referred to as *arbor vitae* or tree of life. Unconscious functions such as heartbeat and breathing are housed in the cerebellum, hypothalamus, and brain stem. The cerebellum controls muscle synergy and helps maintain posture. It receives impulses from the sense organs in the ear that detect body position and send these impulses to the muscles to maintain or correct posture (**Figure 15-4**).

Inside the *spinal cord* is an inner section of gray matter associated with the PNS and an outer section of white matter. The white matter is covered with a myelin

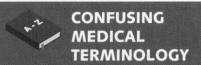

CONFUSING MEDICAL TERMINOLOGY

delusion versus illusion

delusion – a persistent belief in an untruth

illusion – an inaccurate sensory perception, for example, hallucinations

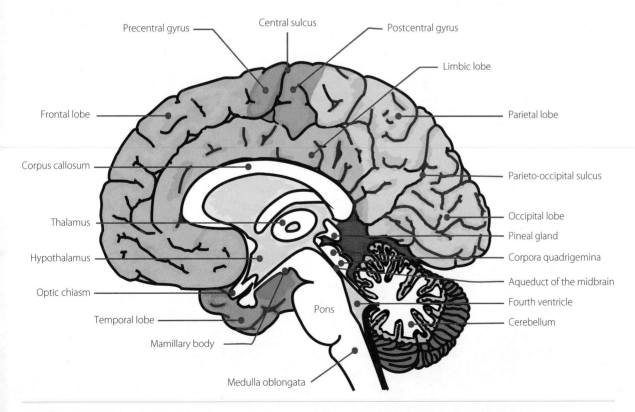

FIGURE 15-4 Side view of the brain showing the limbic lobe, hypothalamus, thalamus, pons, and cerebellum.
© NatthapongSachan/Shutterstock.

sheath and conducts impulses to and from the brain. It carries all the nerves that affect the limbs and lower part of the body (**Figure 15-5**).

The cord of nervous tissue enclosed within the vertebral column is the spinal cord. It controls many of the reflex actions of the body and transmits impulses to and from the brain via ascending and descending tracts.

The Peripheral Nervous System

The PNS is all the nervous tissue found outside the brain and spinal cord. As outlined and defined in Lesson One, it includes the *optic, olfactory, trochlear, trigeminal, abducens, facial, vestibulocular, glossopharyngeal, vagus, hypoglossal,* and *spinal accessory* nerves. Those nerves that control the special senses are discussed in the chapter pertaining to their functions and disorders. The PNS has two subsystems: the *somatic* nervous system (SNS) and the *autonomic* nervous system (ANS). The SNS is the part of the PNS associated with voluntary movement of skeletal muscle, while the ANS is responsible for bodily functions not consciously directed such as breathing, beating of the heart, and digestive processes.

In general, the subdivisions of the ANS (*sympathetic* and *parasympathetic*) exert opposing actions. Activation of the sympathetic portion causes the rate and intensity of reactions to increase, for example, increasing the heart rate, while the parasympathetic will slowly cause the rate and intensity of reactions to decrease, for example, bringing the heart rate back to normal (**Figure 15-6** and **Figure 15-7**).

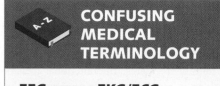

CONFUSING MEDICAL TERMINOLOGY

EEG versus EKG/ECG

EEG – electroencephalogram

EKG/ECG – electrocardiogram

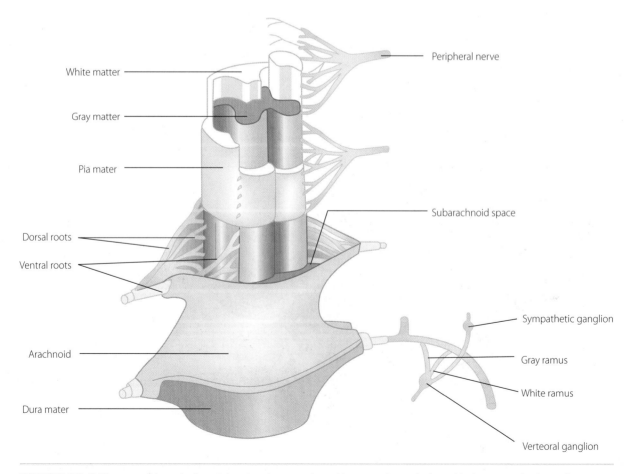

FIGURE 15-5 Diagram of the spinal cord showing three meningeal layers and association with the sympathetic trunk.

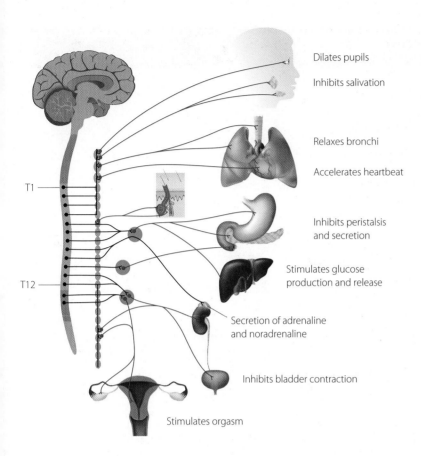

Dilates pupils

Inhibits salivation

Relaxes bronchi

Accelerates heartbeat

Inhibits peristalsis
and secretion

Stimulates glucose
production and release

Secretion of adrenaline
and noradrenaline

Inhibits bladder contraction

T1

T12

Stimulates orgasm

FIGURE 15-6 Sympathetic nervous system.
© Alila Medical Media/Shutterstock.

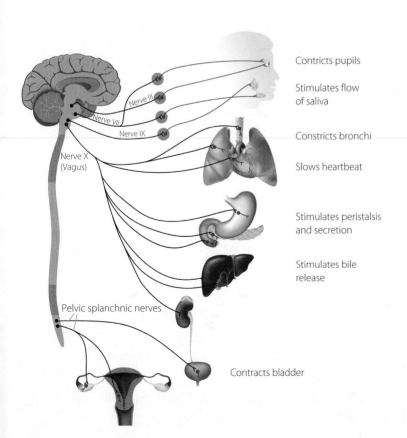

Contricts pupils

Stimulates flow
of saliva

Constricts bronchi

Slows heartbeat

Stimulates peristalsis
and secretion

Stimulates bile
release

Contracts bladder

Nerve III

Nerve VII

Nerve IX

Nerve X
(Vagus)

Pelvic splanchnic nerves

FIGURE 15-7 Parasympathetic nervous system.
© Alila Medical Media/Shutterstock.

LESSON ONE	Materials to Be Learned	

When studying this lesson, refer to Figures 15-1 through 15-7.

PARTS OF THE CENTRAL NERVOUS SYSTEM

The CNS is one of the two main divisions of the NS of the body, consisting of the brain and the spinal cord. The CNS processes information to send to and receive from the PNS and is the main network of coordination and control for the entire body. **Table 15-1** describes terms for parts of the central nervous system.

TABLE 15-1 Parts of the Central Nervous System		
Term	**Pronunciation**	**Definition**
Brain	brān	comprising the forebrain, midbrain, and hindbrain
brain stem	brān stem	the stemlike portion of the brain connecting the cerebral hemispheres with the spinal cord and comprising the pons, medulla oblongata, and midbrain
cerebrum	ser-e-brum	main (largest) portion of the brain, occupying the upper part of the cranial cavity; its two hemispheres, united by the corpus callosum, form the largest part of the CNS in humans
cerebellum	ser´-e-bel-um	situated on the back of the brain stem; consisting of a median lobe (vermis) and two lateral lobes (the hemispheres)
diencephalon	di-en-ceph-a-lon	region of the brain that includes the thalamus, hypothalamus, and the central core of the forebrain
encephalon	en-sef-al-on	the brain
hypothalamus	hyp-o-thal-a-mus	region of the forebrain below the thalamus that coordinates both the autonomic NS and the endocrine system. Regulates body temperature, thirst, hunger, the sleep-wake cycle, and physical expression of emotions (see Figure 15-4)
thalamus	thal-uh-muh-s	part of the brain that processes and relays all sensory and motor signals between the cerebral cortex and the spinal cord, and mediates motor activities, sensation, learning, and memory
Spinal Cord	spi-nal kord	That part of the CNS lodged in the spinal column (see Figure 15-1)
meninges	men-in-jez	the three membranes covering the brain and spinal cord: dura mater, arachnoid, and pia mater
dura mater	du-rah ma-ter	the outermost, toughest of the three meninges (membranes) of the brain and spinal cord (see Figure 15-5)
arachnoid	ah-rak-noid	the delicate membrane interposed between the dura mater and the pia mater (see Figure 15-5)
pia mater	pi-ah ma-ter	the innermost of the three meninges covering the brain and spinal cord (see Figure 15-4)
cerebrospinal fluid	ser´-a-bro-spi-nal floo-id	fluid within the ventricles of the brain, the subarachnoid space in the brain and spinal cord, and the central canal

PARTS OF THE PERIPHERAL NERVOUS SYSTEM

The PNS is composed of nerves and *ganglia*. Ganglia are groups of nerve cells or neurons outside of the CNS. The PNS is divided into two subdivisions: the *somatic* and *autonomic* divisions. The somatic division (SNS) controls voluntary functions and certain reflex actions such as a knee jerk. The autonomic division (ANS) controls the rest of the involuntary functions. The PNS contains both the SNS, which provides voluntary control over skeletal muscle, and the ANS, which controls smooth muscle, cardiac muscle, and gland secretions. The ANS is absolutely essential for survival. **Table 15-2** lists terms that describe parts of the peripheral nervous system.

TABLE 15-2 Parts of the Peripheral Nervous System

Term	Pronunciation	Definition/Function
Cranial Nerves	kra-ne-al nerves	the 12 pairs of nerves emerging from the cranial cavity through various openings in the skull, as follows
abducens	ab-du-sens	muscles of the eye turning the eye outward
accessory	ac-ces-so-ry	neck and back muscles
facial	fa-shal	muscles of the face, ears, and scalp
glossopharyngeal	glos´-o-fah-rin-je-al	pertaining to the tongue, pharynx, and salivary glands
hypoglossal	hi´-po-glos-al	beneath the tongue; associated with chewing, swallowing, and speech
oculomotor	ok´-u-lo-mo-tor	movements of the eye, eyelid, lens and pupils
olfactory	ol-fak-to-re	sense of smell
optic	op-tic	vision
trigeminal	tri-jem-in-al	movements of the upper and lower jaw needed for chewing
trochlear	trock-le-ar	eye movement
vagus	va-gus	muscles needed for speech and swallowing
vestibulocochlear	ves-tib-u-lo-kok-le-er	located in the ear; balance and hearing
Spinal Accessory Nerves		the 31 pairs of nerves without special names that are connected to the spinal cord
Other Components		
parasympathetic	par´-ah-sim´-pah-thet-ik	the part of the ANS bringing body functions back to normal after a stressful situation has ended (see Figure 15-7)
sympathetic	sim´-pah-thet-ik	the part of the ANS assisting the body in emergencies, defense, and survival (see Figure 15-6)

TERMS USED TO DESCRIBE THE NERVOUS SYSTEM

Terms listed in **Table 15-3** are anatomical terms used to describe parts of the NS

TABLE **15-3** Terms Used to Describe the Nervous System

Term	Pronunciation	Definition
cauda equina	kaw-dah e-kwi-na	the collection of spinal roots descending from the lower spinal cord and supplying the rectal area
encephalon	en-sef-ah-lon	the brain
fissure	fish-er	a deep furrow in the brain
foramen magnum	fo-rah-men mag-num	a large opening in the occipital bone through which the spinal cord passes
ganglion	gang-gle-on	a knot; a group of nerve cell bodies located outside the CNS
gyrus (plural: gyri)	ji-rus	convolutions of the cerebrum
hemisphere	hem-i-sfer	either half of the brain; the cerebrum is divided into the left and the right hemispheres that control different functions
limbic system	lim-bik sis-tem	the part of the brain associated with attitudes and emotional behavior
nerve cells (neurons)	nerv selz (new-rons)	conducting cells of the NS consisting of a cell body containing the nucleus and its surrounding cytoplasm, the axon, and dendrites; specialized cells for transmitting impulses
neurilemma (sheath of Schwann)	nu´-ri-lem-ah (Shvan)	the membrane surrounding the peripheral nerves
neurotransmitter	neu-ro-trans-mit-ter	a chemical substance released at the end of a nerve fiber in response to a nerve impulse; neurotransmitters affect sleep, hunger, thinking, memory, movement, and emotions, for example, acetylcholine
plexus	plek-sis	a network of nerves or blood vessels
sulcus (plural: sulci)	sul-kus (sul-ki)	a groove, trench, or furrow on the brain surface (see **Figure 15-2**)
ventricle (brain)	ven-tri-k´-l	interconnected cavities in the brain

CLINICAL DISORDERS OF THE NERVOUS SYSTEM

Table 15-4 lists terms that describe clinical disorders of the nervous system.

TABLE **15-4** Clinical Disorders of the Nervous System

Term	Pronunciation	Definition
amyotrophic lateral sclerosis (ALS)	ah´-mi-o-trof-ic lat-er-al skle-ro-sis	progressive degeneration of the upper and lower motor neurons; usually fatal
anencephaly	an´-en-sef-ah-le	congenital absence of the brain; death occurs in 1–2 days
Bell's palsy	pawl-ze	unilateral facial paralysis of sudden onset caused by lesion of the facial nerve

Term	Pronunciation	Definition
carpal tunnel syndrome	<u>car</u>-pal <u>tun</u>-ell <u>sin</u>-drom	caused by repetitive overuse of the fingers, hands, or wrists, and inflammation of the median nerve in the tunnel. Symptoms are pain, especially at night; treatment involves anti-inflammatory drugs, splints, physical therapy, and ceasing overuse
cerebral palsy (CP)	<u>ser</u>-e-bral <u>pawl</u>-ze	permanent brain damage that occurs during pregnancy, birth, or immediately after birth; those with CP lack muscle control, coordination, and tone as well as posture and balance. It can also impact fine motor skills
cerebrovascular accident (CVA)	ser´-e-bro-<u>vas</u>-ku-lar	a decrease in blood flow supply to the brain and death to that specific portion of the brain; three types of CVA are hemorrhagic stroke, a rupture of cerebral blood vessels; thrombotic stroke, a blood clot in the arteries leading to the brain; and embolic stroke, which occurs when an embolus (fragment of blood clot) lodges in a cerebral vessel and causes occlusion (see Box 15-1)
concussion, also closed head injury (CHI)	kon-<u>kush</u>-un	a violent blow to the head; there may or may not be a loss of consciousness
convulsion (seizure)	kon-<u>vul</u>-shun (se-zhur)	an involuntary contraction or series of contractions of the voluntary muscles; sudden disturbances in mental functions and body movements, some with loss of consciousness
encephalitis	en´-sef-ah-<u>li</u>-tis	inflammation of the brain, usually caused by an infection
epilepsy	<u>ep</u>-i-lep´-se	seizure disorder; cause usually unknown; symptoms managed with medication
fracture (skull)	<u>frak</u>-chur	a break in the bones of the skull; cause can be accidents, falls, gunshot wounds
hematoma	he´-mah-<u>to</u>-mah	blood (clot) outside of blood vessels because of trauma or stroke; if located in the brain, the clot must be dissolved or removed if large enough to cause pressure on the brain
herpes zoster	<u>her</u>-peez <u>zos</u>-ter	"shingles"; an acute inflammatory disease of the spinal nerve (sensory root ganglion) caused by a reactivation of the varicella-zoster virus in someone who has previously had chicken pox. Symptoms are a painful skin rash with blisters
Huntington's chorea	ko-<u>re</u>-ah	chorea is ceaseless rapid, jerky, involuntary movements; Huntington's chorea is a hereditary disease marked by chronic progressive chorea and mental deterioration
hydrocephalus	hi´-dro-<u>sef</u>-ah-lus	"water on the brain"; a congenital or acquired condition marked by dilation of the cerebral ventricles and accumulation of cerebrospinal fluid within the skull; typically, there is enlargement of the head, prominence of the forehead, mental deterioration, and convulsions
meningitis	men´-in-<u>ji</u>-tis	inflammation of the meninges of the brain and spinal cord caused by bacterial, viral, or fungal infection
meningocele (myelomeningocele)	me-<u>ning</u>-go-sel (mi´-e-lo-me-<u>ning</u>-go-sēl)	hernial protrusion of the meninges through a bone defect in the cranium or vertebral column; a severe form of spina bifida

(continues)

TABLE 15-4 (*continued*)

Term	Pronunciation	Definition
migraine (headache)	mī-grān	moderate to severe headache, usually one sided and accompanied by nausea, vomiting, and extreme sensitivity to light and sound
multiple sclerosis (MS)	mul-te-p´-l skle-ro-sis	brain and spinal cord contain areas of degenerated myelin. Symptoms include weakness, incoordination, speech disturbances, and visual complaints
myasthenia gravis (MG)	my-ass-thee-nee-ah grav-iss	a progressive neuromuscular disorder characterized by chronic fatigue and muscle weakness. Onset is gradual, with difficulty speaking and swallowing and weakness of the facial muscles; the weakness may then extend to other muscles enervated by cranial nerves, especially the respiratory muscles
narcolepsy	nar-co-lep-sy	chronic sleep disorder with daytime drowsiness and sudden attacks of sleep which can occur at any time during daytime activities such as talking or working
neuropathy	nu-rop-ah-the	disease or dysfunction of one or more peripheral nerves, typically causing numbness or weakness. Present in various medical conditions
organic brain syndrome (chronic brain syndrome)	or-gan-ik	a general term used to describe decreased mental function due to a medical disease such as Alzheimer's disease or Parkinson's disease; symptoms include changes in memory, behavior, language skills, and ability to carry out activities of daily living
Parkinson's disease (PD)	par-kin-sunz di-sez	a slowly progressive, degenerative, neurologic disorder characterized by resting tremor
petit mal seizures	pet-ee mall seez-yoorz	a minor seizure lasting only a few seconds with momentary clouding of consciousness; the individual may not be aware of the episode. It is more frequent in children
poliomyelitis (polio)	po´-le-o-mi´-e-li-tis	an acute viral disease with fever, sore throat, headache, vomiting, and often stiffness of the neck and back; may be minor or major—causing permanent paralysis; prevented by vaccination since the late 1950s
sciatica	si-at-i-kah	severe pain in the leg along the course of the sciatic nerve; also pain radiating into the buttock and lower limb, most commonly caused by herniation of a lumbar disk
spina bifida	spi-nah bi-fid-a	birth defect of the neural tube (brain and spinal cord) during embryonic development; incomplete closing of the vertebral column and meninges of the spinal column. Results in neurological defects similar to spinal cord injury
spinal cord injuries	spi-nal kord in-ju-rez	a traumatic disruption of the spinal cord that can cause paraplegia and quadriplegia; spinal fractures and dislocations are common in car accidents, falls, and gunshot wounds
subdural hematoma	sub-doo-ral hee-mah-toh-mah	venous bleeding beneath the dura mater, usually a result of a closed head injury. Symptoms include drowsiness, headache, confusion, seizures, and signs of intracranial pressure and paralysis. Treatment involves surgical evacuation of the blood through burr holes in the skull or a craniotomy if the blood has solidified and cannot be aspirated through burr holes

Term	Pronunciation	Definition
Tay-Sach's disease	<u>tay</u>-sacks dih-<u>zeez</u>	an inherited inborn error of metabolism caused by an enzyme deficiency causing altered lipid metabolism that results in accumulation of a specific lipid in the brain, leading to physical and mental retardation. It is a progressive disorder, marked by degeneration of brain tissue, dementia, convulsions, paralysis, blindness, and death
whiplash	<u>hwip</u>-lash	a popular term for an acute cervical sprain; acceleration extension injury of the cervical spine

TERMS USED IN THE DIAGNOSIS AND TREATMENT OF NEUROLOGICAL DISORDERS

Terms in **Table 15-5** are organized into three groups: (1) those documented in the history and physical exam; (2) those used to describe radiological (X-rays) exams; and (3) surgical procedures used either in making a diagnosis or treating symptoms.

TABLE 15-5 Terms Used in the Diagnosis and Treatment of Neurological Disorders

Term	Pronunciation	Definition
History and Physical Exam		
aphasia	a-<u>pha</u>-sia	partial or total loss of the ability to communicate verbally or using written words; caused by a traumatic brain injury, brain tumor, or stroke
ataxia	a-<u>tax</u>-i-a	lack of muscle coordination which may affect voluntary movements such as speaking, swallowing, and walking. Caused by injury or disease of the CNS
Babinski's sign	bah-<u>bin</u>-skez	reflex response; when sole of the foot is stroked, the big toe turns up instead of down (normal in newborn, but pathologic later on)
comatose	<u>com</u>-a-tose	a state of deep unconsciousness for a prolonged period, usually as a result of trauma, stroke, cancer, or infection in the brain
deep tendon reflex (DTR)	<u>ten</u>-don <u>rē</u>-fleks	reflex response (muscle contraction) in response to a sharp tap on a tendon at the insertion of a muscle; used to evaluate the integrity of the spinal cord and peripheral NS
paralysis	pa-<u>ral</u>-y-sis	loss of sensation or voluntary muscle function; usually caused by damage or disorder of the muscles or the nerves supplying the muscles
paresthesia	par´-es-<u>the</u>-ze-ah	an abnormal sensation such as burning or prickling
paresis	<u>par</u>-e-sis	slight or incomplete paralysis
Romberg test	<u>rom</u>-berg	a test of the sense of balance, e.g., the patient may lose balance when standing erect, feet together, and eyes closed
spasticity	<u>spas</u>-tis-ĭ-ty	disorder of the muscles resulting in tight or stiff muscles and the inability to control those muscles; caused by imbalance of signals from the brain and spinal cord to the muscles

(continues)

TABLE **15-5** (continued)

Term	Pronunciation	Definition
stimulus	<u>stim</u>-u-lus	that which can cause a physiological response by an organ or tissue. For example, the ear, and sensory receptors in the skin are sensitive to external stimuli such as sound and touch
tremor	<u>trem</u>-or	unintentional, rhythmic muscle movement with back and forth movements of one or more parts of the body, most commonly of the hands. Caused by disease or trauma to the brain

Radiological Exams

Term	Pronunciation	Definition
angiogram (arteriogram), cerebral	<u>an</u>-je-o-gram (ar-<u>te</u>-re-o-gram´), <u>ser</u>-e-bral	a radiopaque substance is injected into arteries in the neck, then X-ray films are taken; used to evaluate blood vessels in the brain for clots or bleeding
computerized tomography (CT) brain scan; also called CAT scan	kuh-m-<u>pyoo</u>-tuh-rahyz <u>to</u>-mog-ra-phy	three-dimensional view of brain tissue obtained as X-ray beams pass through layers of the brain. A CT scan will show areas of tumors, hemorrhage, blood clots, aneurysms
echoencephalogram	ek´-o-en-<u>sef</u>-ah-lo-gram´	use of ultrasound to show displacement of brain structures
electroencephalogram (EEG)	e-lek´-tro-en-<u>sef</u>-ah-lo-gram´	record of electrical activity of the brain; often used to diagnose epilepsy
magnetic resonance imaging (MRI) of the brain	mag-<u>net</u>-ic <u>res</u>-o-nance <u>im</u>-ag-ing	noninvasive technique using magnetic waves to create an image of the brain; it provides visualization of fluid, soft tissue, and bony structures, and is far more precise and accurate than most diagnostic tools
myelogram (myelography)	<u>mi</u>-e-lo-gram (mi´-e-<u>log</u>-rah-fe)	use of X-ray together with the injection of a special dye to make pictures of the vertebra (bones) and fluid of the spinal column to evaluate for tumors or a herniated disk
pneumoencephalogram (PEG)	nu´-mo-en-<u>sef</u>-ah-lo-gram´	the radiograph obtained by visualization of the fluid-containing structures of the brain after cerebrospinal fluid is intermittently withdrawn by lumbar puncture and replaced by air, oxygen, or helium
positron emission tomography (PET) scan	<u>pos</u>´-i-tron e-<u>mis</u>´-sion <u>to</u>-mog-ra-phy	images of various structures show how the brain uses glucose and gives information about brain function; used to assess for Alzheimer's, stroke, epilepsy, brain tumors and schizophrenia
ventriculography	ven-trik´-u-<u>log</u>-rah-fe	radiography of the cerebral ventricles after introduction of air or other contrast medium

Surgery for Diagnosis or Treatment

Term	Pronunciation	Definition
burr holes	ber	holes made into the skull with a drill creating openings in bone to permit access for biopsy, insertion of drains for relieving pressure, or for monitoring devices
cordotomy	kor-<u>dot</u>-o-me	cutting of nerve fibers of the spinal cord to relieve intractable pain
craniotomy	kra´-ne-<u>ot</u>-o-me	any operation on the cranium, e.g., puncture of the skull and removal of a hematoma to relieve pressure on the brain
laminectomy	lam´-i-<u>nek</u>-to-me	excision of the posterior arch (back side) of a vertebra to view the spinal cord or to relieve pressure

Term	Pronunciation	Definition
lumbar puncture (LP)	lum-bar pungk-chur	spinal tap done to remove spinal fluid for laboratory analysis for white blood cells or a possible source of infection
nerve block	nerv blok	injection of anesthetic into a nerve to produce the loss of sensation to control acute pain
rhizotomy	ri-zot-o-me	cutting the roots of spinal nerves to relieve incurable back pain and muscle spasms
shunt	shunt	to bypass, e.g., using a catheter to drain fluid from brain cavities to the spinal cord
vagotomy	va-got-o-me	surgical transection of the fibers of the vagus nerve; previously used to reduce acid production by the stomach to treat gastric and duodenal ulcers. May be used together with other surgery of the gastrointestinal tract
ventriculography	ven-trik´-u-log-rah-fe	radiography of the cerebral ventricles after introduction of air or other contrast medium

PSYCHIATRIC TERMS

Terms listed in **Table 15-6** are those documented by psychiatrists in a history and physical examination.

TABLE 15-6 Psychiatric Terms

Term	Pronunciation	Definition
aggression	ah-gresh-un	hostile attitude; may be caused by insecurity or inferiority feeling
ambivalence	am-biv-ah-lens	conflicting emotional attitudes toward a goal, e.g., hate and love
amnesia	am-ne-zhe-ah	loss of memory
bipolar disorder	bahy-poh-ler	brain disorder in which the individual experiences extremes in energy, mood, and behavior between mania and depression that interfere with the ability to carry out day-to-day activities; also called manic-depressive illness
brain stimulation therapy	brain stim-u-la-tion ther-a-py	activating different regions of the brain directly with electricity, magnets, or implants to treat neurological and psychiatric disorders. Used to treat symptoms of Parkinson's disease and epilepsy and for depression that does not respond to other treatments
catatonic	cat-a-ton-ic	stupor and motor rigidity and inability to speak or move; observed in schizophrenia
delirium	de-lir-e-um	a mental disturbance of relatively short duration, e.g., illusions, hallucinations, and excitement; may be present in response to medications or a psychiatric disorder
delusion	de-loo-zhun	a false personal belief; often present in schizophrenia and bipolar disorder

(continues)

TABLE 15-6 (continued)

Term	Pronunciation	Definition
hallucination	hah-lu´-si-na-shun	hearing or seeing things not really present
hypochondria	hi´-po-kon-dre-ah	abnormal anxiety about one's health
hysteria	his-te-re-ah	extremely emotional state
major depression	mey-jer dih-presh-uhn	disabling brain disorder that interferes with normal activities of working, eating, sleeping, and enjoying usual activities; most patients require treatment (medications and/or therapy) to overcome symptoms of a depressive episode
malingering	mah-ling-ger-ing	pretending to be ill for personal gain, for example, to be excused from work responsibilities
megalomania	meg´-ah-lo-ma-ne-ah	belief in one's own extreme greatness, goodness, or power
paranoia	par-a-noi-a	mental condition characterized by delusions of persecution, unwarranted jealousy, or exaggerated self-importance that are not consistent with reality
phobia	fo-be-ah	any persistent abnormal dread or fear, for example, of extreme heights, deep water, or open spaces
psychosis	si-ko-sis	a major mental disorder with a loss of contact with reality; characterized by delusions and hallucinations; often part of schizophrenia and bipolar depression
psychotherapy	psy-cho-ther-a-py	"Talk therapy" for treating mental health problems by talking with a psychiatrist, psychologist, or other mental health provider

PSYCHIATRIC CLINICAL DISORDERS

Table 15-7 lists terms used by psychiatrists when making a psychiatric diagnosis.

TABLE 15-7 Psychiatric Clinical Disorders

Term	Pronunciation	Definition
Alzheimer's disease (AD) (presenile dementia)	alts-hi-merz di-sez (pre-se-nīl de-men-she-ah)	progressive mental deterioration in middle or old age, due to generalized degeneration of the brain and the most common cause of premature senility. Early symptoms are forgetfulness, loss of language skills, and changes in behavior; the later stages require complete care
anxiety disorder	anx-i-e-ty dis-or-der	anticipation of a future concern associated with muscle tension and avoidance behavior; can have a negative impact on job performance and personal relationships. Includes generalized anxiety disorder, panic disorder, specific phobias, agoraphobia, social anxiety disorder, and separation anxiety disorder

Term	Pronunciation	Definition
autism spectrum disorder (ASD)	<u>aw</u>-tizm <u>spec</u>-trum dis-<u>or</u>-der	neurodevelopmental disorder characterized by the inability to form social relationships and communicate with others; can cause significant impairment in social, occupational, and other areas of functioning
behavioral disorder	be-<u>hav</u>-ior-al dis-<u>or</u>-der	not being able to focus or control behavior characterized by impulsivity and hyperactivity; also described as Attention Deficit Hyperactivity Disorder (ADHD) in children
mood disorder	mood dis-<u>or</u>-der	mental disorder characterized by a serious change in mood; includes major depressive disorder, bipolar disorder, persistent depressive disorder and seasonal affective disorder (SAD)
psychotic disorder	psy-<u>chot</u>-ic dis-<u>or</u>-der	severe mental disorder with abnormal thinking and perceptions, including delusions and hallucinations; most often present in schizophrenia and in the maniac phase of bipolar disorder
schizophrenia	skit´-so-<u>fre</u>-ne-ah	a chronic, severe, and debilitating brain disorder characterized by visual and auditory hallucinations and delusions as well as disordered thoughts. Most individuals with schizophrenia are not able to hold a job or care for themselves

THE ORIGIN OF MEDICAL TERMS

Table 15-8 describes the origin of medical terms related to the chapter material.

TABLE **15-8** The Origin of Medical Terms		
Word	**Pronunciation**	**Origin and Definition**
laminectomy	lam´-i-<u>nek</u>-to-me	Latin, *lamina* for thin plate + Greek, *-ektomia*, "a cutting out of"
oculomotor	ok´-u-lo-<u>mo</u>-tor	Latin, *ocul* for eye + English, motor + combining vowel, -o-, ocul-o-motor
paranoia	par-a-noi-a	Greek, *para* for irregular; Greek, *noos* for mind; Greek, *paranoos*, distracted
spina bifida	<u>spī</u>-nə ˈ<u>bi</u>-fə-də	Latin, *spina* for spine; Latin, *bifida* for split
schizophrenia	skit´-so-<u>fre</u>-ne-ah	Greek, *skhizein* for split; Greek, *phren* for mind + combining vowel, -o-, schizophrenia
trochlear	<u>trock</u>-le-ar	Latin, block or pulley
vestibulocochlear	ves-tib-u-lo-<u>kok</u>-le-er	Latin, *vestibule* for entrance to another cavity; Greek, *kochlias* for snail with a spiral shell + combining vowel, -o-, vestibule-o-cochlear

ABBREVIATIONS

Abbreviations given in **Table 15-9** are frequently used to describe the NS, including clinical disorders and diagnostic tools.

TABLE **15-9** Abbreviations

Abbreviation	Definition	Abbreviation	Definition
AD	Alzheimer's disease	EEG	Electroencephalogram
ALS	Amyotrophic lateral sclerosis	LP	Lumbar puncture
ANS	Autonomic nervous system	MRI	Magnetic resonance imaging
ASD	Autism spectrum disorder	MG	Myasthenia gravis
CHI	Closed head injury	MS	Multiple sclerosis
CNS	Central nervous system	PEG	Pneumoencephalogram
CP	Cerebral palsy	PET	Positron emission tomography
CT	Computerized tomography	PD	Parkinson's disease
CVA	Cerebral vascular accident	PNS	Peripheral nervous system
DTR	Deep tendon reflex	SNS	Somatic nervous system

BOX 15-1 describes the causes and effects of a stroke.

Box **15-1** Strokes

A blood clot, embolism, or hemorrhage in the brain can cause a stroke. When the primary motor cortex is damaged, there is paralysis of either the left or right side of the body. Damage to the right hemisphere causes paralysis on the left side while damage to the left hemisphere causes paralysis on the right side.

The following box lists three different types of medications that may be prescribed by a physician treating diseases of the neurological system.

PHARMACOLOGY AND MEDICAL TERMINOLOGY

Drug Classification	Anticonvulsant (an-tih-kon-<u>vull</u>-sant)	Antidepressant (an-tih-dee-<u>press</u>-ant)	Hypnotic (hip-<u>notik</u>)
Function	Prevents or relieves convulsions (seizures)	Alleviates mental depression	Induce sleep or semiconsciousness
Word Parts	**anti-** = against; **convulsant** = pertaining to convulsion	**anti-** = against; **depressant** = pertaining to depression	**hypno-** = sleep; **-tic** = pertaining to
Active Ingredients (Examples)	Phenobarbital sodium (Luminal Sodium); diazepam (Valium)	Amitriptyline hydrochloride (Elavil); sertraline (Zoloft)	Flurazepam hydrochloride (Dalmane); zolpidem tartrate (Ambien)

CLINICAL
Note

| Clinic Visit |

CC: Seizures ~ q 2 months

HPI: Sixty-two-year-old white male with long **H/O Sz** and B.P.H. currently on Dilantin 200 mg bid. Prior to arriving @ clinic, the patient was admitted to the hospital for seizures. **EEG** showed "diffuse slow **dysrhythmia** with **paroxysmal** activity which had worsened from previous admission". **CT** and bone scans were unremarkable and patient discharged on Dilantin. The Sz are apparently preceded by a "quiet, withdrawn" aura, the patient has generalized tremulousness, loses consciousness for 4–5 min, with post-ictal depression with **clonic** movements or incontinence.

Physical exam: General—Thin WM has no apparent distress, groomed well

> MS—Alert + **O × 3**
>
> Gait—Slow gait but stable
>
> Toe, Heel and Tandem Gait—Within normal limits
>
> Poor balance on left leg

Assessment: Patient now on 3 meds, all within therapeutic levels and still with seizures q 2 mos. Hesitate to increase meds, infrequency of Sz and do not wish to over sedate patient. Patient seems to be functioning well at home and is not involved in any hazardous activity requiring stricter seizure control which might upset his level of alertness and coordination. Previous workup @ hospital neg. for correctable etiology.

Plan: Maintain patient on present meds with monitoring of compliance and Sz activity by wife.

Direction: For the portions of the clinical note shown by a colored font, provide the definition and/or words for abbreviation.

LESSON TWO | Progress Check

FILL IN

Fill in the blanks to make a complete, accurate sentence:

1. The _____ NS consists of the brain and spinal cord.

2. The _____ NS processes information, coordinates, and controls the body.

3. The _____ NS regulates the activity of cardiac muscle and glands.

4. The interconnected cavities in the brain are called _____.

5. The term used for the network of nerves or blood vessels is _____.

6. A groove or trench on the brain surface is a _____.

7. The _____ system is the part of the brain associated with emotional behavior.

8. _____ refers to a group of nerve cell bodies.

9. Either half of the brain is called a _____.

10. _____ is the medical term for brain.

11. The foramen magnum is _____.

12. The spinal roots that supply the rectal area are called _____.

13. The _____ transmits sensory and motor information back and forth between the CNS and the rest of the body.

14. The outermost membrane of the brain and spinal cord is called _____.

15. _____ is the term for the part of the NS associated with voluntary or conscious movements.

MATCHING: CRANIAL NERVES

Match the nerves on the left to their function on the right:

Nerve
1. Olfactory
2. Optic
3. Trochlear
4. Trigeminal
5. Vestibulochochlear
6. Accessory
7. Hypoglossal

Function
a. Eye movement
b. Movement of the upper and lower jaw
c. Hearing and balance
d. Beneath the tongue
e. Vision
f. Neck and back muscles
g. Sense of smell

MATCHING: INJURY OR DISEASES OF THE NERVOUS SYSTEM

Match the disease state or condition on the left to its definition on the right:

Disease state/condition
1. Bell's palsy
2. Cerebral palsy
3. Concussion
4. Convulsion
5. Hematoma
6. Huntington's chorea
7. Sciatica
8. Parkinson's disease

Definition
a. Unilateral facial paralysis
b. Progressive neurological disorder with tremors
c. Severe leg pain
d. Jerky involuntary movements with mental deterioration
e. Violent blow to the head
f. Paralysis from developmental defects
g. Seizure
h. Blood clot

TRUE OR FALSE: DIAGNOSTIC TOOLS AND TERMS

Check T for statements that are true and F for statements that are false.

T☐ F☐   **1.** Babinski's sign is normal in a newborn but pathologic in an adult.

T☐ F☐   **2.** A craniotomy is the cutting of nerve fibers.

T☐ F☐   **3.** A lumbar puncture is a spinal tap.

T☐ F☐   **4.** An EEG uses ultrasound to diagnose brain dysfunctions.

T☐ F☐   **5.** A myelogram uses dye injections to detect tumors.

T☐ F☐   **6.** A rhizotomy is surgery on the nose.

T☐ F☐   **7.** A delusion is hearing or seeing things that are not present.

T☐ F☐   **8.** Psychosis is a loss of contact with reality in some psychiatric disorders.

T☐ F☐   **9.** The Romberg test determines a person's sense of balance.

T☐ F☐   **10.** An example of a mood disorder is panic disorder.

DEFINITIONS: PSYCHIATRIC TERMS AND CONDITIONS

Define the following terms and abbreviations:

1. AD: _____

2. ASD: _____

3. Delusion: _____

4. Delirium: _____

5. Psychosis: _____

6. Hypochondria: _____

7. Megalomania: _____

8. Paranoia: _____

9. Phobia: _____

10. Schizophrenia: _____

11. Malingering: _____

12. Hallucination: _____

SPELLING AND DEFINITION: THE NERVOUS SYSTEM

Circle the letter of the correctly spelled term and then define the term:

1. **(a)** Cerebrum   **(b)** Cerebrim   **(c)** Cherubim   **(d)** Cerabrem
   Definition: _____

2. **(a)** Meniges   **(b)** Meninjes   **(c)** Meninges   **(d)** Meneongis
   Definition: _____

3. **(a)** Akraknoid   **(b)** Arachnoid   **(c)** Arachnid   **(d)** Arakenid
   Definition: _____

4. **(a)** Trochanter   **(b)** Trocklear   **(c)** Trichlear   **(d)** Trochlear
   Definition: _____

5. **(a)** Olfactory   **(b)** Audifactory   **(c)** Occulofactory   **(d)** Optifactory
   Definition: _____

6. **(a)** Hypogloseal   **(b)** Hypoglossal   **(c)** Hyperglossary   **(d)** Hydroglosal
   Definition: _____

7. **(a)** Anoncephaly   **(b)** Anoncephalon   **(c)** Anencephaly   **(d)** Acephalic
   Definition: _____

8. **(a)** Hydrocephalus   **(b)** Hidrocephalon   **(c)** Hydroceptaly   **(d)** Hidrosephaly
   Definition: _____

9. **(a)** Menogenocele   **(b)** Myeongocele   **(c)** Menelomingocele   **(d)** Meningocele
   Definition: _____

10. **(a)** Poliomyelitis   **(b)** Poliomylitis   **(c)** Poliomilitis   **(d)** Poliomyleitis
   Definition: _____

IDENTIFYING WORD PARTS

For each of the medical terms, list the root word and the prefix and/or suffix.

Word	Root Word	Prefix	Suffix
1. Anencephaly			
2. Aphasia			
3. Ataxia			
4. Comatose			
5. Encephalon			
6. Encephalitis			
7. Hydrocephalus			
8. Megalomania			
9. Meningitis			
10. Meningocele			

CHAPTER 16

Genitourinary and Reproductive Systems

© teekid/iStock/Getty Images

OBJECTIVES

After completing this chapter and the exercises, the student should be able to:

1. Identify the organs and describe the location and functions of the following systems: urinary system, male reproductive system, and female reproductive system.
2. Identify and define clinical disorders affecting the following systems: urinary system, male reproductive system, and female reproductive system.
3. Identify and describe methods used for the diagnosis and treatment of diseases of the following systems: urinary system, male reproductive system, and female reproductive system.
4. Identify three secondary sex characteristics that occur in the male and female bodies at the onset of puberty.
5. Identify six sexually transmitted diseases of the male and female reproductive systems.
6. Identify and describe the stages of pregnancy and childbirth including methods used for evaluation and intervention.

GENITOURINARY AND REPRODUCTIVE SYSTEMS

Urinary System

All living things produce waste, and humans are no exception. Waste cannot accumulate in an organism without causing harm. Waste excretion occurs by several avenues. In humans, excretion of waste occurs in the lungs, skin, liver, intestines, and kidneys. Of all the organs that participate in removing waste, the kidneys are one of the most important because they relieve the body of the greatest variety of dissolved wastes.

If the kidneys fail, there is no way for all the waste products to be eliminated from the body. Death will follow unless a kidney transplant replaces the failing kidney or the impurities are filtered out by dialysis (artificial kidney).

ALLIED HEALTH PROFESSIONS

Radiologic Technologists and Radiation Therapists

Radiologic technologists take X-rays and administer nonradioactive materials into patients' bloodstreams for diagnostic purposes. They also are referred to as radiographers and produce X-ray films (radiographs) of parts of the human body for use in diagnosing medical problems. They prepare patients for radiologic examinations by explaining the procedure, removing jewelry and other articles through which X-rays cannot pass, and positioning patients so that the parts of the body can be appropriately radiographed. To prevent unnecessary exposure to radiation, these workers surround the exposed area with radiation protection devices such as lead shields or they limit the size of the X-ray beam. Radiographers position radiographic equipment at the correct angle and height over the appropriate area of a patient's body. Using instruments similar to a measuring tape, they may measure the thickness of the section to be radiographed and set controls on the X-ray machine to produce radiographs of the appropriate density, detail, and contrast. They place the X-ray film under the part of the patient's body to be examined and make the exposure. They then remove the film and develop it.

Treating cancer in the human body is the principal use of radiation therapy. As part of a medical radiation oncology team, radiation therapists use machines—called linear accelerators—to administer radiation treatment to patients. Linear accelerators, used in a procedure called external beam therapy, project high-energy X-rays at targeted cancer cells. As the X-rays collide with human tissue, they produce highly energized ions that can shrink and eliminate cancerous tumors. Radiation therapy is sometimes used as the sole treatment for cancer, but is usually used in conjunction with chemotherapy or surgery.

INQUIRY

American Society of Radiologic Technologists: www.asrt.org

Data from Cross, Nanna, McWay, Dana. *Stanfield's Introduction to the Health Professions*, 7th ed. Burlington, MA: Jones & Bartlett Learning; 2017.

The urinary system consists of the organs that produce urine and eliminate it from the body. It is a major organ system in the maintenance of homeostasis.

The *urinary system* consists of two *kidneys*, which produce urine; two *ureters*, which carry urine to the urinary bladder for temporary storage; and the *urethra*, which carries urine to the outside of the body through an external *urethral orifice* (**Figure 16-1**). Lesson One defines and illustrates the system along with associated structures.

The kidney has many important functions. Among them are the following:

1. Elimination of organic wastes
2. Regulation of concentration of important ions
3. Regulation of acid–base balance
4. Regulation of red blood cell (RBC) production
5. Regulation of blood pressure
6. Some control of blood glucose and blood amino acids
7. Elimination of toxic substances
8. Acts as an endocrine gland

The kidneys (**Figure 16-2**) are bean-shaped, dark red organs, approximately 5 inches long and 1 inch thick (about the size of a clenched fist). They are located high on the posterior abdominal wall adjacent to the last two pairs of ribs. They are *retroperitoneal*. Each is capped by an *adrenal* gland. Each kidney is surrounded by three layers of connective tissue. The *renal fascia* (outside covering) anchors the kidney to the surrounding structures and maintains its position. The *perirenal* fat is adipose tissue inside the renal fascia to cushion the kidney. The *renal capsule* is the smooth, transparent membrane that directly covers the kidney and can be easily stripped from it. For a detailed explanation of the internal structure of the kidney, the structure of a nephron, and blood supply to the kidney, the student is referred to anatomy and physiology texts.

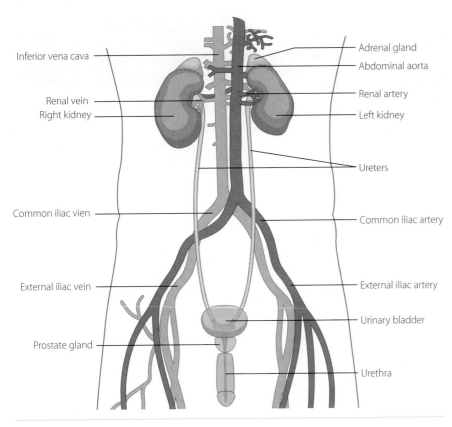

FIGURE 16-1 Urinary system with blood vessels.

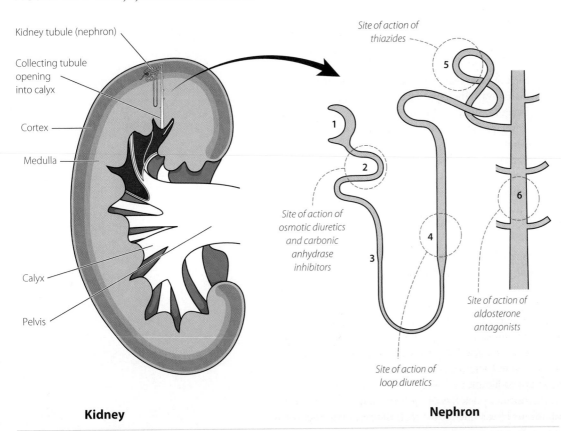

FIGURE 16-2 Cross-section of a kidney and enlarged view of the nephron.

Reproductive System

The *reproductive* systems in males and females are concerned primarily with perpetuation of the species. In that respect, they differ from all other organ systems of the body, which are concerned with *homeostasis* and survival of the human body. Reproduction begins when the germ cells unite in a process called fertilization. In the female, the germ cell is the *ovum* (plural: *ova*); in the male, it is the *spermatozoon* (plural: *spermatozoa*).

The male and female reproductive systems are detailed in **Figures 16-3** and **16-4**. The male and female organs are defined in Lesson One.

Male Reproductive System

The male reproductive system's function is to produce, nourish, and transport sperm from the penis into the female vagina during intercourse (*copulation*) and to produce the male hormone testosterone.

The primary male organs are the *gonads*, which are called *testes* (singular *testis* or *testicle*). They are responsible for the production of *spermatozoa* and *testosterone*. The accessory organs of the reproductive system are a series of ducts called *seminal vessels* and the *prostate gland*. The *scrotum, penis*, and two *spermatic cords* support them.

The spermatozoon is a mature germ cell. It is microscopic in size and looks like a translucent tadpole. It has a flat elliptical head section that contains the hereditary material, the chromosomes, and a long tail with which it propels itself in a rapid, lashing movement. The sex chromosome carried by the sperm determines the sex of the offspring. When mature, the sperm are carried in the semen.

From puberty on, the male reproductive organs produce and release billions of spermatozoa throughout the lifetime of the male. They also secrete testosterone, a male hormone, which is responsible for the secondary bodily changes that take place at puberty such as pubic hair, beard, and deepening of the voice.

Female Reproductive System

Reproduction can only begin when the germ cells from the male (spermatozoa) unite with the germ cells from the female (ova). The reproductive role of the female is to produce eggs (ova) capable of being fertilized and to provide a safe, nutrient-filled environment in which the fetus develops for 9 months if fertilization takes place. The ability to reproduce begins at puberty when mature ova can be released from the ovary and secondary sex characteristics appear, such as breast development, growth of pubic hair, widening of the pelvis ("developing hips," a sight not always welcome to young girls), and menstruation. Body build and stature difference between the male and female become pronounced. The hormones from the ovaries that play important roles in these processes are *estrogen* and *progesterone*. Other sex hormones are secreted by the pituitary gland and adrenal glands.

If fertilization occurs any time between puberty and cessation of the menses (*menopause*), the fertilized egg will grow and develop in the uterus. If fertilization does not occur, the uterine lining will shed through a bloody discharge, which is menstruation. The female has all of the eggs at birth she will produce in her lifetime, so this cycle repeats itself monthly throughout the childbearing years. At the end of her reproduction cycle, menstruation stops and she no longer discharges eggs from the ovaries. This is known as menopause or climacteric. She also has a decrease in hormone production. Medical terminology in relation to menopause is not given in the chapter. A brief explanation of this condition follows:

Menopause is cessation of menstrual cycles. It is considered complete after *amenorrhea* (absence of menstruation) for 1 year. The *climacteric* is the period during which the cycles are irregular before they stop.

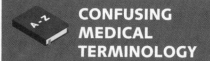

CONFUSING MEDICAL TERMINOLOGY

ureter/o versus **uter/o** versus **urethr/o**

ureter/o – ureter, e.g., ureterotomy (u-reter-<u>ot</u>-to-me) refers to incision of a ureter

uter/o – uterus, e.g., uterus (yoo-ter-<u>uhs</u>) refers to part of the reproductive organ of a woman

urethr/o – urethra, e.g., urethrocystitis (u-re-thro-sis-<u>ti</u>-tis) refers to inflammation of the bladder and urethra

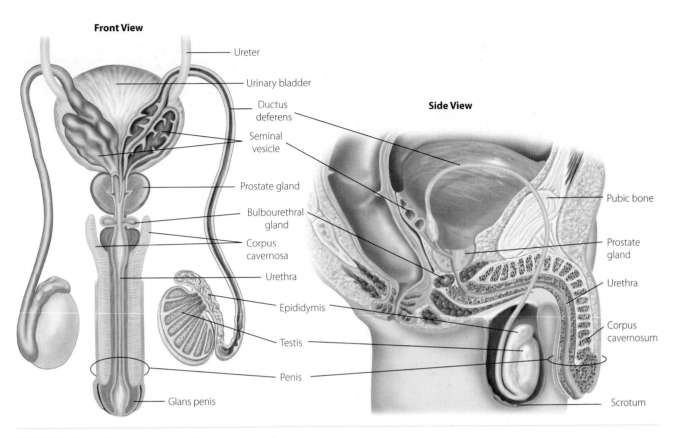

FIGURE 16-3 Midsagittal section of the male reproductive system.

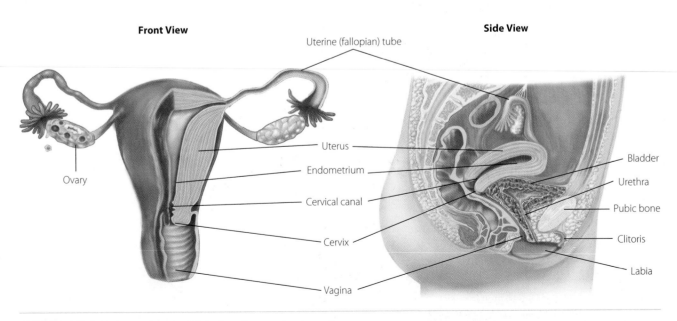

FIGURE 16-4 Midsagittal section of the female reproductive system.

The symptoms of menopause are related to decreased levels of estrogen and progesterone, which affect a number of organ systems and body chemistry:

1. Mammary glands, reproductive organs, and external genitalia decrease in size.
2. Vaginal lining thins and vaginal secretions become alkaline.
3. Vasodilation of blood vessels in the skin results in hot flashes and excessive perspiration in 75–80 percent of women during the climacteric.
4. Some women experience irritability, insomnia, headache, joint pains, and heart palpitations.
5. In approximately 25 percent of women, the accelerated loss of bone mass owing to diminished estrogen leads to osteoporosis. This is more likely to occur in small women with less bone mass. Diets low in calcium, especially during childbearing years, are another risk factor that promotes osteoporosis.

Female anatomy consists of external and internal genitalia. The external genitalia are the *mons pubis, labia majora, clitoris, labia minora, vestibule, urinary meatus, vaginal orifice, Bartholin's glands,* and *peritoneum.* Collectively, they are called the *vulva* or *pudendum.*

The internal genitalia consist of the *vagina, uterus, fallopian tubes,* and *ovaries.* The female also has mammary glands (breasts), and although they are not part of the reproductive process, they are part of the reproductive system because they are responsible for the production of milk (lactation).

Urology is a surgical specialty of diseases of the male and female urinary tract and the male reproductive organs. *Nephrology* is a specialty with a focus on kidney disease, including kidney dialysis. *Gynecologists* are physicians who specialize in the care of the female reproductive system, while *obstetricians* specialize in the care of women during pregnancy and childbirth. Most physicians combine obstetrics and gynecology in their practice. Nurse *Midwives* also provide women's care, including care during childbirth.

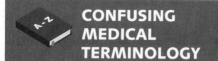

CONFUSING MEDICAL TERMINOLOGY

-uria versus urea

-uria – urinary condition, urination, urine, e.g., polyuria (poly-<u>ee</u>-yoo-r-ee-uh) refers to the passing of an excessive quantity of urine, as in diabetes; also a suffix

urea – chemical waste product, e.g., urea in urine; a medical noun

---

LESSON ONE | **Materials to Be Learned**

URINARY SYSTEM: ORGANS AND STRUCTURES

Table 16-1 describes the organs and structures of the urinary system.

TABLE **16-1** Urinary System: Organs and Structures

Organ or Structure	Pronunciation	Definition
Bowman's capsule (renal capsule)	<u>boh</u>-muhnz <u>cap</u>-suhl	cup-shaped end of renal tubule containing the glomerulus
calyx	<u>ka</u>-liks	cup-shaped part of the renal pelvis through which urine passes from the renal tubules
cortex	<u>kawr</u>-teks	the outer layer of the kidney
glomerulus	gloh-<u>mer</u>-yah-luhs	collection of coiled intertwined capillaries located in the kidney cortex
kidneys	<u>kid</u>-nez	two organs on the posterior abdominal wall that filter the blood, excreting the end products of body metabolism in the form of urine

Organ or Structure	Pronunciation	Definition
meatus	mee-<u>ay</u>-tus	an opening or tunnel through any part of the body, as in the urinary meatus, which is the external opening of the urethra
medulla	me-<u>dul</u>-ah	the inner layer of the kidney
nephron	<u>nef</u>-ron	unit of the kidney which filters blood and excretes urine; consisting of the glomerulus and tubules
renal artery	<u>ree</u>-nal <u>ar</u>-teh-ree	one of a pair of large arteries branching from the abdominal aorta to supply blood to the kidneys, adrenal glands, and the ureters
renal pelvis	<u>ree</u>-nal <u>pel</u>-vis	the funnel-shaped expansion of the upper end of the ureter
renal tubule	<u>ree</u>-nal <u>toob</u>-yool	long, twisted tube leading from glomerulus to collecting tubules
renal vein	<u>ree</u>-nal vain	one of two large veins that carries blood from the kidneys to the inferior vena cava
ureter	u-<u>re</u>-ter	the tubular structure through which urine passes from the kidney to the bladder
urethra	yoo-<u>ree</u>-thruh	the passage through which urine is discharged from the bladder to the body exterior
urinary bladder	<u>yoor</u>-uh-ner-ee <u>blad</u>-er	musculomembranous sac that stores urine, receiving it through the ureters and discharging it through the urethra
urinary meatus	<u>yoor</u>-uh-ner-ee me-<u>a</u>-tus	opening of the urethra to the exterior

TERMS USED IN THE DIAGNOSIS AND TREATMENT OF UROLOGICAL DISORDERS

Terms in **Table 16-2** are organized into three groups: (1) those documented in the history and physical exam; (2) those used to describe radiological (X-ray) exams; and (3) procedures used to make a diagnosis or for treatment.

TABLE **16-2** Terms Used in the Diagnosis and Treatment of Urological Disorders		
Term	**Pronunciation**	**Definition**
History and Physical Exam		
albuminuria	al-bu´-mi-<u>nu</u>-re-ah	abnormal presence of albumin (protein) in the urine
anuria	ah-<u>nu</u>-re-ah	no urine produced
azoturia	az´-o-tu-<u>re</u>-ah	excess urea (or other nitrogen compounds) in urine
bacteriuria	back-tee-ree-<u>yoo</u>-ree-ah	bacteria in the urine
bladder distention	<u>blad</u>-der dis-<u>ten</u>-shun	full urinary bladder

(continues)

TABLE **16-2** (continued)

Term	Pronunciation	Definition
blood chemistries	blud <u>kem</u>-is-treez	blood tests for kidney function, especially blood urea nitrogen (BUN) and creatinine
blood urea nitrogen (BUN)	blud u-<u>re</u>-ah <u>ni</u>-tro-jin	the urea (in terms of nitrogen) concentration in serum or plasma; an important indicator of renal function
calculus (renal; plural: calculi)	<u>kal</u>-ku-lus (<u>re</u>-nal)	kidney stone(s)
continent	<u>kon</u>-ti-nent	able to control urination (and/or defecation)
chronic kidney disease (CKD)	<u>kron</u>-ik <u>kid</u>-nee dih-<u>zeez</u>	also kidney failure; kidney fails to function normally to remove toxic body waste from the blood, especially nitrogen (urea), water, sodium, and potassium
cystitis	sis-<u>ti</u>-tis	inflammation of the urinary bladder
diuresis	di´-u-<u>re</u>-sis	increased excretion of urine
dysuria	dis-<u>u</u>-re-ah	painful or difficult urination
enuresis	en´-u-<u>re</u>-sis	uncontrolled urination while sleeping (bedwetting); more common in children
"floating kidney"	<u>flot</u>-ing <u>kid</u>-ne	a kidney not securely fixed in the usual location because of birth defect or injury
frequency (urgency)	<u>fre</u>-kwen-se (<u>ur</u>-jen-se)	desire to urinate at short intervals, but discharging small amounts because of reduced bladder capacity
glomerulonephritis	glo-mer´-u-lo-ne-<u>fri</u>-tis	nephritis with inflammation of the capillary loops in the renal glomeruli
glycosuria	glye-kohs-<u>yoo</u>-ree-ah	high level of glucose in the urine; symptom of uncontrolled diabetes
hematuria	hem´-ah-<u>tu</u>-re-ah	the presence of blood in the urine
hydronephrosis	hi-dro-ne-<u>fro</u>-sis	backup of urine into the renal pelvis because of an obstruction in the ureter; can cause kidney infection and kidney failure
incontinent	in-<u>kon</u>-ti-nent	inability to control urination (and/or defecation)
ketonuria	kee-toh-<u>noo</u>-ree-ah	excessive amounts of ketone bodies in the urine; found in uncontrolled diabetes
KUB		abbreviation for kidney, ureter, and bladder; term used in charting history and physical exam
micturate	mik-<u>tu</u>-rāt	urinate
nephrolithiasis	nef´-ro-li-<u>thi</u>-ah-sis	a condition marked by the presence of renal calculi (stones)
nephroptosis	nef´-rop-<u>to</u>-sis	downward displacement of a kidney
nocturia, nycturia	nok-<u>tu</u>-re-ah, nik-<u>tu</u>-re-ah	excessive urination at night
oliguria	ol´-i-<u>gu</u>-re-ah	excreting a small amount of urine
peritonitis	pair-ih-ton-<u>eye</u>-tis	inflammation of the peritoneum (the membrane lining the abdominal cavity)

Term	Pronunciation	Definition
polydipsia	pol-ee-<u>dip</u>-see-ah	excessive thirst; caused by high blood and urine levels of glucose and uncontrolled diabetes
pyelitis	pi´-e-<u>li</u>-tis	inflammation of the renal pelvis
pyuria	pi-<u>u</u>-re-ah	bacteria in the urine; sign of urinary tract infection
uremia	u-<u>re</u>-me-ah	the retention of toxic body waste in blood; result of renal failure
urethritis	u´-re-<u>thri</u>-tis	inflammation of the urethra
urinary tract infection (UTI)	<u>yoor</u>-uh-ner-ee trakt in-<u>fek</u>-shun	an infection of any or all parts of the urinary tract, including the bladder, kidneys, ureters, or urethra
void	void	to empty the bladder, to urinate

Radiological Exams

intravenous pyelogram (IVP)	in´-trah-<u>ve</u>-nus <u>pi</u>-e-lo-gram	examination of the structures and function of the urinary system
retrograde pyelogram	<u>re</u>-tro-grād <u>pi</u>-e-lo-gram´	examination of the structures of the collecting system of the kidneys; used to locate an obstruction in the urinary tract
scan (renal)	skan (<u>re</u>-nal)	an image produced after the patient is injected with a radioactive substance; determines kidney shape and function
ultrasonography	ul´-trah-so-<u>nog</u>-rah-fe	imaging body structures by recording the echoes of high frequency sound waves reflected by body tissues on paper or an electronic record

Treatment

catheterization	kath´-e-ter-i-<u>za</u>-shun	passage of a catheter (tube) into the bladder to relieve bladder distention; used if there is an obstruction in the urinary tract
cystoscopy	sis-<u>tos</u>-ko-pe	visual examination of the urinary tract with a cystoscope
dialysate	dye-al-ih-<u>sayt</u>	a solution of water and electrolytes that passes through the artificial kidney to remove excess fluids and wastes from the blood, also called "bath." Used in kidney dialysis to treat kidney failure
dialysis	di-<u>al</u>-i-sis	the process of using an artificial kidney to filter waste materials, water, nitrogen, and electrolytes from the body for those with kidney failure
intake and output (I & O)		the amount of fluids ingested and excreted in a given period of time, measured, and charted; used to monitor kidney function
nephrorrhaphy	nef-<u>ror</u>-ah-fe	suture of the kidney
renal transplant	<u>re</u>-nal trans-<u>plant</u>	surgically transferring a healthy kidney from a donor to another person to replace a diseased kidney
ureterostomy	u-re´-ter-<u>os</u>-to-me	creation of a new outlet for a ureter through the abdominal wall to the outside when there is an obstruction of the urinary tract or if the bladder has been removed because of disease or injury

(continues)

TABLE **16-2** (*continued*)

Term	Pronunciation	Definition
urinalysis (UA)	u´-ri-<u>nal</u>-i-sis	analysis of urine for nitrogen (urea) and creatinine to evaluate kidney function and for bacteria to evaluate for urinary tract infection
testape	tes-<u>tap</u>	special paper strips inserted in a glucose meter to measure blood glucose levels to manage diabetes

REPRODUCTIVE SYSTEM

Male Reproductive Organs
Table 16-3 describes the male reproductive organs.

TABLE **16-3** Male Reproductive Organs

Organ	Pronunciation	Definition
accessory glands	ak-<u>ses</u>-o-re glandz	the pair of seminal vesicles, bulbourethral glands, and a single prostate gland
bulbourethral glands	buhl-boh-yoo-<u>ree</u>-thruhl glandz	pea-sized glands at the root of the penis that secrete lubricating fluid during intercourse; also called Cowper's glands
ductus deferns (plural)/vas deferens	<u>duc</u>-tus <u>def</u>-er-enz/vas <u>def</u>-er-enz	narrow tubular structures for excretion of semen and spermatozoa from the epididymis to the ejaculatory duct in the prostate gland
ejaculatory duct vesicle	e-<u>jak</u>-u-<u>la</u>-tor´-e duk <u>ves</u>-i-cul	the duct formed by union of the ductus deferens and the duct of the seminal vesicle
epididymis	ep´-i-<u>did</u>-i-mis	a duct bordering the testes for storage, transit, and maturation of spermatozoa
external genitalia	eks-<u>ter</u>-nal jen´-i-<u>ta</u>-le-ah	scrotum and penis
glans penis	glanz <u>pee</u>-nis	tip of the penis (**Figure 16-5**)
gonad	<u>goh</u>-nad	male sex glands called the testes (plural) or testicle (singular)
penis	<u>pee</u>-nis	the organ of copulation; surrounds the urethra
perineum	per-uh-<u>nee</u>-uhm	area between the scrotum and anus
prepuce	<u>pree</u>-pyoos	fold of skin covering the glans penis at birth; foreskin
prostate gland	pross-<u>tayt</u> gland	gland surrounding the neck of the bladder and urethra; contributes secretions that enhance sperm motility and neutralizes acidic vaginal secretions
scrotum	<u>scrow</u>-tum	two-compartment sac outside the body that houses the testes
seminal duct	<u>sem</u>-in-al duk	the passages for transferring spermatozoa and semen
seminal vesicles	<u>sem</u>-in-al <u>vess</u>-ih-kls	glands that secrete a thick, yellowish fluid, known as seminal fluid, into the ductus deferens
testis (plural: testes)	<u>tes</u>-tis (<u>tes</u>-tez)	one of the pair of male gonads that produce semen and the male hormone testosterone
urethra	yoo-<u>ree</u>-thruh	opening for sperm and urine passage to the outside of the body

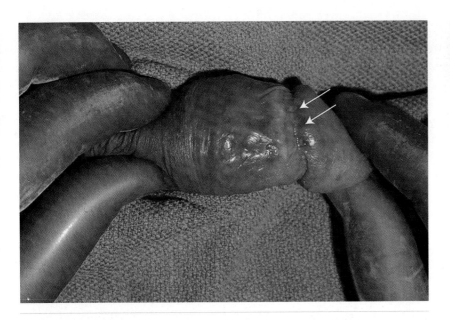

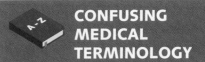

CONFUSING MEDICAL TERMINOLOGY

vesic/o versus vesicul/o

vesic/o – urinary bladder, e.g., vesicotomy (ves-ih-<u>kot</u>-o-me) refers to incision of the bladder

vesicul/o – seminal vesicle, blister, little bladder, e.g., vesiculectomy (veh-sik-u-<u>lek</u>-to-me) refers to excision or surgical removal of a vesicle (in this case, the seminal vesicle)

FIGURE 16-5 Superficial ulcers on the shaft of the penis as a result of genital herpes.

Courtesy of Leonard V. Crowley, MD, Century College.

Female Reproductive Organs

Table 16-4 describes the organs of the female reproductive system.

TABLE **16-4** Female Reproductive Organs

Organ	Pronunciation	Definition
Bartholin's glands	<u>bar</u>-teh-linz glandz	small mucus-secreting glands located near the vagina
clitoris	klit´-<u>or</u>-is	erectile tissue at junction of labia majora and labia minora; equivalent to male penis
cervix	<u>ser</u>-viks	neck-like section at lower end of uterus
Internal Genitalia		
hymen	<u>high</u>-men´	thin elastic connective tissue covering the vaginal opening
fallopian tubes (oviducts)	fah-<u>loh</u>-pee-an toobs (<u>oh</u>-vih-duks)	ducts in which fertilization occurs and passageway for ova to the uterus
ovary	oh-<u>vay</u>-ree	the female gonad: either of the paired female sex glands in which ova are formed and released, and which produce the female hormones
uterus	<u>yoo</u>-ter-us	cavity opening into the vagina below and into a fallopian tube on either side; organ for nourishing the fetus
vagina	vaj-<u>in</u>-nah	birth canal and receptacle for copulation

(continues)

TABLE 16-4 (continued)

Organ	Pronunciation	Definition
External Genitalia		
adnexa	ad-nek-sah	structures next to the uterus, including the fallopian tubes, ovaries, and ligaments of the uterus
areola	ah-ree-oh-lah	the darker pigmented, circular area surrounding the nipple of each breast; also known as the "areola mammae" or the "areola papillaris"
labia majora	lay-bee-ah mah-jor-ah	two outer folds of skin on either side of the vaginal orifice
labia minora	lay-bee-ah mih-nor-ah	two thin folds of skin within the folds of the labia majora
mammary glands	mam-oh-ree glandz	female breasts; considered accessory glands, they are necessary for breastfeeding the infant (lactation)
mons pubis	monz pew-biss	mound of fatty tissue over the pubis
perineum	par-ih-nee-um	area between vaginal orifice and anus
vulva	vull-vah	term which refers to the external genitalia, including the mons pubis, labia majora, clitoris, labia minora, vestibule, urinary meatus, vaginal orifice, Bartholin's gl ands, and the perineum

CLINICAL CONDITIONS OF THE REPRODUCTIVE SYSTEMS

Clinical Conditions of the Male Reproductive System

Terms in **Table 16-5** are organized into three groups: (1) those documented in the history and physical exam; (2) those used to describe radiological (X-ray) exams; and (3) terms used to describe surgery.

TABLE 16-5 Clinical Conditions of the Male Reproductive System

Clinical Condition	Pronunciation	Definition
History and Physical Exam		
benign prostatic hypertrophy (BPH)	bi-nīn pros-tat-ic hi-per-tro-fe	enlargement of the prostate gland, common among men by the age of 50 years
cryptorchidism	krip´-tor-ki-dizm	undescended testicle(s)
epididymitis	ep´-i-did´-i-mi-tis	inflammation of the epididymis; commonly caused by STIs
hydrocele	hi-dro-sel´	fluid collected around the testes; can cause swelling of the scrotum
orchitis	or-ki-tis	inflammation of a testis; can be caused by bacterial infection, especially STIs
varicocele	var-i-ko-sel´	enlargement of veins in the bag of skin that hold the testes; also varicose veins
Surgical Treatment		
balanoplasty	bal-ah-noh-plas-tee	surgical repair of the glans penis
circumcision	ser´-kum-sizh-un	removal of foreskin or prepuce of the penis; usually done in newborn male infants

Clinical Condition	Pronunciation	Definition
orchiectomy	or´-ke-<u>ek</u>-to´-me	surgical removal of one or both testes; most often done to treat cancer of the prostate; since the testes produce sperm, surgical removal of both testes will result in infertility
orchiopexy	<u>or</u>-ke-o-pek´-se	surgery to release an undescended testis in the scrotum
prostatectomy	pros´-tah-<u>tek</u>-to´-me	surgical removal of all or part of the prostate; used to treat prostate cancer or benign prostatic hyperplasia
vasectomy	vah-<u>sek</u>-to-me	male sterilization by cutting or tying the ductus deferens; used as a method of birth control

Clinical Conditions of the Female Reproductive System

Terms in **Table 16-6** are organized into three groups: (1) terms documented in the history and physical exam; (2) those used to describe radiological (X-ray) exams; and (3) terms used to describe surgery.

TABLE 16-6 Clinical Conditions of the Female Reproductive System

Clinical Condition	Pronunciation	Definition
History and Physical Exam		
Bartholin's cyst or abscess	<u>bar</u>-tel-inz sist or <u>ab</u>-ses	chronic or acute inflammation of Bartholin's gland
colposcopy	kol-<u>pos</u>-ko-pe	examination of the cervix by means of a colposcope
cystocele	<u>sis</u>-to-sel	hernia of the bladder into the vagina
endometriosis	en´-do-me´-tre-<u>o</u>-sis	an abnormal condition in which cells of the inner lining of the uterus spread into the peritoneal cavity and attach to the ovaries and fallopian tubes; can cause abdominal pain and infertility
fibroids	<u>fi</u>-broidz	benign tumor (leiomyoma) of the uterus
fistula	<u>fis</u>-tu-lah	an abnormal passage between two internal organs, vesicovaginal (between the bladder and vagina) fistula; results in leaking of urine into the vagina
hydrosalpinx	hi´-dro-<u>sal</u>-pinks	fluid collecting in the uterine tube, causing distention
laparoscopy	lap´-ah-<u>ro</u>-sko´-pe	laparoscopic visualization of the peritoneal cavity
miscarriage	mis´-<u>kar</u>-ij	spontaneous abortion, usually occurs before 14 weeks of pregnancy
monilia (moniliasis)	mo´-<u>nil</u>-e-ah (mon´-i-<u>li</u>-ah-sis)	yeast-like fungal infection of the vagina; may also be described as *Candida vaginitis*
pelvic examination	<u>pel</u>-vic eg´-zam´i-<u>na</u>-tion	a diagnostic procedure in which the external and internal genitalia are physically examined using inspection and palpation
pelvic inflammatory disease (PID)	<u>pel</u>-vic in-<u>flam</u>-a-to-ry di-<u>sez</u>	any inflammatory condition of the female pelvic organs, especially one caused by bacterial infection; complication of STIs

(continues)

TABLE 16-6 (continued)

Clinical Condition	Pronunciation	Definition
prolapse of uterus	<u>pro</u>-laps of <u>u</u>-ter-us	downward displacement of the uterus into the vagina; complication of childbirth or aging
salpingitis	sal´-pin-<u>ji</u>-tis	inflammation of one or both fallopian tubes
vaginal speculum	<u>vaj</u>-i-nal <u>spek</u>-u-lum	an instrument used to dilate the vagina during a pelvic examination
Radiological Exams		
hysterosalpingogram	his´-ter-o-sal-<u>ping</u>-go-gram	an X-ray film of the uterus and the fallopian tubes to allow visualization of the cavity of the uterus and the passageway of the tubes
Surgical Treatment		
abortion (AB)	ah´-<u>bor</u>-shun	intentional expulsion from the uterus of the products of conception before the fetus is viable or able to live outside the mother's body
colporrhaphy	kol-<u>por</u>-ah-fe	suture of the vagina; to correct cystocele and rectocele
dilatation and curettage (D&C)	dil´-ah-<u>ta</u>-shun ku´-re-<u>tahzh</u>	dilating the uterine cervix and using a curette to scrape the endometrium of the uterus; to diagnose disease, to correct vaginal bleeding, or to produce abortion
hysterectomy	his´-te-<u>rek</u>-to-me	surgical removal of the uterus; often done to treat excessive bleeding secondary to uterine fibroids
tubal ligation	<u>tu</u>-bal li-<u>ga</u>-shun	sterilization by "tying" both fallopian tubes; used for birth control

SEXUALLY TRANSMITTED INFECTIONS

Sexually transmitted infections (STIs) occur in both men and women and are the most communicable diseases in the world, especially in young people between the ages of 15 and 24 years of age. Specific viruses, bacteria, and protozoan parasites cause STIs and the diseases are spread through sexual contact with body fluids such as blood, semen, and vaginal secretions. STIs may be contracted during vaginal, oral, or anal intercourse or by direct contact with infected skin. The human immunodeficiency virus (HIV) can also be transmitted through sharing of needles by drug users, from the placenta of the infected mother to the baby during birth, and through breast milk of an infected mother when nursing the baby.

There may be no symptoms in the early stages of STIs; unfortunately, untreated STIs can have serious complications. For example, gonorrhea and chlamydia in women can cause pelvic inflammatory disease (PID), ectopic pregnancy, and infertility. Also, in some types of human papillomavirus (HPV) complications are genital warts and cervical cancer. Either bacterial vaginosis (BV) or trichomoniasis during pregnancy can result in infants of low birth weight. Untreated HIV can develop into the more serious acquired immune deficiency syndrome (AIDS).

Antiviral medications can prevent the progression of HIV to full-blown AIDS and STIs caused by bacteria can be treated effectively with antibiotics when diagnosed. However, since STIs are often asymptomatic in the early stages, these diseases often go untreated and the incidence of STIs in the United States continues to be extremely high. **Table 16-7** describes common causes of sexually transmitted infections.

TABLE **16-7** Sexually Transmitted Infections

Term	Pronunciation	Definition
acquired immunodeficiency syndrome (AIDS)	ac-quir-ed im-mu-no-de-fi-cien-cy syn-drome	a fatal disease caused by the human immunodeficiency virus (HIV), which destroys the body's immune system; AIDS can be prevented by antiviral medications for those diagnosed with HIV
bacterial vaginosis(BV)	bac-te-ri-al vag-i-no-sis	caused by changes in the balance between "good" and "bad" bacteria in the vagina; transmitted between female partners but not heterosexual partners. Complications are low birth weight infants
Chlamydia trachomatis	klah´-mid-ee-ah tra-cho-ma-tis	bacterial infection that invades the urethra of men and the vagina and cervix of women; asymptomatic in the early stages, which makes possible the spread of chlamydia as the partners are unaware they have it
genital herpes	jen-ih´-tal her-peez	caused by type 2 herpes simplex virus (HSV-2), although it may be caused by HSV-1, the virus associated with oral infections (cold sores). Remissions and relapses occur and no drug is known to be effective as a cure (**Figure 16-6** shows herpes of the female exterior genitalia)
Neisseria gonorrhea	nahy-seer-ee-uh gon-oh´-ree-ah	bacterial infection causing inflammation of the mucous membranes of the genital tract; spread by intercourse with an infected partner or is passed from an infected mother to her infant during birth
human papillomavirus (HPV)	hyoo-mun pa-pih-loh-muh-vy-rus	some forms of the virus can cause genital warts or cervical cancer; the disease can be prevented by the HPV vaccine
syphilis	sif-ih´-lis	caused by spirochete bacteria; the first sign of the disease is a chancre (hard ulcer) on the external genitalia a few weeks after exposure; usually on the penis of the male and on the labia of the female. The disease goes through a latent period with no symptoms, but later stages of the disease cause damage to all organs
Trichomoniasis vaginalis ("trich")	trich-o-mo-ni-a-sis vaj-e-´na-les	infection caused by a protozoan parasite; common symptoms are itching and burning of external genitals and a vaginal discharge with a "fishy" odor; complications include premature birth

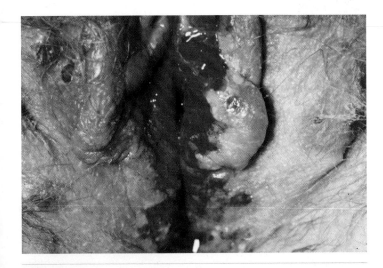

FIGURE 16-6 Multiple ulcers of the vulva (female external genitalia) as a result of herpes.

TERMS USED TO DESCRIBE PREGNANCY AND BIRTH

In this section, **Figure 16-7** illustrates the position of the fetus in the abdominal cavity during pregnancy and **Table 16-8** defines terms used to describe pregnancy and birth.

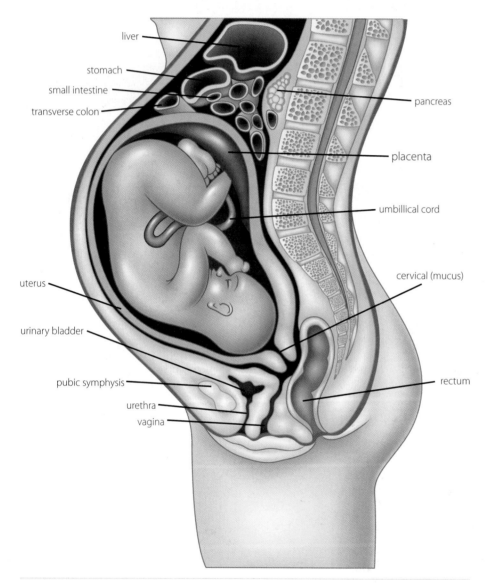

liver
stomach
small intestine
transverse colon

pancreas

placenta

umbillical cord

cervical (mucus)

uterus

urinary bladder

pubic symphysis
urethra
vagina

rectum

FIGURE 16-7 Anatomy of a normal pregnant female.

TABLE **16-8** Terms Used to Describe Pregnancy and Birth

Term	Pronunciation	Definition
Terms Used to Describe Time Periods of Pregnancy		
antepartum	an-te-<u>par</u>-tum	period from conception to onset of labor
conception	con-<u>cep</u>-tion	fertilization of an ovum by a sperm in the fallopian tube followed by implantation in the uterus
gestation	jes-<u>ta</u>-shun	period from conception to birth
intrapartum	in-tra-<u>par</u>-tum	period from onset of labor through first hour after delivery
parturition	par-tu-<u>ri</u>-tion	process of giving birth
postpartum	post-<u>par</u>-tum	six-week period following childbirth
prenatal	pre-<u>na</u>-tal	before birth
trimester	tri-<u>mes</u>-ter	division of pregnancy into periods of 12–14 weeks, the first trimester is weeks 1–12
Terms Used to Describe the Anatomical Components of Pregnancy		
amnion (BOW)	<u>am</u>-ne-on	amniotic sac; bag of waters
amniotic fluid	am-nee-<u>ot</u>-ik fluid	surrounds the unborn baby (fetus) during pregnancy; the fluid is contained in the amniotic sac
fetus	<u>fe</u>-tus	an unborn human baby more than 8 weeks after conception (see Figure 16-7)
placenta	plah-<u>sen</u>-tah	organ for exchange of nutrients and wastes between mother and fetus; called the afterbirth (see Figure 16-7)
umbilical cord	um-<u>bil</u>-i-cal cord	connects the embryo or fetus with the placenta of the mother (see Figure 16-7)
Terms Used in History and Physical Exam to Describe Previous and Current Pregnancies		
artificial insemination	ar-ti-<u>fi</u>-cial in-sem-i-<u>na</u>-tion	depositing of seminal fluid containing sperm within the vagina or cervix other than by sexual intercourse
ectopic pregnancy (extrauterine)	ek-<u>top</u>-ik (eks´-trah-<u>u</u>-ter-in)	pregnancy outside the uterus, usually in the fallopian tube
EDC		expected date of confinement (due date)
fetal heart tones (FHT, fht)	<u>fe</u>-tal hart tonz	the fetal heart sounds heard through the mother's abdomen in pregnancy
Goodell's sign	<u>goo</u>-dels	the softening of the uterine cervix, a probable sign of pregnancy
gravida	<u>grav</u>-i-dah	a pregnant woman; gravid means "pregnant"
in vitro fertilization (IVF)	n <u>vit</u>-ro fer-til-i-<u>za</u>-tion	the fertilization of an ovum outside the uterus

(continues)

TABLE **16-8** (continued)

Term	Pronunciation	Definition
linea nigra	lin-ee-ah nig-rah	a darkened vertical midline appearing on the abdomen of a pregnant woman, connecting the distance between the umbilicus and the symphysis pubis
LMP		last menstrual period; used to calculate due date
multigravida	mul-ti-grav-i-dah	a woman who has had more than one pregnancy
multipara	mul-tip-ah-rah	a woman who has borne more than one viable infant
Nagele's rule	nay-geh-leez	formula for calculating when the baby is due or the date of birth: subtract 3 months from the first day of the last normal menstrual period and add 7 days to that date to arrive at the estimated due date
obstetrical index (OB index)	ob-stet-ri-cal in-deks	the number of pregnancies, term deliveries, abortions, and stillbirths a woman has experienced
pelvimeter (pelvimetry)	pel-vim-e-ter (pel-vim-e-tre)	an instrument used to measure the capacity and diameter of the pelvis for delivery
primipara	pri-mip-ah-rah	a woman bearing her first viable child
quickening	kwik-en-ing	the first movement of the fetus felt by the woman, usually between 18 and 20 weeks' gestation
toxemia	tok-se-me-ah	also known as pre-eclampsia; characterized by a sharp rise in blood pressure, loss of large amounts of the protein albumin, and edema or swelling of the hands, feet, and face. Delivery of the infant usually resolves the condition in the mother

Terms Used to Describe Diagnostic Tools of Pregnancy

amniocentesis	am´-ne-o-sen-te-sis	taking a sample of amniotic fluid during pregnancy by inserting a hollow needle through the abdominal wall; for diagnosis of genetic defects or possible obstetric complications
culdocentesis	kull-doh-sen-tee-sis	use of a needle to aspirate fluid for examination or diagnosis; the needle is passed through the vagina into the cul-de-sac area (area immediately behind the vagina)
ultrasonography	ull-trah-son-og-rah-fee	noninvasive method of using reflected sound waves to detect the presence of the embryo or fetus

Terms Used to Describe Childbirth

bloody show	blud-e sho	appearance of blood forerunning labor
breech birth	breech birth	when a baby is born with buttocks or feet first instead of head first; often requires delivery by C-section
caesarean (C-section)	si-zar-i-en	a surgical procedure in which the abdomen and uterus are incised and a baby is delivered

Term	Pronunciation	Definition
cephalopelvic disproportion (CPD)	sef´-ah-lo-<u>pel</u>-vik dis-pruh-<u>pawr</u>-shuhn	a condition in which the fetal head is too large for the mother's pelvis
dystocia	dis-<u>to</u>-se-ah	abnormal labor or childbirth
effacement	eh-<u>face</u>-ment	the thinning of the cervix to enlarge the diameter of its opening during childbirth in the normal processes of labor
epidural anesthesia	epi-<u>du</u>-ral an´-es-<u>the</u>-ze-ah	regional anesthesia used to block pain in the lower region of the body during a vaginal birth delivery or C-section; pain medications are injected into the lower spine to block nerve impulses and prevent pain
episiotomy	e-piz´-e-<u>ot</u>-o-me	surgical incision into the perineum and/or vagina to aid a difficult delivery and prevent rupture of tissues
forceps delivery	<u>for</u>-seps de-<u>liv</u>-er-e	delivery in which forceps (instrument with two spoon-shaped blades) is inserted through the vagina to grasp the head of the fetus and pull it through the birth canal. Currently, C-section is used with difficult births because of possible injury to the baby with use of forceps
induction	in-<u>duk</u>-shun	labor is initiated artificially with medication; done if the gestational period is 41–42 weeks or there are medical risks to the mother or fetus
lochia	<u>lo</u>-ke-ah	a vaginal discharge during the first week or two after childbirth
premature rupture of membranes (PROM)	pre-ma-<u>ture</u> <u>rup</u>-ture of <u>mem</u>-branes	spontaneous rupture of amniotic sac before the onset of labor
presentation	prez´-en-<u>ta</u>-shun	the position of a baby in utero with reference to the part of the baby that is directed toward or into the birth canal
stillbirth (SB)	<u>stil</u>-birth	birth of a baby without signs of life at or after 24 weeks of pregnancy; death can occur in late pregnancy or during birth

Terms Used to Describe the Newborn Infant

Term	Pronunciation	Definition
Apgar score	<u>ap</u>-gar skôr	the evaluation of an infant's physical condition, usually performed 1 and 5 minutes after birth, based on a rating of five factors that reflect the infant's ability to adjust to extrauterine life
Coombs' test	kumz test	a blood test to diagnose hemolytic anemias in a newborn
NICU		neonatal intensive care unit
meconium	me-<u>ko</u>-ne-um	dark green mucilaginous material in the intestine of the full-term fetus, expelled as first stool
neonatal period	ne´-o-<u>na</u>-tal	the first 4 weeks after birth
vernix caseosa	<u>ver</u>-niks ca-see-<u>o</u>-suh	a "cheesy" white substance on the skin of the newborn

THE ORIGIN OF MEDICAL TERMS

Table 16-9 explains the Greek or Latin origin of several terms studied in this chapter.

TABLE **16-9** The Origin of Medical Terms

Word	Pronunciation	Origin and Definition
amniocentesis	am´-ne-o-sen-te-sis	Greek, *amnion*, membrane around a fetus; + Greek, *kentēsis* a puncture, from *kentein* to prick
antepartum	an-te-par-tum	Latin, *ante*, before; + Latin, *partus*, a bringing forth, equivalent to par (ere) to bear
colporrhaphy	kol-por-ah-fe	Greek, *Kolpos*, fold or hollow + Greek, *rhaphe*, suture
dystocia	dis-to-se-ah	Greek, *dus*, abnormal; + Greek, *tokos*, childbirth + *ia*, condition
hysterosalpingogram	his´-ter-o-sal-ping-go-gram	Greek, *hustera*, womb; + Greek, *salpingo*, trumpet; + Greek, *gram*, a diagram
inseminate	in-sem-i-nate	Latin, *in*, into + Latin, *sēmināre* to plant or sow from Latin, *semin*, seed
neonatal	ne´-o-na-tal	Greek, *neo*, new + Latin, *nātālis*, belonging to one's birth
nephrolithiasis	nef´-ro-li-thi-ah-sis	Greek, *nephros*, kidney; + Greek, *litho*, stone; + Greek, *iasis*, pathological or morbid condition

ABBREVIATIONS

These abbreviations in **Table 16-10** are frequently used to describe the genitourinary and reproductive systems, including clinical disorders and diagnostic tools

TABLE **16-10** Abbreviations

Abbreviation	Definition	Abbreviation	Definition
AB	abortion	HPV	human papillomavirus
AIDS	acquired immunodeficiency syndrome	IVP	intravenous pyelogram
BV	bacterial vaginosis	KUB	kidney, ureter, and bladder
BOW	bag of waters	LMP	last menstrual period
BPH	benign prostrate hypertrophy	NICU	neonatal intensive care unit
BUN	blood urea nitrogen	OB	obstetrics; obstetrician
CKD	chronic kidney disease	PROM	Premature rupture of membranes
CPD	cephalopelvic disproportion	PID	pelvic inflammatory disease
D & C	dilation and curettage	SB	stillbirth
EDC	expected date of confinement	STIs	sexually transmitted infections
FHT	fetal heart tones	TRICH	trichomoniasis
GYN	gynecology; gynecologist	UTI	urinary tract infection
HIV	human immunodeficiency virus		

BOX 16-1 is a discussion of possible causes of chronic kidney disease.

Box 16-1 Chronic Kidney Disease

Kidney disease in children may be the result of a birth defect or an infection. Adults most at risk for developing Chronic Kidney Disease (CKD) are those with uncontrolled high blood pressure, diabetes, or heart disease. Once someone has CKD, either an artificial kidney or transplanted kidney is necessary to properly filter the blood to remove toxic wastes to prevent death.

The following box lists three different types of medications that may be prescribed by a physician treating diseases of the urinary and reproductive systems.

PHARMACOLOGY AND MEDICAL TERMINOLOGY

Drug Classification	antifungal (an-tih-<u>fung</u>-gal)	anti-infective (antibiotic) (an-tih-in-<u>fek</u>-tiv)	diuretic (dye-yoor-<u>ret</u>-ik)
Function	destroys or inhibits the growth of fungi	stops or controls the growth of infection-causing microorganisms	increases urine excretion
Word Parts	**anti-** = against; **fung/o** = fungus; **-al** = pertaining to	**hyper-** = excess; **infective** = pertaining to infection	pertaining to an increase in urination
Active Ingredients (Examples)	miconazole (Monistat); nystatin (Mycostatin); clotrimazole (Gyne-Lotrimin)	metronidazole (Flagyl); doxycycline hyclate (Vibramycin)	furosemide (Lasix); hydrochlorothiazide (Hydro-Diuril)

CLINICAL
Note

OB DELIVERY NOTE

A 25-year-old **G1**, **P0** moving to P1 African American female with **IUP** at 36 6/7 weeks with **EDC** at 2 1/7 weeks. Patient presents with 80 percent **effacement** and 4 cm dilated. Pregnancy uncomplicated. Patient reported bloody show 48 hours prior to **PROM**

Labor: PROM and moderate variable decels

Delivery: **NSVD**

Infant: Viable female **APGAR** 9 at 1 minute and 9 at 5 minutes

Anesthesia: Epidural

Episiotomy: Second-degree midline, no laceration

Placenta: Complete spontaneous

EBL: 300 cc

Note: Patient to post anesthesia recovery stable condition. Baby to well-baby nursery.

Direction: For the portions of the clinical note shown by a colored font, provide the definition and/or words for abbreviation.

LESSON TWO	Progress Check

LISTS: THE URINARY AND REPRODUCTIVE SYSTEMS

1. List the organs of the urinary system:

a. Two _____

b. Two _____

c. One _____

d. One _____

2. List three important functions of the urinary system:

a. _____

b. _____

c. _____

3. Describe the most important function of the reproductive system.

a. _____

MULTIPLE CHOICE: ANATOMY OF THE KIDNEY

Circle the letter of the correct answer:

1. Which of the following statements describes the cortex?
 a. Membranous sac containing urine
 b. Outer layer of the kidney
 c. Upper end of the ureter
 d. The renal pelvis

2. The urinary bladder receives urine through the _____ and discharges it through the _____.
 a. ureter, nephron
 b. bladder, urethra
 c. medulla, meatus
 d. ureter, urethra

3. The functional unit of the kidney that produces urine is called a:
 a. ureter
 b. bladder
 c. nephron
 d. urethra

4. The medulla is:
 a. the inner part of the kidney
 b. the outer layer of the kidney
 c. the renal pelvis
 d. the urinary meatus

COMPARE AND CONTRAST: THE URINARY SYSTEM

Explain the *differences* in the following conditions of the urinary tract:
Example: Calculi/cystitis: Calculi are kidney stones, but cystitis is inflammation of the urinary bladder.

1. Albuminuria/anuria: _____

2. Enuresis/diuresis: _____

3. Incontinence/urinary retention: _____

4. Hydronephrosis/nephrolithiasis: _____

5. Nycturia/oliguria/dysuria: _____

6. Pyelitis/glomerulonephritis: _____

MATCHING: TREATMENT OF THE URINARY SYSTEM

Match the treatment of the urinary system with its definition:

Procedure
1. Dialysis
2. IVP
3. I & O
4. UA
5. UTI
6. Catheterization
7. Cystoscopy
8. Retrograde pyelogram
9. Renal transplant
10. Ureterostomy

Definition
a. Urinalysis
b. Creation of a new outlet for urine through the abdominal wall
c. Examination of structures of the collecting system of the kidneys
d. Use of an artificial kidney to filter and remove waste products from the blood
e. Intake and output (of fluids)
f. Intravenous pyelogram
g. Surgically transferring a healthy kidney from a donor to someone with a diseased kidney
h. Urinary tract infection
i. Passage of a tube into the bladder to relieve bladder distention and remove urine
j. Visual examination of the urinary tract with a cystoscope

MATCHING: SURGICAL PROCEDURES OF THE MALE REPRODUCTIVE SYSTEM

Match the surgical procedure of the male reproduction system with its definition:

Procedure
1. Circumcision
2. Orchiopexy
3. Orchiectomy
4. Prostratectomy
5. Vasectomy

Definition
a. Cutting or tying the ductus deferens
b. Excision of the prostate gland
c. Removal of the foreskin
d. Release of undescended testicle(s)
e. Removal of one or both testes

MATCHING: SURGICAL PROCEDURES OF THE FEMALE REPRODUCTIVE SYSTEM

Match the surgical procedure of the female reproduction system with its definition:

Procedure
1. Abortion
2. Colporrhaphy
3. Hysterectomy
4. Oophorectomy
5. Tubal ligation

Definition
a. Removal of one or more ovaries
b. "Tying" both fallopian tubes
c. Removal of products of conception from the uterus before the fetus can survive
d. Suture of the vagina to repair a tear, cystocele, or rectocele
e. Removal of the uterus

COMPLETION: MALE AND FEMALE REPRODUCTIVE SYSTEMS

Write in the medical term for each of the following meanings:

1. _____ : A male gonad that supplies sperm to the semen

2. _____ : The scrotum, penis, vulva, clitoris, and urethra

3. _____ : Extension of the epididymis and part of the ejaculatory duct

4. _____ : Gland surrounding the neck of the bladder in males

5. _____ : The gland that is used for storage and maturation of spermatozoa

6. _____ : Passage way for spermatozoa and semen

7. _____ : A female gonad that produces eggs

8. _____ : Tube where fertilization occurs

9. _____ : Female organ that nourishes the fetus

10. _____ : Birth canal and receptacle for coitus

DEFINITIONS: PREGNANCY AND CHILDBIRTH

These medical terms are specific to pregnancy and childbirth. Name the term that means:

1. _____ : Taking a sample of amniotic fluid

2. _____ : Evaluation of an infant's condition at birth

3. _____ : The fetal head is too large for the mother's pelvis

4. _____ : Abnormal labor or childbirth

5. _____ : A pregnancy outside the uterus

6. _____ : Period from conception to birth

7. _____ : A pregnant woman

8. _____ : First 4 weeks after birth (infant)

9. _____ : Six-week period after birth (mother)

10. _____ : The afterbirth

TRUE OR FALSE: SEXUALLY TRANSMITTED INFECTIONS

Check T before statements which are true and F before statements which are false.

T ❑ **F** ❑   **1.** STIs are easy to treat because the symptoms are so severe.

T ❑ **F** ❑   **2.** HPV can be prevented by inoculating preteens with the HPV vaccine.

T ❑ **F** ❑   **3.** Genital herpes can be effectively treated with antibiotics.

T ❑ **F** ❑   **4.** BV is the result of changes in the normal bacterial flora in the vagina.

T ❑ **F** ❑   **5.** Some STIs can be transmitted from an infected woman to her infant during childbirth.

T ❑ **F** ❑   **6.** Complications of STIs in pregnant women are low birth weight infants and premature births.

T ❑ **F** ❑   **7.** Trichomoniasis is a common STI caused by a parasite.

T ❑ **F** ❑   **8.** Untreated syphilis causes damage to the heart, brain, and other organs in the late stage of the disease.

T ❑ **F** ❑   **9.** Complications of untreated HPV are genital warts and cancer of the cervix.

T ❑ **F** ❑   **10.** A common complication of untreated STIs in women is PID and infertility.

IDENTIFYING WORD PARTS

For each of the medical terms, list the root word and the prefix and/or suffix.

Word	Root Word	Prefix	Suffix
1. Azoturia	_____	_____	_____
2. Cryptorchidism	_____	_____	_____
3. Endometriosis	_____	_____	_____
4. Episiostomy	_____	_____	_____
5. Incontinent	_____	_____	_____
6. Inseminate	_____	_____	_____
7. Laparoscopy	_____	_____	_____
8. Neonatal	_____	_____	_____
9. Primapara	_____	_____	_____
10. Postpartum	_____	_____	_____

© teekid/iStock/Getty Images

Musculoskeletal System

OBJECTIVES

After completing this chapter and the exercises, the student should be able to:

1. Locate and name the major bones of the body by labeling the diagram provided.
2. Locate and name the major muscles of the body by labeling the diagram provided.
3. Classify the joints found in the musculoskeletal system.
4. Identify the types of bone fractures.
5. Identify and describe the types of muscles.
6. Define and explain various pathologic conditions of the musculoskeletal system.
7. Identify important diagnostic and treatment methods used for the musculoskeletal system.

THE MUSCULOSKELETAL SYSTEM

The musculoskeletal system includes the bones, muscles, and joints. All have important functions in the body. The human skeleton consists of 206 bones. Bones provide internal structural support, giving shape to our bodies and enabling us to stand upright. Some bones protect internal organs. The rib cage, for example, protects the lungs and heart and the skull protects the brain. The skeleton plays an important role in purposeful movement as the site of attachment for tendons of many skeletal muscles. The skeletal muscles' action on bones results in movement or stabilizes the skeleton. Bones are home to cells that give rise to red blood cells, white blood cells, and platelets (hematopoiesis). They are a storage depot for fat, which is necessary for cellular energy production, and a reservoir for minerals, especially calcium and phosphorus. Bones release and absorb calcium as needed to help maintain normal blood levels. Calcium is essential to muscle contraction, and disturbances in calcium levels can impair their function.

The adult human skeleton contains about 206 bones that make up the solid framework of the body. The skeleton is completed in certain areas by cartilage. The skeleton is organized into the *axial* skeleton, the *appendicular* skeleton, and the joints between bones; *Axis* and *appendicular*, are defined in Table 17-1 in Lesson One.

ALLIED HEALTH PROFESSIONS

Athletic Trainers, Orthotists, and Prosthetists

Athletic trainers help prevent and treat injuries for people of all ages and all skill levels. Clients include a wide range from high school to professional athletes as well as those who participate in recreational sports. Professional ballet dancers and figure skaters depend on the athletic trainer when they experience an injury. Athletic trainers specialize in the prevention and treatment of bone and muscle injuries; they provide instruction on the proper use of exercise equipment as well as exercises to improve balance and strength to prevent injuries. When there is an injury, the trainer supervises an exercise program that will promote healing of the injury and allow the athlete to return to her/his usual activities. Athletic trainers work for physicians, high schools, colleges and universities, and professional sports teams.

Orthotists and prosthetists fit artificial limbs and orthopedic braces for individuals with a musculoskeletal or neurological condition. An orthotist designs and fits corrective braces or supports for body parts that need straightening. Examples are a child with cerebral palsy who requires leg braces to be able to walk or an elderly woman with a neck injury who requires a neck brace to allow healing. A prosthetist designs and adjusts artificial limbs for amputees, for example, for someone who has lost the lower leg as a result of a car accident. A pedorthist creates or modifies footwear to help people maintain or regain as much mobility as possible, for example, for someone who has broken an ankle. These professionals evaluate patients and take measurements so that the medical devices are properly designed and will fit the patient. They often prepare a mold of the body part that will be fitted with a brace or artificial limb as well as select the material for the device. This often requires several sessions with the patient to test and adjust the device. After the device is properly fitted, the orthotists and prosthetists will provide instructions on how to use and care for the device and will provide repair and adjustment as needed. Orthotists and prosthetists practice in a variety of healthcare settings, including outpatient clinics, hospitals, and private offices. They also work in rehabilitation and nursing home facilities as well as veterans' facilities.

INQUIRY

American Academy of Orthotists and Prosthetists: www.opcareers.org
National Athletic Trainers' Association: www.nata.org

Data from Cross, Nanna, and McWay, Dana. *Stanfield's Introduction to the Health Professions*, 7th ed. Burlington, MA: Jones & Bartlett Learning; 2017.

The axial skeleton is composed of 80 bones that make the long axis of the body and protect the organs of the heart, neck, and torso.

1. The *vertebral column* has 26 vertebrae separated by intervertebral disks.
2. The *skull* is balanced on the vertebral column.
    a. *Cranial* bones enclose and protect the brain.
    b. *Facial* bones give shape to the face or contain teeth.
    c. Six *auditory* (ear) *ossicles* transmit sound.
    d. The *hyoid* supports the tongue and larynx.
3. The *thoracic* cage includes the ribs and sternum.

The appendicular skeleton is composed of 126 bones that make up arms, legs, and the pectoral and pelvic girdles that anchor them to the axial skeleton. The functions of the skeletal system are:

1. To support and shape the body.
2. To provide movement: Bones and joints act as levers. As the muscles that are anchored to bones contract, the force applied to the levers results in movement.
3. For protection: The skeletal system protects the soft delicate organs of the body.
4. For blood cell formation (*hematopoiesis*): The red bone marrow is the site of production of red blood cells (*erythrocytes*), white blood cells (*leukocytes*), and *platelets* of the blood.
5. For storage of minerals, primarily calcium phosphate and calcium carbonate: The bones contain 99 percent of the body's calcium. Calcium and phosphorus in the bone are withdrawn as needed for other body functions. They must be replenished through diet.

Muscles, whether attached to bones or to internal organs and blood vessels, are responsible for movement. Most muscles cross one or more joints, and when they contract they cause movement. Internal movement is the contraction and relaxation of visceral muscles, for example, of the digestive tract. Some muscles steady the joints, helping to maintain an upright posture against the pull of gravity. Other muscles anchored to the bones of the skull and face allow us to frown, smile, open and close our eyes, and move our lips. Muscles also produce enormous amounts of heat as a by-product of metabolism.

Muscle tissue constitutes 40–50 percent of body weight. It consists predominantly of contractile cells called muscle fibers. Through contraction, muscles produce movement and do work.

Muscles have these properties: *contractility, excitability* (response when stimulated by nerve impulses), *extensibility* (stretch beyond their relaxed length), and *elasticity* (return to their original length). Mammals are the only animals with facial muscles, and the human body contains the same number of muscles from birth to death.

There is special classification and terminology related to muscles. These are explained and defined in Lesson One. The functions of the muscular system are:

1. Movement
2. Body support and maintenance of posture
3. Heat production

The energy sources for muscle contraction are an interesting part of muscle physiology involving the citric acid cycle. Additional energy sources are formed by the metabolism of glucose and fatty acids through anaerobic (glycolytic pathway) and aerobic reactions. The value of exercise in weight control can be verified with these facts.

Many injuries, diseases, and disorders affect the musculoskeletal system. These are defined in Lesson One. Lessons to be learned are separated into sections for better identification and clarity:

1. Head and body bones, joints, and accessories
2. Body muscles
3. Pathological conditions of the musculoskeletal system and the procedures and tests used to diagnose and treat them (medical management).

An *orthopedist* is a physician who specializes in diseases and injuries of bones and joints, while a *podiatrist* specializes in diseases of the foot, ankle, and lower leg. Both orthopedists and podiatrists perform surgery as part of a treatment plan. A *rheumatologist* is a physician who specializes in nonsurgical treatment of autoimmune diseases of the bones, joints, and connective tissue.

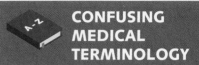

CONFUSING MEDICAL TERMINOLOGY

-metry versus metr/o

-metry – the process of measurement, e.g., osteometry (os-<u>teo</u>-met-re) refers to measurement of the bone

metr/o – uterus, e.g., menometrorrhagia (men-o-me-<u>tro</u>-ra-je-a) refers to excessive menstrual uterine bleeding

LESSON ONE	Materials to Be Learned

The musculoskeletal system serves the following functions in the body:

1. *Support and protection*: The forms and shapes of the body are maintained and vital organs are protected from injury
2. *Movement*: Body movement is made possible by a coordination of different components of the musculoskeletal system
3. *Red blood cell turnover*: Marrow from the large bones serves as the site for turnover (destruction and rebuilding) of red blood cells
4. *Storage*: Bones store minerals and muscles store nutrients for energy production

THE SKELETAL SYSTEM

Figures 17-1 through **17-3** show the anterior and posterior views of the human skeleton, bones of the skull, and bones of the vertebral column, respectively.

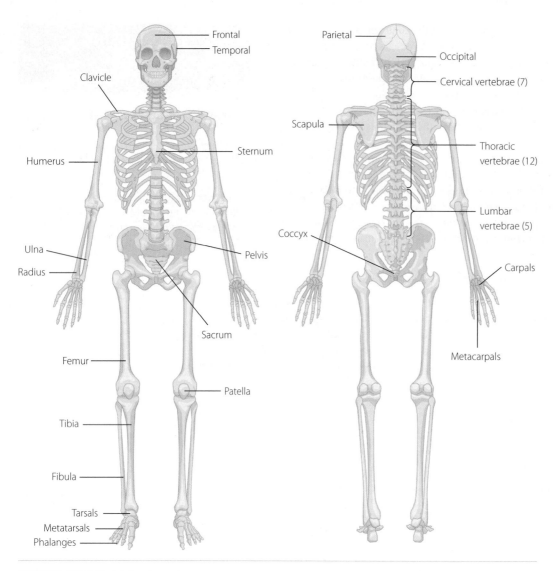

FIGURE 17-1 Skeletal system.

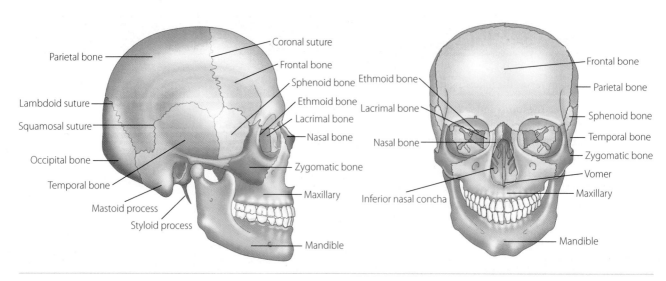

FIGURE 17-2 The skull.

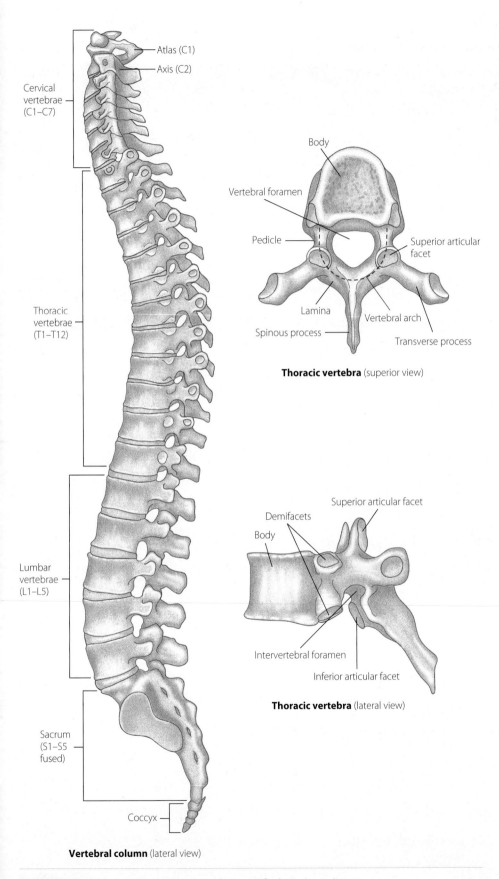

Atlas (C1)
Axis (C2)
Cervical vertebrae (C1–C7)

Thoracic vertebrae (T1–T12)

Lumbar vertebrae (L1–L5)

Sacrum (S1–S5 fused)

Coccyx

Vertebral column (lateral view)

Body
Vertebral foramen
Pedicle
Lamina
Spinous process
Superior articular facet
Vertebral arch
Transverse process

Thoracic vertebra (superior view)

Demifacets
Body
Superior articular facet
Intervertebral foramen
Inferior articular facet

Thoracic vertebra (lateral view)

FIGURE 17-3 The vertebral column and features of selected vertebrae.

Divisions of the Skeletal System
Table 17-1 describes the two main divisions of the skeletal system.

TABLE 17-1 Divisions of the Skeletal System

Main Division	Pronunciation	Definition
appendicular skeleton	ap´-en-<u>dik</u>-u-lar <u>skel</u>-i-tn	bones of the upper and lower limbs attached to the pectoral and pelvic girdles that anchor them to the axial skeleton
axial skeleton	<u>ak</u>-si-el <u>skel</u>-i-tn	imaginary line that passes through the center of the body traversing the length of the body; includes bones of the skull, thorax, and vertebral column

Bones of the Axial Skeleton
Table 17-2 lists bones of the axial skeleton.

TABLE 17-2 Bones of the Axial Skeleton

Medical Name	Pronunciation	Definition
Head Bones		
ethmoid	<u>eth</u>-moid	the upper nasal bone between the eyes; the bone is light and spongy
frontal	<u>frun</u>-tal	forehead
hyoid	<u>hahy</u>-oid	point of attachment for muscles in the mouth and throat
lachrymal	<u>lak</u>-ruh-muhl	two bones that house the tear ducts
mandible	<u>man</u>-di-b´-l	large bone constituting the lower jaw
maxilla	mak-<u>sil</u>-ah	one of a pair of large bones forming the upper jaw
nasal	<u>ney</u>-zuhl	two bones that shape the nose
occipital	ok-<u>sip</u>-i-tal	the cuplike bone at the back of the skull
palatine	<u>pal</u>-uh-tahyn	forms the hard palate (roof of the mouth)
parietal	pah-<u>ri</u>-e-tal	bone of the skull (top of the head)
sphenoid	<u>sfe</u>-noid	bone at the base of the skull, anterior to the temporal bones
temporal	<u>tem</u>-po-ral	large bones forming part of the temples
turbinate	<u>ter</u>-bi-nat	cone-shaped nasal bone
vomer	<u>voh</u>-mer	lower part of the nasal septum
zygomatic	zahy-guh-<u>mat</u>-ik	two bones, one on each side of the face, which form the high part of the cheek bones and outer eye socket
Vertebral Column		
coccyx	<u>kok</u>-siks	small triangular bone forming the lower extremity of the spinal column; common name is tailbone
cervical vertebrae	<u>sur</u>-vi-kuh-l <u>vur</u>-tuh-bruh	vertebrae C1-C7 in the neck or top portion of the vertebral column (see Figure 17-3)

Medical Name	Pronunciation	Definition
lamina (plural: laminae)	lam-i-nah lam-i-nee	the flattened part of the vertebral arch (thinnest part of a vertebra)
lumbar vertebrae	luhm-ber vur-tuh-bruh	vertebrae L1-L5 at the bottom of the vertebral column or lower back just above the sacrum (see Figure 17-3)
sacrum	sak-ruh-m	triangular structure of five fused vertebrae at the base of the vertebral column
thoracic vertebrae	thaw-ras-ik vur-tuh-bruh	vertebrae T1-T12 between the cervical and lumbar vertebrae or in the area where ribs are attached (see Figure 17-3)
Rib Cage		
ribs	ribs	a series of curved bones that are articulated with the vertebrae and occur in pairs, 12 on each side of the vertebrate body, certain pairs being connected with the sternum and forming the thoracic wall
sternum	ster-num	the elongated, flattened bone forming the middle portion of the thorax (breastbone)

Bones of the Appendicular Skeleton

Table 17-3 describes bones of the appendicular skeleton.

TABLE 17-3 Bones of the Appendicular Skeleton

Part	Pronunciation	Definition
Upper Limbs		
carpals	kahr-puh-l	wrist bones; two rows of four bones each
humerus	hu-mer-us	upper arm bone, consisting of a body, a head, and the condyle
metacarpals	met-uh-kahr-puh-ls	five long bones in the hand that attach to the wrist (carpal) at one end and the phalanges at the other end
phalanges	fuh-lan-jeez	finger bones
radius and ulna	ra-de-us and ul-nah	the radius is the larger of the two bones of the forearm; the ulna is the bone on the medial or little finger side of the forearm, lying parallel with the radius
Lower Limbs		
femur	fe-mur	the thigh bone, extending from the pelvis to the knee
fibula and tibia	fib-u-lah and tib-e-ah	the fibula is the smallest of the bones of the leg; the tibia is the second longest bone of the skeleton, located at the medial side of the leg
metatarsals	met-uh-tahr-suh-ls	five bones between the ankle and the toes (phalanges)
phalanges	fuh-lan-jeez	bones in the toes
tarsals	tahr-suh-ls	seven bones of the ankle that connect the tibia and fibula to the foot

(continues)

TABLE **17-3** (continued)		
Part	**Pronunciation**	**Definition**
Pectoral Girdle		
clavicle	klav-i-k´-l	a long, curved, horizontal bone just above the first rib (collar bone)
scapula	skap-u-lah	shoulder blade
Pelvic Girdle		
pelvis	pel-vis	includes the right and left hip bones: the sacrum and the coccyx; all bones are fused together to form the pelvic girdle. The lower limbs of the axial skeleton are attached to the pelvis

Joints and Accessory Parts

Joints are *articulations* between two or more bones. Joints are made of connective tissue and are separated by cartilage which prevents bones from touching. They connect the bones of the skeleton and are classified by the degree of movement permitted. Immovable joints permit no movement. Skull bones, for example, are held together by immovable joints, as is the pubic symphysis that is formed by the two pubic bones. Freely movable joints allow movement such as joints of the ankle, elbow, shoulders, and hips. The synovial joint is considered the most freely moving joint, because it contains synovial fluid which prevents friction and direct contact between the ends of bones. Examples are the ball and socket hip joint or the joint between the pelvis and the femur. The joints between vertebrae are separated by cartilage, which serves as a cushion to prevent bone from touching bone. Intervertebral joints allow slight movement so that we can bend or curl up in our beds. **Table 17-4** describes different types of joints and accessory parts.

TABLE **17-4** Joints and Accessory Parts		
Part	**Pronunciation**	**Definition**
Types of Joints		
ball and socket	bawl and sok-et	a joint in which the globular head of an articulating bone is received into a cuplike cavity, e.g., the hip and shoulder; surrounded by synovial fluid and considered movable
diarthroidal	dahy-ahr-throh-dee-uh-l	a joint that permits maximal motion, as the shoulder, knee, or hip joint
hinge	hinj	hinge joint, e.g., an elbow or interphalangeal joints between phalanges of the fingers and toes; surrounded by synovial fluid and considered movable
intervertebral	in-ter-ver-te-bral	cartilage between the spinal vertebrae provide a cushion between bones; considered slightly moveable
sutures	su-cherz	lines of junction between the bones of the skull; considered an immovable joint

Part	Pronunciation	Definition
Fluid Between Joints to Reduce Friction		
bursa (plural: bursae)	ber-sah (ber-see)	a fluid-filled sac located between tendons and bones of the knee or elbow; the fluid allows for free movement of the joint and prevents friction
synovial fluid	si-no-ve-al	the transparent, viscid fluid found in joint cavities, bursae, and tendon sheaths; the fluid allows for free movement of the joint and prevents friction between the ends of bones
Accessory Parts		
aponeurosis	ap´-o-nu-ro-sis	a flattened tendon, connecting a muscle with the parts it moves
fascia (plural: fasciae)	fash-e-ah (fash-shee-ee)	a sheet of fibrous tissue holding muscle fibers together
ligament	lig-ah-ment	a band of fibrous tissue connecting bones or cartilage
meniscus (plural: menisci)	me-nis-kus (me-nis-ki)	a crescent-shaped fibrocartilage in the knee joint
tendon	ten-don	a fibrous cord of connective tissue attaching the muscle to bone or cartilage
theca	the-kah	a case or sheath of a tendon

Bone Processes, Depressions, and Holes

Bone processes are enlarged tissues that extend out from the bones to serve as attachments for muscles and tendons. The bone head is the rounded end of a bone separated from the body of the bone by a neck. Many bones have a small rounded process called a tubercle for attachment of tendons or muscles. Below the neck of the femur is a large bony process called a trochanter, and at the end of the bone is a rounded knuckle-like projection that fits into the fossa (bone depression) of another bone to form a joint.

Bone depressions are the openings or cavities in a bone that help to join one bone to another and are the passageway for the blood vessels and nerves. As noted earlier, the fossa is a shallow cavity in or on a bone. The foramen is an opening for blood vessels and nerves. A fissure or suture is a deep, narrow, slit-like opening. A sinus is a hollow space in a bone, for example, the paranasal sinuses.

Refer to **Table 17-5** for terms and definitions related to bone processes, depressions, and holes.

TABLE **17-5** Bone Processes, Depressions, and Holes

Structure	Pronunciation	Definition
acetabulum	as´-e-tab-u-lum	the cup-shaped cavity (socket) receiving the head of the femur
foramen (plural: foramina)	fo-ra-men (fo-ram-i-nah)	holes in a bone for large vessels and nerves to pass through
fossa (plural: fossae)	fos-ah (fos-ee)	a hollow or depressed area

(continues)

TABLE **17-5** (continued)

Structure	Pronunciation	Definition
groove	groov	a narrow, linear hollow or depression in bone
malleolus	mah-<u>le</u>-o-lus	a rounded process, such as the protuberance on either side of the ankle joint, at the lower end of the fibula or the tibia
olecranon	o-<u>lek</u>-rah-non	bony projection of the ulna at the elbow
prominence	<u>prom</u>-i-nens	protrusion or projection
sinus	<u>si</u>-nus	a recess, cavity, or channel such as one in the bone, e.g., nasal sinus
tuberosity	too´-be-<u>ros</u>-i-te	an elevation or protuberance, especially of a bone

THE MUSCULAR SYSTEM

Basically, there are three categories of muscles in the body:

1. Heart or cardiac muscle.
2. Striated or striped muscles, e.g., skeletal muscles. These muscles are voluntary muscles that a person has control over.
3. Nonstriated or nonstriped muscles, e.g., smooth muscles. These muscles are involuntary and there is no way to have control over them, e.g., movement of the stomach and intestine.

Body muscles are identified as:

1. *Function*: A muscle name has two parts: the first part is a word root, ending in a suffix (-or or -ens); the second part is the name of the affected body structure. An example is the extensor carpi or extension of the wrist.
2. *Points of origin and attachment*: The muscle name joins the names of points of origin and attachment with a word terminal (-eus or -is). An example is the sternoclavicularis for sternum and clavicle.
3. *Form or position*: The muscle name contains a descriptive word and the name of the muscle location. An example is the pectoralis minor for small chest muscle.
4. *Resemblance to an object for which the muscle is used*: An example is the buccinator. This refers to the cheek muscle, which is used in blowing a trumpet.

Figure 17-4 shows the human muscular system and **Figure 17-5** shows, specifically, the muscles of the head. In addition, **Figure 17-6** shows, specifically, the muscles in the neck, thorax, and the arm.

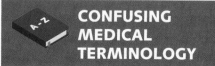

CONFUSING MEDICAL TERMINOLOGY

myel/o versus myel/o

myel/o – bone marrow, e.g., myeloma (<u>mi</u>-el-o-mah) refers to the tumor of the bone marrow (its cells) of the spinal cord

myel/o – spinal cord, e.g., polioencephalomeningomyelitis (<u>po</u>-le-o-en-sef-al-o-men-in-jo-mi-<u>el</u>-i-tis) refers to inflammation of the gray matter of the brain, the membrane, and the spinal cord

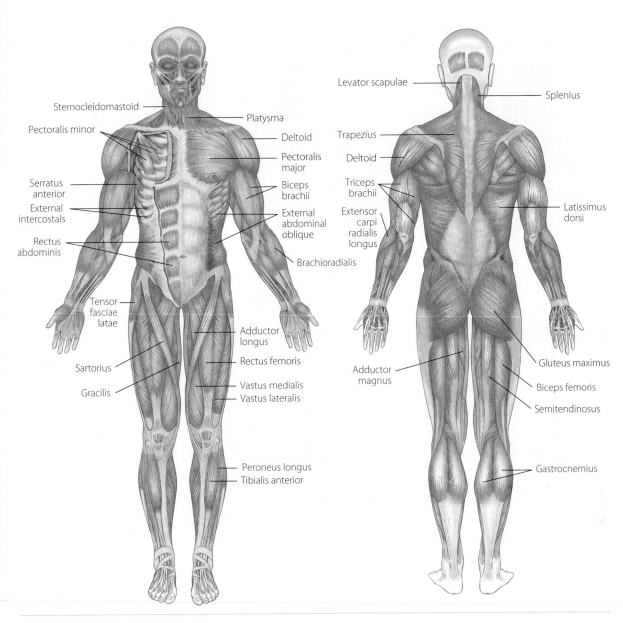

FIGURE 17-4 The muscular system, anterior and posterior views.

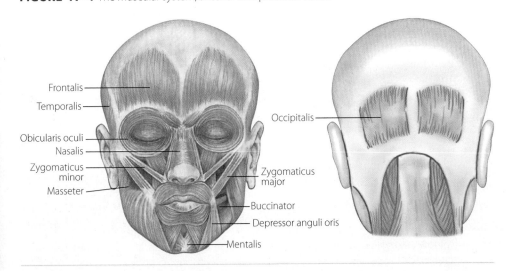

FIGURE 17-5 Muscles of the head.

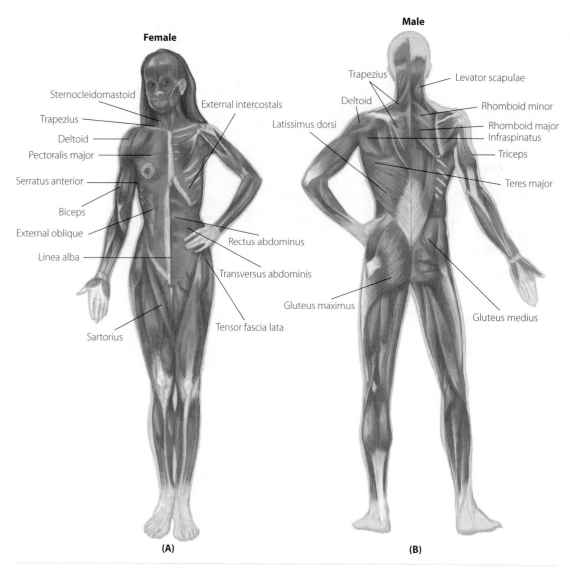

FIGURE 17-6 (A) Anterior aspect of the muscles of the neck, thorax, and arm. **(B)** Posterior aspect of the muscles of the neck, thorax, and arm.

Muscles of the Body

Table 17-6 describes muscles of the body.

TABLE **17-6** Muscles of the Body		
Medical Term	**Pronunciation**	**Definition**
Major Types of Muscle Tissue		
cardiac muscle	<u>kar</u>-de-ac <u>muhs</u>-uhl	specialized muscle found in the walls of the heart; involuntary muscles, controlled by the autonomic nervous system
skeletal muscle	<u>skel</u>-i-tl <u>muhs</u>-uhl	also called striated (striped) or voluntary muscles; muscles attached to skeletal bones except for face, eyes, tongue, and throat; under conscious control
smooth muscle	smooth <u>muhs</u>-uhl	muscles found in the wall of the stomach, intestine, blood vessels, and respiratory tract; also called involuntary or visceral muscle; under unconscious control

Medical Term	Pronunciation	Definition
Head and Facial Muscles		
buccinator	buck-sin-<u>ay</u>-tor	fleshy part of the cheek; used to smile, blow outward, and whistle
masseter	mass-<u>see</u>-ter	muscle at angle of jaw; used for biting and chewing
orbicularis occuli	or-<u>bick</u>-yoo-<u>lar</u>-iss <u>ock</u>-yool-eye	body of the eyelid, opens and closes the eye, wrinkles forehead
orbicularis oris	or-<u>bick</u>-yoo-<u>lar</u>-iss <u>or</u>-iss	muscle surrounding the mouth; closes and purses the lips
temporal	<u>tem</u>-por-al	muscle above the ear; used for opening and closing the jaw
Other Muscles of the Body		
biceps brachii	bye-<u>seps</u> bray-<u>kee</u>-eye	muscle extending from scapula to radius; used to flex lower arm and turn palm of hand upward
deltoid	<u>dell</u>-toyd	muscle covering the shoulder joint; extends from clavicle and scapula to humerus, and abducts the shoulder
gastrocnemius	gas-trok-<u>nee</u>-mus	main calf muscle; attaches to heel bone; flexes the foot and the knee
gluteus maximus	gloo-tee-us <u>max</u>-ih-mus	fleshy part of the buttocks; extends from ilium to femur; extends and rotates hip laterally
hamstring	<u>ham</u>-string	muscle in posterior thigh used for flexing knee, as in kneeling, and for hip extension
latissimus dorsi	lah-<u>tis</u>-ih-mus <u>dor</u>-see	muscle extending from lower vertebrae to humerus; used for adduction of the shoulder joint
pectoralis major	peck-tor-<u>ray</u>-lis	large, fan-shaped muscle across front of the chest; adducts, flexes, and rotates the shoulder joint inward
quadriceps femoris	<u>kwod</u>-rih-seps fem-<u>or</u>-is	anterior thigh muscle; part of a five-muscle group that extends the knee and flexes the hip
sternomastoid	stir-no-<u>mass</u>-toyd	muscle extending from sternum to side of the neck; used for turning the head
trapezius	trap-<u>pee</u>-zee-us	triangular muscle extending from back of shoulder to clavicle; used to raise shoulders
triceps brachii	<u>tri</u>-seps bray-<u>kee</u>-eye	muscle extending from scapula to ulna; responsible for extending the elbow

Types of Joint Movements

Table 17-7 describes different types of joint movements. Visual representation of movements is shown in **Figure 17-7**.

TABLE **17-7** Types of Joint Movements

Movement	Pronunciation	Definition
abduction	ab-<u>duk</u>-shun	to draw away from the axial (median) line
adduction	ad-<u>duk</u>-shun	to draw toward the axial (median) line
circumduction	cir-cum-<u>duc</u>-tion	moving a part so that one end follows a circular path while the other end remains stationary; e.g., moving the lower arm while the elbow is stationary
eversion	e-<u>ver</u>-sion	turning the foot so the plantar surface (sole) faces laterally
inversion	in-<u>ver</u>-sion	turning the foot so the plantar surface (sole) faces medially

TABLE **17-7** (continued)		
Movement	**Pronunciation**	**Definition**
extension	ek-<u>sten</u>-shun	movement by which the two ends of any jointed part are drawn away from each other; straightening
flexion	<u>flek</u>-shun	bending
protraction	pro-<u>trac</u>-tion	moving a bone forward, e.g., moving the mandible (jaw) out
retraction	re-<u>trac</u>-tion	moving a bone backward, e.g., moving the mandible (jaw) in
pronation	pro-<u>na</u>-shun	the prone position (palm down, face down)
supination	su´-pi-<u>na</u>-shun	palm or face upward

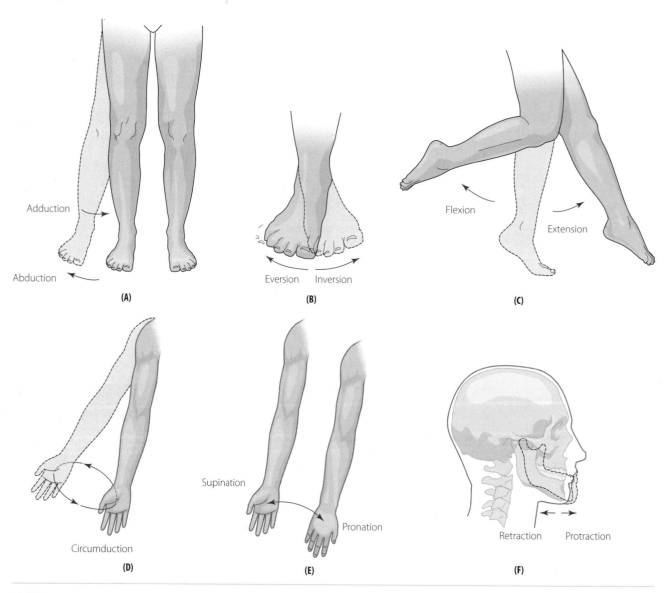

FIGURE 17-7 Movements of diarthroidial joints: **(A)** abduction-adduction, **(B)** eversion-inversion, **(C)** flexion-extension, **(D)** circumduction, **(E)** supination-pronation, and **(F)** protraction-retraction.

Physiological State of Muscles

Table 17-8 describes different physiological states of muscles.

TABLE **17-8** Physiological State of Muscles		
Condition	**Pronunciation**	**Definition**
atrophy	<u>at</u>-ro-fe	wasting away of muscle from disuse
contracture	kon-<u>trak</u>-chur	permanent contraction of a muscle
hypertrophy	hi-<u>per</u>-tro-fe	muscle enlargement from overuse
paralysis	pah-<u>ral</u>-i-sis	loss of muscular contraction because of nerve damage
paresis	pah-<u>re</u>-sis	slight or incomplete paralysis
tone	tōn	normal degree of vigor and tension in a muscle; muscles partially contracted

BONE INJURIES

Figure 17-8 and **Table 17-9** describe bone injuries. In addition, **Figure 17-9** shows how bone injuries are treated.

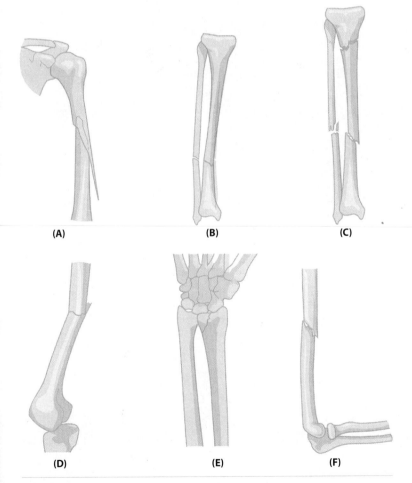

(A)   (B)   (C)

(D)   (E)   (F)

FIGURE 17-8 Types of bone fractures: **(A)** Longitudinal, through upper shaft of right humerus, **(B)** Spiral of tibia and fibula, **(C)** comminuted, of tibia and fibula, **(D)** transverse, through lower shaft of femur, **(E)** impacted, and **(F)** pathologic, through area of destruction secondary to metastatic carcinoma.

TABLE 17-9 Bone Injuries

Type	Pronunciation	Definition
dislocation	dis-lo-<u>ca</u>-tion	bones at joint forced out of alignment because of injury
fracture	<u>frak</u>-chur	the breaking of a bone; there are many types (see Figure 17-8)
skull fracture	skul <u>frak</u>-chur	a fracture of the bony structure of the head
spondylolisthesis	spon´-di-lo-lis-<u>the</u>-sis	forward displacement of a vertebra over a lower segment; a type of dislocation
subluxation	sub´-luk-<u>sa</u>-shun	partial bone dislocation
torn ligament, tendon, or cartilage	<u>lig</u>-ah-ment, <u>ten</u>-don, <u>kar</u>-ti-lij	a complete or partial tear of a ligament, tendon, or cartilage; common sports injury

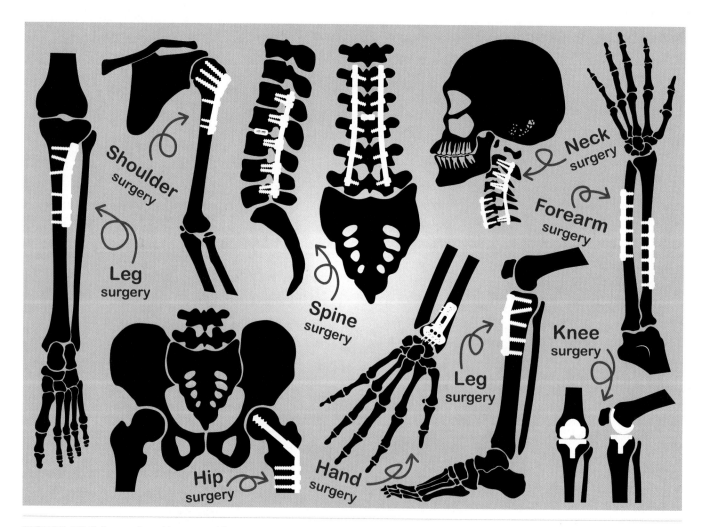

FIGURE 17-9 Bones aligned by external fixation with rods and screws placed on the outside of the bone to hold in place during healing.

© Puwadol Jaturawutthichai/Shutterstock.

CLINICAL DISORDERS

Table 17-10 describes clinical disorders of bone and muscle. **Figures 17-10** through **17-14** are examples of bone disorders.

TABLE **17-10** Clinical Disorders

Disorder	Pronunciation	Definition
achondroplasia	a-chon-dro-pla-sia	a genetic disorder affecting the normal growth of cartilage, resulting in dwarfism characterized by a normal torso but short arms and legs
bursitis	ber-si-tis	inflammation of a bursa
collagen disease	kol-ah-jen di-zez	a group of diseases with widespread pathologic changes in connective tissue, e.g., systemic lupus erythematosus
gout	gowt	a hereditary form of arthritis caused by accumulation of uric acid crystals in the great toe and fingers (see Figure 17-10)
herniated nucleus pulposus	her-ne-at´-ed nu-kle-us pul-po-sus	a rupture of the fibrocartilage surrounding an intervertebral disc, releasing the nucleus pulposus that cushions the vertebrae above and below
juvenile rheumatoid arthritis (JRA)	ju-ve-nile roo´mah-toid ar-thri-tis	autoimmune condition in which the immune system attacks the joints resulting in inflammation, pain, swelling, and possible joint damage. Must be diagnosed before age 16 to be considered juvenile arthritis
kyphosis	ki-fo-sis	humpback or hunchback; a spinal deformity
Legg-Calvé-Perthes disease	leg-kal-vay-per-tes di-zez	osteochondrosis of the head of the femur in children
lordosis	lor-do-sis	exaggerated forward curvature of the lumbar spine
Lyme disease	līm di-zēz	inflammatory disease characterized first by a rash and flu-like symptoms, and later by possible arthritis and neurological and cardiac disorders; caused by bacteria and transmitted by deer ticks
mastoiditis	Mas-toid-it-is	inflammation of the mastoid (bone); complication of otitis media (ear infection)
muscular dystrophy	mus-ku-lar dis-tro-fe	genetic disease with progressive atrophy of skeletal muscles
myositis	mi´-o-si-tis	inflammation of a voluntary muscle
Osgood-Schlatter disease	oz-good-shlat-er di-zez	inflammation of the tibial tubercle caused by chronic irritation and seen primarily in muscular, athletic adolescents; characterized by swelling and tenderness over the tibial tubercle that increases with exercise
osteoarthritis (OA)	os-te-o-ar-thri-tis	degeneration of joint cartilage and underlying bone causing pain and stiffness, especially in the hip, knee, and thumb joints; also degenerative joint disease (DJD) (see Figure 17-11)
osteochondritis	os´-te-o-kon-dri-tis	inflammation of bone and cartilage
osteochondrosis	os´-te-o-kon-dro-sis	disease of the bone and cartilage
osteomalacia	os´-te-o-mah-la-she-ah	softening of the bones resulting from vitamin D deficiency

(continues)

TABLE **17-10** (continued)

Disorder	Pronunciation	Definition
osteomyelitis	os´-te-o-mi´-e-li-tis	inflammation of bone and marrow caused by bacterial invasion
osteoporosis	os´-te-o-po-ro-sis	porous condition of bones; occurs primarily in postmenopausal women
plantar fasciitis	plan-tur fash-ee-ahy-tis	inflammation of the plantar fascia, the thick band of tissue that runs across the bottom of the foot and connects the heel bone to the toes
rheumatic fever	rheu-mat-ic fe-ver	can occur after strep throat infection with group A streptococcus, especially in children, if not treated adequately with antibiotics. Symptoms include red, swollen, painful, and tender joints in the knees, ankles, elbows, and wrists
rheumatoid arthritis (RA)	roo´mah-toid ar-thri-tis	disorders marked by inflammation, degeneration, or metabolic derangement of the connective tissue structures, especially the joints; accompanied by pain, stiffness, or limitation of motion (see Figures 17-12 and 17-13)
rickets	rik-ets	vitamin D deficiency, especially in infancy and childhood, causing soft and curved bones of the legs due to lack of bone mineralization
sarcoma (osteogenic)	sar´-ko-mah (os´-te-o-jen-ik)	a malignant tumor of bone
scoliosis	sko´-le-o-sis	lateral curvature of the spine (see Figure 17-14)
spondylitis (ankylosing)	spon´-di-li-tis (ang´-ki-lo-sing)	inflammation of the vertebrae, commonly progressing to eventual fusion of the involved joints
systemic lupus erythematosus (SLE)/lupus	sis-tem-ik loo-pus er-i´-the-ma-to-sus	a chronic inflammatory disease affecting many systems of the body, most often the joints and muscles, causing pain and fatigue
tendinitis	ten´-di-ni-tis	inflammation of a tendon

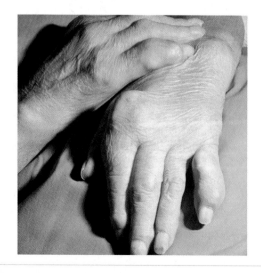

FIGURE 17-10 Deformities of hands caused by accumulation of uric acid crystals (tophi) in and around finger joints.

Courtesy of Leonard V. Crowley, MD, Century College.

Normal Joint   **Destruction of Cartilage**

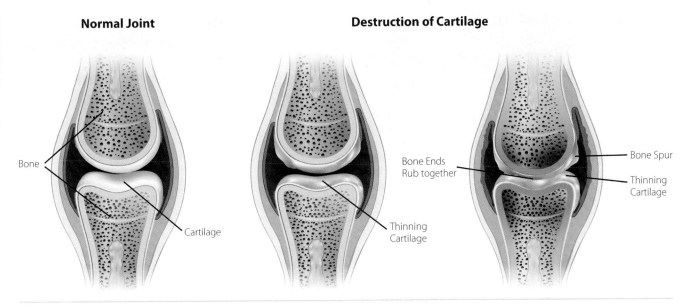

FIGURE 17-11 Osteoarthritis of the knee joint.

© Tefi/Shutterstock.

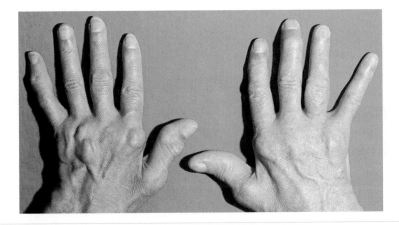

FIGURE 17-12 Rheumatoid arthritis, early manifestations, illustrating swelling of knuckle joints (metacarpophalangeal joints) as a result of inflammation and ulnar deviation of fingers.

Courtesy of Leonard V. Crowley, MD, Century College.

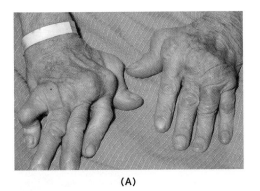

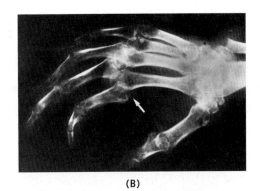

(A)   (B)

FIGURE 17-13 (A) Advanced joint deformities caused by rheumatoid arthritis. **(B)** Radiograph illustrating destruction of articular surfaces and anterior dislocation of the base of index finger as a result of joint instability.

Courtesy of Leonard V. Crowley, MD, Century College.

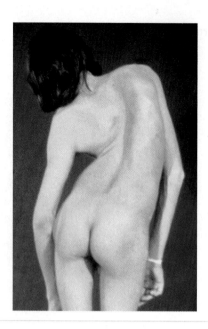

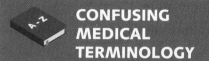

CONFUSING MEDICAL TERMINOLOGY

ile/o versus ili/o (ileum versus ilium)

ile/o – part of intestine, e.g., ileum (il-<u>ee</u>uhm) refers to part of the small intestine; e.g., ileorectal (il-<u>e</u>-o-rek-tal) refers to pertaining to the ileum and the rectum

ili/o – part of the hipbone, e.g., ilium (il-<u>ee</u>-uhm) refers to pertaining to the hip bone (pelvic); iliofemoral (il-e-o-<u>fem</u>-or-al) refers to pertaining to the large thigh bone (femur) and the hip bone

FIGURE 17-14 Severe scoliosis, which causes marked asymmetry of trunk and greatly reduces the size of the thoracic cavities, interfering with the pulmonary function.

Courtesy of Leonard V. Crowley, MD, Century College.

BOX 17-1 explains the symptoms and treatment of scoliosis and **BOX 17-2** compares tissue injury and location for sprain and strain.

Box 17-1 Spinal Fusion for the Treatment of Adolescent Idiopathic Scoliosis

Adolescent idiopathic scoliosis develops during rapid growth in preteens as an abnormal curvature of the spine resulting in one shoulder appearing higher than the other. The curvature can become more severe if untreated and cause backaches, breathing difficulties, and the ability to participate in sports. In adults, scoliosis can cause long-term complications because of crowding of the heart and lungs, resulting in heart failure. The condition is treated in teens to prevent potential health problems. Spinal fusion surgery is the current treatment in which permanent rods are placed alongside the spine and screwed into place to correct the spinal curve and stabilize the spine (see Figures 17-9 and 17-14).

Data from American Academy of Orthopaedic Surgeons. Patient Story: Adolescent Idiopathic Scoliosis. Internet: http://orthoinfo.aaos.org/topic.cfm?topic=A00742

Box 17-2 Sprain or Strain, What Is the Difference?

A sprain is a stretch or tear of a *ligament* (a band of fibrous tissue that connects two or more bones at a joint), while a strain is a stretch or tear of either a muscle or a *tendon* (the fibrous cords of tissue that connect muscle to bone). Common sites for a sprain are the ankle, knee and thumb. The two most common sites for a strain are the lower back and the hamstring muscle (the back of the thigh).

Data from Mayo Foundation for Medical Education and Research (MFMER). Sprains and Strains. Internet: https://www.mayoclinic.org/diseases-conditions/sprains-and-strains/basics/definition/con-20020958

TERMS USED IN THE DIAGNOSIS AND TREATMENT OF MUSCULOSKELETAL DISORDERS

Table 17-11 lists terms used in the diagnosis and treatment of musculoskeletal disorders.

TABLE 17-11 Terms Used in the Diagnosis and Treatment of Musculoskeletal Disorders

Procedure	Pronunciation	Definition
Laboratory Tests		
antistreptolysin O (ASO)	an-ti-strep-to-<u>ly</u>-sin	serum test for antibodies against streptolysin O, produced by group A streptococcus bacteria. Causes strep throat; complication of infection is rheumatic fever with symptoms of swelling and pain in the joints
antinuclear antibodies (AN)	an-ti-<u>nu</u>-cle-ar anti-bode-s	serum test used as screening for autoimmune diseases
C-reactive protein (CRP)	C re-<u>ac</u>-tive <u>pro</u>-tein	protein present in blood serum in inflammatory conditions, including autoimmune disorders
rheumatoid factor (RF)	<u>roo</u>-mah-toid <u>fac</u>-tor	autoantibody (antibody directed against an organism's own tissues) found in rheumatoid arthritis
sed rate (erythrocyte sedimentation rate [ESR])	e-<u>ryth</u>-ro-cyte sed-uh-muh-n-<u>tey</u>-shuh-n rate	blood test for inflammatory activity; screening test for autoimmune diseases
Radiological Exams		
electromyogram (electromyography)	e-lek-tro-<u>mi</u>-o-gram (e-lek´-tro-mi-<u>og</u>-rah-fe)	the film record made and the study of muscular contraction
magnetic resonance imaging (MRI)	mag-<u>net</u>-ic <u>res</u>-o-nance <u>im</u>-ag-ng	noninvasive diagnostic tool that uses a magnetic field and radio waves to create 3-D images of the skeletal system, especially bones and joints
myelogram	mi-<u>e</u>-lo-gram	the film produced by radiography of the spinal cord after injection of a dye into the spinal cavity
myogram	mi-<u>o</u>-gram	a record produced by myography; same as electromyogram
Surgery for Diagnosis or Treatment		
amputation	am-pu-<u>ta</u>-shun	Removal of a limb or other appendage of the body because of trauma or disease
arthrocentesis	ar-thro-sen-<u>te</u>-sis	puncture of a joint cavity to remove fluid
arthroplasty	<u>ar</u>-thro-plas-ty	surgery to relieve pain and restore range of motion by realigning or reconstructing a joint; e.g., of the wrist, knee, or hip
arthroscopy	ahr-thros-<u>kuh</u>-pe	examination of the interior of a joint with an endoscope
arthrotomy	ar-throt-<u>o</u>-me	surgical creation of an opening into a joint such as for drainage
external fixation	eks-<u>ter</u>-nal fik-<u>sa</u>-shun	the process of making a bone immovable; a rod and screws are placed on the outside of the bone (see Figure 17-9)

(continues)

TABLE **17-11** (continued)

Procedure	Pronunciation	Definition
fracture reduction	frak-chur re-duk-shun	the correction of a fracture, luxation
joint replacement (arthroplasty)	joint re-place-ment	replacement of a damaged joint with an artificial joint to relieve chronic pain caused by osteoporosis or rheumatoid arthritis; most commonly for the knee or hip
kyphoplasty	kī-fo-plas-tē	treatment of a compression fracture of the vertebrae by inserting a balloon into the spine to create a space for injecting a bone cement mixture; done to stabilize the vertebrae to prevent pinching of the spinal cord and pain
laminectomy with discectomy	lam-i-nek-to-me dis-kek-to-me	laminectomy is the excision of the lamina or spongy tissue between the discs in the spine; discectomy is the excision of an injured disc; procedures used to relieve the symptoms of a herniated disc (see Figure 17-3)
meniscectomy	men-i-sek-to-me	excision of a meniscus, e.g., the fibrocartilage of the knee joint
transplantation	re-plan-ta-shun	insertion of donor organ or tissue, e.g., meniscus transplant in someone with a torn meniscus
spondylosyndesis	spon-di-lo-sin-de-sis	surgical procedure in which vertebrae are joined; spinal fusion
Other Treatments		
electrical stimulation	e-lek-tri-kal stim-u-la-shun	a process used to heal fractures more quickly
Traction	trak-shun	the act of drawing or pulling to align a bone or bones after a fracture

THE ORIGIN OF MEDICAL TERMS

Table 17-12 explains the Greek or Latin origin of several terms used in this chapter.

TABLE **17-12** The Origin of Medical Terms

Word	Pronunciation	Origin and Definition
acetabulum	as´-e-tab-u-lum	Latin, *acetum*, vinegar (small cup for vinegar) + Latin, *bulum*, vessel + Latin, *abulum*, denoting a container
bursa	ber-sah	Latin, *bursa mucosa*, mucus pouch from Medieval Latin, *bursa*, bag, purse from Greek, *byrsa*, hide, skin, wineskin, drum
carpal	kahr-puh-l	Latin, *carpālis*, from Greek *karpos*, wrist
gastrocnemius	gas-trok-nee-mus	Latin, *gastrocnēmius*, from Greek *gastroknēmiā*, calf of the leg *gastro-*, belly (from its belly-like shape) + Greek, *knēmē*, leg
hyoid	hahy-oid	Greek, *hyoeides*, shaped like the letter upsilon (υ)
latissimus dorsi	lah-tis-ih-mus dor-see	Latin, *musculus latissimus dorsi*, broadest muscle of the back

Word	Pronunciation	Origin and Definition
masseter	mass-<u>see</u>-ter	Greek, *masētēr*, from Greek, *masasthai*, to chew
meniscus	me-<u>nis</u>-kus	Greek, *mēniskos*, crescent, diminutive of *mēnē*, moon
spondylitis	spon´-di-<u>li</u>-tis	Greek, *spóndyl(os)*, vertebra + *-itis*, inflammation
sternum	<u>ster</u>-num	Greek, *sternon*, chest

ABBREVIATIONS

These abbreviations are frequently used to describe the musculoskeletal system, including clinical disorders and diagnostic tools (**Table 17-13**).

TABLE **17-13** Abbreviations

Abbreviation	Definition	Abbreviation	Definition
ANA	antinuclear antibodies	OA	osteoarthritis
ASO	antistreptolysin O	ORIF	open reduction internal fixation
CRP	C-reactive protein	RA	rheumatoid arthritis
DJD	degenerative joint disease	RF	rheumatoid factor
JRA	juvenile rheumatoid arthritis	SLE (LE)	systemic lupus erythematosus (lupus erythematosus)
MRI	magnetic resonance imaging	SR (ESR)	sedimentation rate (erythrocyte sedimentation rate)

The following box lists two different categories of medications that may be prescribed by a physician treating musculoskeletal diseases.

PHARMACOLOGY AND MEDICAL TERMINOLOGY

Drug Classification	skeletal muscle relaxant (<u>skell</u>-eh-tal muscle rih-<u>lak</u>-sant)	nonsteroidal anti-inflammatory drug (NSAID) (non-ste-<u>roid</u>-l anti in-<u>flam</u>-uh-tawr-ee)
Function	relieves muscle tension	reduces pain, inflammation, and swelling
Word Parts	**skelet/o** = skeleton; **-al** = pertaining to; **muscul/o** = muscle; **-e** = noun ending	**anti-** = against; **inflammatory** = pertaining to inflammation.
Active Ingredients (examples)	dantrolene sodium (Dantrium); carisoprodol (Soma); cyclobenzaprine-hydrochloride (Flexiril)	acetylsalicylic acid (aspirin, Bayer Children's Aspirin); ibuprofen (Advil, Motrin, Nuprin) naproxen (Aleve)

CLINICAL
Note

ORTHOPEDIC FOLLOW-UP NOTE

CC: Post-op follow-up for left femur fracture

HPI: Status postsurgery

Seventy-six-year-old white female: Patient underwent **open reduction** and **internal fixation** of left **supracondylar femur fracture** and now returns for follow-up.

X-ray: Fixation in place, mild **osteopenia**, no significant change since surgery

Exam: Wound healed well

Extension of left knee: 20 degrees short of full **ROM**

Flexion of left knee: Greater than 90 degrees

IMP: Patient improving well, to return for follow-up in 6 weeks. X-ray of left knee at that time

Direction: For the portions of the clinical note shown by a colored font, provide the definition and/or words for abbreviation.

LESSON TWO | **Progress Check**

LIST: THE MUSCULOSKELETAL SYSTEM

List the four major functions of the musculoskeletal system and one example of each.

1. _____

2. _____

3. _____

4. _____

MATCHING: LOCATIONS OF BONES

Match medical terms for bones of the axial skeletal system listed on the left with their locations listed on the right.

Medical Term	**Common Term**
1. Palatinte	**a.** Lower jaw
2. Frontal	**b.** Upper jaw
3. Temporal	**c.** Bone at base of the skull
4. Parietal	**d.** Nasal bone
5. Occipital	**e.** Upper nasal spongy bone between the eyes
6. Mandible	**f.** Hard palate (roof of the mouth)
7. Maxilla	**g.** Forehead
8. Sphenoid	**h.** Top of the skull
9. Turbinate	**i.** Bones at the temple
10. Ethmoid	**j.** Cuplike bone at the base of the skull

MULTIPLE CHOICE: BONES

Circle the letter of the correct answer:

1. The clavicle is:
    a. the rib bone
    b. the collar bone
    c. the breastbone
    d. the thigh bone

2. The sternum is:
    a. the collar bone
    b. the breastbone
    c. the thigh bone
    d. the nasal bone

3. The femur is:
    a. the thigh bone
    b. the nasal bone
    c. the breastbone
    d. a bone in the forearm

4. The radius and ulna are:
    a. leg bones
    b. shoulder blades
    c. bones in the forearm
    d. thigh bones

5. The fibula and tibia are:
    a. bones in the forearm
    b. breastbones
    c. thigh bones
    d. leg bones

6. The number of vertebrae in the vertebral column is:
    a. 18
    b. 22
    c. 26
    d. 30

7. The longitudinal axis is commonly called:
    a. the tailbone
    b. the backbone
    c. the lower leg
    d. the upper arm

8. The bone that goes from pelvis to knee is the:
    a. coccyx
    b. humerus
    c. femur
    d. tibia

9. The radius is to the ulna as the:
    a. maxilla is to the mandible
    b. clavicle is to the sternum
    c. occipital is to the parietal
    d. tibia is to the fibula

10. Carpal bones are:
    a. wrist bones
    b. hand bones
    c. ankle bones
    d. finger and toe bones

NAME THE STRUCTURE: JOINTS AND ACCESSORY PARTS

Name the following joints and accessory parts from the word pool given below the descriptions:

1. _____ : A fluid-filled sac located in tissues.

2. _____ : A sheet of fibrous tissue holding muscles together.

3. _____ : Flattened part of the vertebral arch.

4. _____ : Band of fibrous tissue.

5. _____ : A flattened connecting tendon.

6. _____ : Elbows, knees, and fingers.

7. _____ : Lines of junction between the bones of the skull.

8. _____ : Hip and shoulder joints.

9. _____ : Fibrous cord of connective tissue.

10. _____ : Crescent-shaped fibrous cartilage in the knee.

Word Pool: Aponeurosis, ball and socket, bursa, fascia, hinge joint, lamina, ligament, meniscus, sutures, tendons

MATCHING: MUSCLES

Match the muscle conditions at the left to their definitions on the right:

Muscle Condition
1. Atrophy
2. Hypertrophy
3. Tone
4. Paralysis
5. Contracture

Definition
a. Permanent drawing together
b. Loss of contraction caused by nerve damage
c. Wasting from disuse
d. Enlargement from overuse
e. Normal vigor and tension

MATCHING: MUSCULOSKELETAL INJURY

Match the musculoskeletal injury to its clinical name:

Musculoskeletal Injury
1. Common sports injury
2. Partial dislocation
3. Displacement of a vertebra
4. Broken bone anywhere
5. Broken bone in the head

Clinical Name
a. Subluxation
b. Spondylolisthesis
c. Skull fracture
d. Torn ligament
e. Fracture

MATCHING: MUSCULOSKELETAL INFLAMMATION

The musculoskeletal system is prone to many types of inflammation. Match the condition listed at the left to its *location* in the right column:

Musculoskeletal Inflammation
1. Arthritis
2. Bursitis
3. Myositis
4. Osteochondritis
5. Osteomyelitis
6. Spondylitis
7. Tendonitis
8. Plantar fasciitis
9. Mastoiditis

Location
a. In a tendon
b. In the bone and bone marrow
c. In the mastoid bone
d. In the plantar fascia
e. In the bone and cartilage
f. In a bursa
g. In a joint
h. In a voluntary muscle
i. In a vertebrae

COMPARE AND CONTRAST: MUSCULOSKELETAL DISEASES

Explain the differences in the following clinical disorders:
Example: Osgood-Schlatter disease/Legg-Calvé-Perthes disease: Osgood-Schlatter disease is inflammation of the tibia caused by chronic irritation; Legg-Calvé-Perthes disease is inflammation of the head of the femur in children.

1. Kyphosis/lordosis _____
2. Osteomalacia/rickets _____
3. Lyme disease/rheumatic fever _____
4. Muscular dystrophy/myositis _____
5. Osteomyelitis/osteoporosis _____
6. Sarcoma/scoliosis _____
7. Juvenile rheumatoid arthritis/rheumatoid arthritis _____
8. Closed fracture/open fracture _____
9. Complicated fracture/comminuted fracture _____
10. Impacted fracture/incomplete fracture _____

IDENTIFYING WORD PARTS

For each of the medical terms, list the root word and the prefix and/or suffix.

Word	Root Word	Prefix	Suffix
1. Abduction			
2. Acetabulum			
3. Articulation			
4. Arthroplasty			
5. Bursitis			
6. Fasciitis			
7. Intervertebral			
8. Lordosis			
9. Osteomalacia			
10. Subluxation			

© teekid/iStock/Getty Images

Eyes and Ears

OBJECTIVES

After completing this chapter and the exercises, the student should be able to:

1. Identify and label the structures of the eyes and ears.
2. Describe the functions of the eyes and ears.
3. Define and explain various pathologic conditions affecting the eyes and ears.
4. Identify important diagnostic tools and treatment for conditions of these special sense organs.
5. Use correctly spelled terminology to build medical words related to structure, function, and pathologic conditions of these special sense organs.
6. Define commonly used abbreviations.

EYES AND EARS

Eyes and ears are part of special senses that stem from the peripheral nervous system.

The Eye

The eye (**Figure 18-1**) is an optical system that focuses light rays on photoreceptors, which change light energy to nerve impulses. Human eyes are spherical organs located in bony orbits, or eye sockets, cavities formed by the bones of the skull. The eye is embedded in orbital fat for insulation and protection. It is attached to the orbit by six muscles, the extrinsic eye muscles, which control eye movement. Small tendons connect these muscles to the outermost layer of the eye. Structures of the eye include:

1. The *sclera* is the tough, white outer layer of the eyeball that protects the interior of the eye. At the front of the eye, the sclera forms a domed transparent orb called the *cornea*. The cornea has a curved surface that focuses light coming into the eye.
2. The *uvea* is the vascular layer below the sclera. It supplies blood to muscles and nerves within the eye and gives the eye its color. It contains three structures: the choroid, the ciliary body, and the iris.

ALLIED HEALTH PROFESSIONS

Dispensing Opticians, Ophthalmic Laboratory Technicians, Pharmacy Technicians, and Pharmacy Aides

Dispensing opticians fit eyeglasses and contact lenses, following prescriptions written by ophthalmologists or optometrists. They examine written prescriptions to determine corrective lens specifications. They recommend eyeglass frames, lenses, and lens coatings after considering the prescription and the customer's occupation, habits, and facial features. Dispensing opticians measure clients' eyes, including the distance between the centers of the pupils and the distance between the eye surface and the lens. Dispensing opticians prepare work orders that give ophthalmic laboratory technicians the information needed to grind and insert lenses into a frame.

Ophthalmic laboratory technicians make prescription eyeglasses or contact lenses. These technicians cut, grind, edge, and finish lenses according to specifications provided by dispensing opticians, optometrists, or ophthalmologists, and may insert lenses into frames to produce finished glasses. The technician reads prescription specifications, selects standard glass or plastic lens blanks, and then marks them to indicate where the curves specified on the prescription should be ground.

Next, the technician examines the lens through a lensometer to make sure that the degree and placement of the curve is correct. Then the lenses are cut and the edges beveled to fit the frame and dipped in solution to tint or coat the lenses. The final lens is placed into the glass frame for the final product.

Pharmacy technicians, assistants, and/or aides help licensed pharmacists provide medication and other healthcare products to patients. Pharmacy technicians usually perform more complex tasks than assistants do, although in some states their duties and job titles overlap. Technicians typically perform routine tasks, such as counting and labeling, to help prepare prescribed medication for patients.

However, a pharmacist must check every prescription before it can be given to a patient. Technicians refer any questions regarding prescriptions, drug information, or health matters to the pharmacist. Pharmacy assistants or aides usually have fewer, less complex responsibilities than pharmacy technicians do. Aides and assistants are often clerks or cashiers who primarily answer telephones, handle money, stock shelves, and perform other clerical duties.

Pharmacy aides also perform administrative duties in pharmacies. They work closely with pharmacy technicians. Aides refer any questions regarding prescriptions, drug information, or health matters to a pharmacist.

INQUIRY

American Board of Opticianry: www.abo.org
National Contact Lens Examiners: www.abo-ncle.org
Pharmacy Technician Certification Board: www.ptcb.org
Institute for the Certification of Pharmacy Technicians: www.nationaltechexam.org
National Pharmacy Technician Association: www.pharmacytechnician.org

Data from Cross, Nanna, and McWay, Dana. *Stanfield's Introduction to the Health Professions*, 7th ed. Burlington, MA: Jones & Bartlett Learning; 2017.

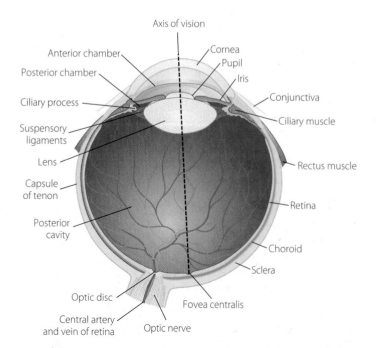

FIGURE 18-1 Transverse section showing the structure of the eye.

3. The *choroid*, a darkly pigmented layer of tissue, houses many tiny blood vessels and acts to absorb light within the eye. This prevents blurring of visual images. The *ciliary body*, an extension of the choroid, enables the eye to focus on objects of varying distances. Another extension of the choroid is the *iris*. Pigmentation of the iris is what determines the eye color. At the center of the iris is an opening called the *pupil*. The pupil of the eye expands and contracts, regulating the amount of light entering the eye.

4. On the inner surface of the choroid is the *retina*, light-sensitive receptor cells. The retina contains rods and cones that detect color stimuli (*photopigments*), which it sends to the brain for interpretation.

5. The *optic nerve* carries impulses from the retina to areas of the brain that are responsible for processing visual information.

6. Although not involved in vision directly, the eyelids and eyelashes protect the eyeball from physical trauma. A thin membrane known as *conjunctiva* lines the inside of each eyelid.

7. The *lacrimal* glands of the eye produce tears, which keep the eye lubricated.

The Ear

The ear (**Figure 18-2**) has three distinct and anatomically separate sections: the outer, middle, and inner ears.

The middle ear lies within the temporal bones of the skull. It contains three tiny bones, the auditory ossicles. They are named for their shapes. Starting from the outside, they are the *malleus* (hammer), *incus* (anvil), and *stapes* (stirrup). The malleus is connected to the *tympanic membrane*.

The middle ear cavity opens to the pharynx via the *Eustachian tube*, also called the auditory tube. The Eustachian tube serves as a pressure valve. Yawning and swallowing open the tube to equalize pressure within the middle ear.

The inner ear is a mazelike structure that occupies a large cavity in the temporal bone. It consists of bony and membranous structures surrounded by fluid. It contains two sensory organs—the *cochlea*, a snail shell-shaped bony structure that houses the organs of hearing, and the *vestibular apparatus*.

The *cochlea* is a hollow, bony spiral containing three fluid-filled canals: the *upper vestibular canal*, the *middle cochlear canal*, and the *lower tympanic canal*.

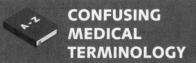

CONFUSING MEDICAL TERMINOLOGY

core/o versus corne/o

core/o – pupil (also pupill/o), e.g., coreoplasty (<u>kor</u>-ree-o-plas-te), also called coroplasty, refers to plastic surgery to correct a deformed or occluded pupil of the eye

corne/o – cornea, e.g., corneal (<u>kor</u>-ne-al) refers to pertaining to the cornea of the eye

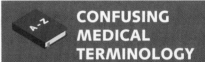

CONFUSING MEDICAL TERMINOLOGY

oral versus aural

oral – pertaining to the mouth

aural – pertaining to the ear

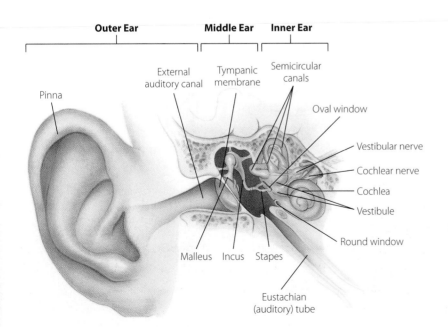

FIGURE 18-2 Frontal diagram of the outer ear, middle ear, and inner ear.

The *organ of Corti* contains the receptor cells, tiny hair cells that are stimulated by sound vibrations. The sound vibrations are then converted to nerve impulses that are transmitted to the brain for interpretation.

To summarize briefly how we hear, let us create a pathway of sound waves through the ear by structure and function:

1.   The outer ear auricle (*pinna*) funnels sound waves into the external auditory canal, which directs it to the tympanic membrane (eardrum) causing it to vibrate.
2.   The middle ear, which contains the eardrum *ossicles*, the malleus, incus, and stapes, vibrate when struck by the sound waves and transmit the sound to the cochlea in the inner ear by causing the oval window to vibrate the fluids within the canals.
3.   The cochlea converts the fluid waves to nerve impulses. The semicircular canals, the *sacculi* and *utricle*, detect head movement and linear acceleration and are often described as the *organ of balance*.
4.   The auditory nerve fibers that lie close to the hair cells of the organ of Corti pick up the sound wave impulses and transmit them to the cerebral cortex of the brain, where they are interpreted and we are able to hear.

-   *Opticians* specialize in examining the eye when prescription lens are needed.
-   *Ophthalmologists* are physicians who specialize in diseases and treatment of the eye.
-   *Otolaryngologists* are physicians who specialize in the diagnosis and management of diseases of the ears, including hearing loss, balance disorders, and congenital disorders of the inner and outer ear.

All the structures and functions pertaining to the eyes and ears are defined and illustrated throughout the chapter. Major disorders and diseases are also defined and discussed.

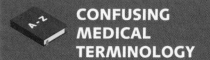

CONFUSING MEDICAL TERMINOLOGY

mallei versus malleoli

mallei (mal-<u>ee</u>-ahy) – the outermost of a chain of three small bones in the middle ear of mammals; also called hammer

malleoli (mah-le´-o-<u>lahy</u>) – two rounded processes on the distal tibia and fibula

---

LESSON ONE	Materials to Be Learned

STRUCTURES OF THE EYE

Figure 18-1 and **Table 18-1** describe the anatomic parts of the eye.

TABLE **18-1** Structures of the Eye

Structure	Pronunciation	Definition
aqueous humor	<u>a</u>-kwe-us <u>hu</u>-mor	watery liquid in the chamber in front of the lens; it circulates through the anterior chamber of the eye
canal of Schlemm	kah-<u>nal</u> of shlem	opening through which aqueous humor must flow out or pressure in the eye increases, resulting in glaucoma
canthus (plural: canthi)	<u>kan</u>-thus	the angle at either end of the fissure between the eyelids
choroid	<u>ko</u>-roid	the middle, vascular coat of the eye, between the sclera and the retina
ciliary muscle	<u>sil</u>-e-er´-e <u>mus</u>-el	eye muscle capable of changing lens shape during contraction and relaxation
conjunctiva	kon´-junk-<u>ti</u>-vah	membrane lining the eyelids and covering the eyeball

Structure	Pronunciation	Definition
cornea	<u>kor</u>-ne-ah	transparent anterior part of the eye; barrier against dirt, germs, and other particles that can harm the eye; responsible for focusing light on the retina
fovea	<u>fo</u>-vea	depression in the retina that contains only cones (not rods); area of highest visual acuity
fundus	<u>fun</u>-dus	the back portion of the interior of the eyeball, visible through the pupil by use of the ophthalmoscope
iris	<u>i</u>-ris	pigmented membrane behind the cornea, perforated by the pupil
lacrimal glands/tear glands	lac-ri-<u>mal</u> glands	lie in the upper, outer corner of the bony eye socket into small ducts behind the upper lid
lens	lenz	transparent body separating the posterior chamber and constituting the refracting mechanism of the eye
meibomian gland	mei-<u>bo</u>-mian gland	gland in the eyelids that discharges an oily lubricant through tiny openings in the edges of the lids
orbit	<u>or</u>-bit	bony eye socket
photoreceptor	pho-to- re-<u>cep</u>-tor	light-sensitive cells (cones and rods) in the retina; cones are located in the central retina and control color vision; rods are located outside the *fovea* and control black/white and low-light vision
pupil	<u>pu</u>-pil	opening in the center through which light enters the eye
retina	<u>ret</u>-i-nah	innermost layer of the eyeball containing elements for reception and transmission of visual stimuli; converts light into electrical impulses that travel through the optic nerve to the brain
sclera	<u>skle</u>-rah	tough white outer coat of the eyeball
trabecula	tra-<u>bec</u>-u-la	tissue lying between the anterior chamber of the eye and the canal of Schlemm; allows drainage of aqueous humor
vitreous humor	<u>vit</u>-re-us <u>hu</u>-mor	jellylike transparent substance in the posterior chamber

EYE DISORDERS

Figure 18-3 shows retinoblastoma, an eye disorder. **Table 18-2** is a list of various other disorders of the eye.

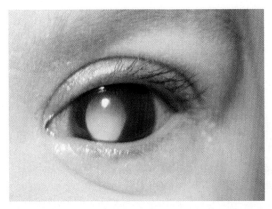

FIGURE 18-3 Retinoblastoma of an eye that appears as a pale mass of tissue seen through the dilated pupil.

TABLE **18-2** Eye Disorders

Disorder	Pronunciation	Definition
age-related macular degeneration (AMD)	age-re-<u>la</u>-ted <u>mac</u>-u-lar de-gen-er-<u>a</u>-tion	deterioration of the macula of the eye, resulting in a severe loss of central vision in the affected eye
amblyopia/lazy eye	am´-ble-<u>o</u>-pe-ah	undeveloped central vision in one eye that leads to the use of the other eye as the dominant eye; strabismus is most common cause. Symptoms are closing one eye to see
astigmatism	ah-<u>stig</u>-mah-tism	condition characterized by irregular cornea and lens of the eye; corrected with lenses
blepharitis	blef´-ah-<u>ri</u>-tis	inflammation of the eyelids
cataract	<u>kat</u>-ah-rakt	condition of aging; opaque (not clear) lens of the eye blocks light from focusing on the retina causing blurred vision; caused by clumping of protein within the lens
chalazion	kah-<u>la</u>-ze-on	a small eyelid mass resulting from chronic inflammation of a meibomian gland
color blindness	<u>kul</u>-er <u>blind</u>-nes	popular term for any deviation from normal perception of color; three different kinds of cones that respond to blue, green, and red light; red-green color blindness is the most common, followed by blue-yellow color blindness
conjunctivitis/pink eye	kon-junk´-ti-<u>vi</u>-tis	inflammation of the conjunctiva; can be caused by viral or bacterial infections, allergies, or environmental pollutants
corneal dystrophies	<u>cor</u>-ne-al <u>dys</u>-tro-phies	loss of clarity due to a buildup of material that clouds the cornea; depending on the severity of the disorder, light is blocked from focusing on the retina, causing impaired vision
corneal ulcer	<u>kor</u>-ne-al <u>ul</u>-ser	a local inflammation of the cornea caused by injury or inflammation
dacryoadenitis	dak´-re-o-ad´-e-<u>ni</u>-tis	inflammation of a lacrimal gland
dacryocystitis	dak-re-o-sis-<u>ti</u>-tis	inflammation of the lacrimal sac
dacryolith	<u>dak</u>-re-o-lith´	a lacrimal calculus (stone)
diabetic retinopathy	<u>dye</u>-ah´-bet-ic´ <u>reh</u>-tin-op´-ah-thee´	scarring of the capillaries of the retina as a consequence of diabetes mellitus (DM); retinal effects include abnormal dilation of the retinal veins, hemorrhage, microaneurysms, and neovascularization (new blood vessels forming near the optic disk causing leakage of blood). Can cause a decline in vision and blindness
diplopia	di-<u>plo</u>-pi-a	double vision; caused by strabismus
dry eye		caused by aging, certain medications, and health conditions; inadequate tears to keep the eye surface adequately lubricated; symptoms are scratchy, stinging or burning of the eyes, and blurred vision
exopthalmos	ex-oph-<u>thal</u>-mos	protrusion of the eyeball from the orbit; caused by injury or a tumor; if bilateral, may be caused by hyperthyroidism
floaters (in vitreous)/spots before the eyes	<u>flo</u>-ters	Deposits in the vitreous of the eye usually move about and are probably a benign degenerative change; also seen in hypertension

Disorder	Pronunciation	Definition
foreign body in the eye	for-in bod-e	any object not belonging to the eye; hazards depending on circumstances
glaucoma	glaw-ko-mah	eye disease characterized by an increase in intraocular pressure related to alterations in circulation of vitreous humor, causing pathologic changes and blindness if untreated
hemorrhage (subconjunctival)	hem-o-rij (sub´-kon-junk-ti-val)	blood escaping from the vessels and bleeding from beneath the conjunctiva
herpes zoster/shingles (ophthalmic)	her-pez zos-ter shin-gles (of-thal-mic)	caused by the same virus that causes chicken pox. The virus can remain dormant in the body and appear later as shingles which can cause blindness; receiving the shingles vaccination reduces the chances of getting shingles
hyperopia/farsightedness	hi´-per-o-pe-ah	difficulty with vision at a close range; if severe, can cause blurring at any distance
hypertropia	hy-per-tro-pi-a	condition of strabismus; deviating eye turns upward
injury	in-ju-re	eye injuries include foreign bodies, contusions, lacerations, burns, and more
intraocular pressure (IOP)	in-tra-oc-u-lar pres-sure	pressure of fluid within the eye; with aging, the trabecular meshwork may become sclerotic and obstructed, preventing the normal flow of aqueous humor and causing an increase in the intraocular pressure or glaucoma
iritis	i-ri-tis	inflammation of the iris
keratitis	ker-a-ti-tis	inflammation of the cornea; can be caused by viral or bacterial infections, allergies, or excessive exposure to sunlight
keratoconus	ker-ah-to-ko-nus	conical protrusion of the central part of the cornea
meibomian cyst	mi-bo-me-an	a small localized swelling of the eyelid resulting from obstruction and retained secretions of the meibomian glands; a nonmalignant condition; often requires surgery for correction
myopia/nearsightedness	my-o-pi-a/near-sight-ed-ness	able to see close objects clearly, but objects at a distance appear blurry
nystagmus	nis-tag-mus	involuntary rapid movement (horizontal, vertical, rotary, or mixed, i.e., of two types) of the eyeball
papilledema	pap´-il-e-de-mah	edema of the optic disk
presbyopia	pres-be-o-pe-ah	diminution of accommodation of the lens of the eye caused by loss of elasticity, normally occurring with aging; farsightedness
pterygium/surfer's eye	te-rig-e-um/sur-fers eye	growth of pink, fleshy tissue on the conjunctiva; caused by exposure to UV light, dust, wind, or dry eyes
ptosis	to-sis	drooping of upper eyelid
refractive error	re-frac-tive error	the shape of the eye prevents a clear image from being focused on the retina causing any of these: myopia, hyperopia, presbyopia, and astigmatism; can be corrected with eyeglasses or contact lens

(continues)

TABLE **18-2** (continued)

Disorder	Pronunciation	Definition
retinal detachment (RD)	<u>ret</u>-i-nal de-<u>tach</u>-ment	separation of retina from choroid; caused by retinal tear and seeping of vitreous fluid underneath the retina; cryotherapy is used to reattach the retina
retinitis	ret´-i-<u>ni</u>-tis	inflammation of the retina
retinoblastoma	ret´-i-no-blas-<u>to</u>-mah	a tumor arising from the retinal cells (see Figure 18-3)
retinopathy	ret´-i-<u>nop</u>-ah-the	any disease of the retina
retinopathy of prematurity (ROP)	ret´-i-<u>nop</u>-ah-the pre-ma-<u>tu</u>-ri-ty	abnormal development of retinal blood vessels in some premature infants (born before 31 weeks); when severe, can cause the retina to detach from the wall of the eye and possibly blindness
strabismus/cross-eyed	strah-<u>biz</u>-mus	deviation of the eye from normal; inability to maintain binocular vision due to muscle imbalance in one eye; affected eye turns in, out, up, or down
stye	sti	red bump that forms on or in the lower or upper eyelid as the result of a blocked gland; other symptoms are swelling of the eyelid
trachoma	trah-<u>ko</u>-mah	contagious disease of the conjunctiva and cornea, producing photophobia, pain, and lacrimation; caused by a bacterium called *Chlamydia trachomatis*. Disease of developing nations where poverty, crowded living conditions, and poor sanitation allow spread of the disease
uveitis	u´-ve-<u>i</u>-tis	inflammation of the uvea (iris and blood vessels)
xerophthalmia	xe-roph-<u>thal</u>-mi-a	dry, thickened condition of the eyeball; caused by severe vitamin A deficiency in developing countries; can cause ulceration of the cornea and ultimately blindness

TERMS USED IN THE DIAGNOSIS AND TREATMENT OF EYE DISORDERS

Table 18-3 defines terms used in the diagnosis and treatment of eye disorders.

TABLE **18-3** Terms Used in the Diagnosis and Treatment of Eye Disorders

Term	Pronunciation	Definition
History and Physical Exam		
accommodation	ah-kom´-o-<u>da</u>-tion	normal adjustment of the eye for seeing objects at various distances
anisocoria	an´-i-so-<u>ko</u>-re-ah	inequality in size of the pupils of the eyes
best corrected visual acuity (BCVA)	best cor-<u>rect</u>-ed <u>vis</u>-ual acu-i-ty	best vision achieved with correction with glasses or contact lens, as measured on the standard Snellen eye chart
CC		with correction (glasses or lenses)
diopter	di-<u>op</u>-ter	unit of measure for lenses
emmetropia	em´-e-<u>tro</u>-pe-ah	normal vision
esotopia/cross-eyed	es-o-<u>tro</u>-pi-a	form of strabismus; one or both eyes deviate inward

Term	Pronunciation	Definition
exotropia/walleyed	ex-o-<u>tro</u>-pi-a	form of strabismus; one or both eyes deviate outward
oculus dexter (OD)	<u>oc</u>-u-lus <u>dex</u>-ter	right eye
oculus sinister (OS)	<u>oc</u>-u-lus <u>sin</u>-is-ter	left eye
oculus unitas (OU)	<u>oc</u>-u-lus <u>u</u>-ni-tas	both eyes
peripheral vision	pe-<u>rif</u>-er-al <u>vizh</u>-un	vision at the outer edges when the eyes are looking straight ahead
PERRLA (or PERLA)	<u>per</u>-la	acronym for pupils equal, round, react to light, accommodation
refractive error	re-<u>frak</u>-tiv er-ror	the determination of the refractive errors of the eye and their correction with glasses or lenses
SC		without correction (glasses or lenses)
visual acuity (VA)	<u>vis</u>´ual <u>acu</u>´ity	clarity or clearness of vision
20/20 vision		a person who can read what the average person can read at 20 feet has 20/20 vision
Diagnostic Tools		
amsler grid	<u>am</u>-sler grid	grid with a pattern that resembles a checkerboard; used to screen for macular degeneration which affects central vision. Wavy, instead of straight lines, will appear for those who have the disorder
cryoprobe	<u>kri</u>-o-prob	an instrument for applying extreme cold to tissue
cystitome	<u>sis</u>-ti-tome	an instrument for opening the lens capsule
electronystagmography	e-lek´-tro-nis´-tag-<u>mog</u>-rah-fe	recordings of eye movements to provide objective documentation of induced and spontaneous nystagmus
intravenous fluorescein angiography (IVFA)	in-tra-<u>ve</u>-nous fluo-<u>res</u>-ce-in an-gi-<u>og</u>-ra-phy	imaging test in which a fluorescent vegetable dye is given intravenously; provides a detailed analysis of blood flow in the retina and choroid; used to diagnose diabetic retinopathy, macular degeneration, and other eye disorders
fundoscope/ ophthalmoscope	<u>fun</u>-dus-skōp/of-<u>thal</u>-mo-skōp	an instrument containing a perforated mirror and lenses used to examine the interior of the eye (fundus)
lensometer	lenz-<u>om</u>-e-ter	device for obtaining eyeglass prescriptions
gonioscopy	go´-ne-<u>os</u>-ko-pe	instrument for demonstrating ocular motility and rotation
keratometer	ker-a-<u>tom</u>-e-ter	instrument for measuring curvature of the anterior surface of the cornea
laser	<u>la</u>-zer	transfers light of various frequencies into an extremely intense, small beam of radiation; used as a tool in diagnosis and surgery
ocular and orbit ultrasonography/ ultrasound	<u>oc</u>-u-lar <u>or</u>-bit ul-tra-so-<u>nog</u>-ra-phy/<u>ul</u>-tra sound	sound waves pass through the eye and *orbit* and are electronically converted into 2-D graphics. Used to detect abnormalities of the eye and orbit: vitreous hemorrhage, detachment of the retina, ocular tumors, or cysts, alterations in corneal or ocular shape
Snellen eye chart	<u>snel</u>-len eye chart	one of several charts used in testing visual acuity; letters, numbers, or symbols are arranged on the chart in decreasing size from top to bottom

(continues)

TABLE 18-3 (*continued*)

Term	Pronunciation	Definition
slit lamp	slit lamp	used for examining conjunctiva, lens, vitreous humor, iris, and cornea; a high-intensity beam of light is projected through a narrow slit and a cross section of the illuminated part of the eye is examined through a magnifying lens
tonometer	to-<u>nom</u>-e-ter	instrument for measuring intraocular pressure
tonometry	to-<u>nom</u>-e-tre	measurement of tension or pressure, e.g., intraocular pressure
Treatment Including Surgery		
cataract extraction	<u>kat</u>-ah-rakt eks-<u>trak</u>-shun	a surgical excision of the lens of the eye and placement of intraocular lens
cryoextraction	kri´-o-eks-<u>trak</u>-shun	application of extremely low temperature for the removal of a cataractous lens
cryoretinopexy	kri´-o-<u>ret</u>-i-no-pex-ee	fixation of a detached retina using extremely low temperature instead of the laser beam
dacryocystotomy	dak´-re-o-sis-<u>tot</u>-o-me	incision of the lacrimal sac and duct
enucleation	e-nu´-kle-<u>a</u>-shun	surgical removal of the eye
eye bank	eye bank	storage for donor organs; eye donations provide tissue for corneal transplant surgery
guide dogs		trained dogs for the blind; also called seeing eye dogs
intraocular lens (IOL)	in-tra-<u>oc</u>-u-lar lens	artificial lens implanted after eye surgery to remove cataracts
iridectomy	ir´-i-<u>dek</u>-to-me	excision of part of the iris
iridencleisis	ir´-i-den-<u>kli</u>-sis	excision of part of the iris in glaucoma
keratoplasty/corneal graft	<u>ker</u>-ah-to-plas´-te/<u>cor</u>-ne-al graft	plastic surgery of the cornea; removal of the damaged portion of the cornea and the insertion in its place of a piece of cornea of the same size and shape from donor tissue
laser photocoagulation	<u>la</u>-zer fo´-to-ko-ag´-u-<u>la</u>-shun	using the laser beam to treat retinal detachment
miotic (or myotic)	mi-<u>ot</u>-ik	a drug that causes contraction of the pupil
mydriatic	mid´-re-<u>at</u>-ik	a drug that dilates the pupil
photorefractive keratectomy (PRX)	pho-to-re-<u>frac</u>-tive ker-a-<u>tec</u>-to-my	laser surgery used to reshape the cornea to correct myopia, hyperopia, or astigmatism
pterygium surgery	te-<u>rig</u>-e-um <u>ser</u>-jer-e	surgery to remove pink, fleshy tissue on the conjunctiva
radial keratotomy (RK)	radial ker-a-<u>tot</u>-o-my	surgical procedure on the cornea to correct myopia (distance vision)
trabeculectomy	trah-bek´-u-<u>lec</u>-to-me	excision of fibrous bands or connective tissue (*trabeculum*) to relieve pressure caused by glaucoma
vitrectomy	vi-<u>trek</u>-to-me	aspiration of vitreous fluid and replacement with saline solution

STRUCTURES OF THE EAR

Figure 18-2 and **Table 18-4** review the anatomical parts of the ear.

TABLE **18-4** Structures of the Ear		
Structure	**Pronunciation**	**Definition**
acoustic meatus	ah-koos-tik me-a-tus	opening or passage in the ear
eustachian tube	u-stay-shen tube	a tube lined with mucous membrane that joins the nasopharynx and the tympanic cavity; equalizes air pressure
external/outer ear	ex-ter-nal ou-ter ear	outer portion of the ear, including the auricle (or pinna) and ear canal extending to the tympanic membrane
inner ear	in-ner ear	the vestibule, semicircular canals, and cochlea, composing the membranous labyrinth
middle ear	mid-dle ear	separated from the external ear by the tympanic membrane; transmits sound waves between the middle and inner ears through a chain of three tiny bones: malleus, incus, and stapes
tympanic membrane/ eardrum	tim-pan-ik mem-brane/ear-drum	the thin partition between the external acoustic meatus and the middle ear
tympanum	tim-pan-um	eardrum (middle ear)

EAR DISORDERS

Table 18-5 describes common ear disorders.

TABLE **18-5** Ear Disorders		
Disorder	**Pronunciation**	**Definition**
acoustic neuroma	ah-koos-tic new-rom-ah	a benign tumor arising from the acoustic nerve in the brain that causes tinnitus, vertigo, and decreased hearing; small tumors may be surgically resected or removed by radiation therapy
auditory neuropathy	au-di-to-ry neu-rop-a-thy	hearing disorder in which sound enters the inner ear normally but the transmission of signals from the inner ear to the brain is impaired
cholesteatoma	koh-les-tee´-ah-toh-mah	collection of skin cells and cholesterol in a sac within the middle ear; can lead to conductive hearing loss; symptoms include weakness of facial muscles, vertigo, and earache
conduction deafness	kon-duk-shun def-nes	hearing loss that occurs when the conduction of sound waves through the external and middle ear to the inner ear is impaired
deafness	def-nes	lacking the sense of hearing; hearing impairment
eustachian salpingitis	u-stay-shen sal´-pin-ji-tis	inflammation of the eustachian tubes

(continues)

TABLE **18-5** (*continued*)		
Disorder	**Pronunciation**	**Definition**
furunculosis	fu-rung´-ku-<u>lo</u>-sis	a bacterial skin infection (boils) affecting the ear canal
impacted cerumen	im-<u>pak</u>-ted se-<u>roo</u>-men	cerumen (earwax) impacted firmly into the ear
labyrinthitis	lab´-i-rin-<u>thi</u>-tis	infection or inflammation of the labyrinth (inner ear); otitis interna; causes dizziness and loss of balance. Often associated with an upper respiratory infection such as the flu and is a temporary condition
mastoiditis	mas´-toi-<u>di</u>-tis	inflammation of the mastoid antrum and cells (of the temporal bone)
Meniere's disease	men´-e-<u>ārz</u> di-<u>zez</u>	buildup of fluid in the compartments of the inner ear called the labyrinth; symptoms are vertigo, tinnitus, and feeling of congestion in the ear; treated with medications
myringitis	mir´-in-<u>ji</u>-tis	inflammation of the tympanic membrane (eardrum)
otitis externa	o-<u>ti</u>-tis ex-<u>ter</u>-na	inflammation of the external ear
otitis media	o-<u>ti</u>-tis me-<u>di</u>-a	inflammation of the middle ear
otosclerosis	o´-to-skle-<u>ro</u>-sis	new bone tissue in the middle ear that immobilizes the stapes, resulting in conductive hearing loss
presbycusis	pres´-bĭ-<u>ku</u>-sis	progressive hearing loss associated with aging; progressive degeneration of cochlear structures and central auditory pathways; begins with the high frequencies, then progresses to sounds of middle and low frequencies
sensorineural deafness/ nerve deafness	<u>sen</u>-soh´-ree-<u>noo</u>-ral <u>def</u>-nes	results from physical damage to the hair cells, the vestibulocochlear nerve, or the auditory cortex; caused by aging, extremely loud noise, some antibiotics, or other medical conditions
tinnitus	ti-<u>ni</u>-tus	a noise (ringing) in the ears
vertigo	<u>ver</u>-ti-go	a sensation of rotation or dizziness

TERMS USED IN THE DIAGNOSIS AND TREATMENT OF EAR DISORDERS

Table 18-6 describes terms used in the diagnosis and treatment of ear disorders.

TABLE **18-6** Terms Used in the Diagnosis and Treatment of Ear Disorders		
Term	**Pronunciation**	**Definition**
History and Physical Exam		
auris dextra (AD)	<u>au</u>-ris <u>dex</u>-tra	right ear
auris sinstra (AS)	<u>au</u>-ris <u>sin</u>-is-ter	left ear

Term	Pronunciation	Definition
auris unitas (AU)	<u>au</u>-ris u-<u>ni</u>-tas	both ears
auris uterque (AU)	<u>au</u>-ris <u>uter</u>-que	each ear
auditory (or acoustic)	<u>aw</u>-di-to´-re (ah-<u>koos</u>-tik)	pertaining to the ear; sense of hearing

Diagnostic Tools

audiometer	aw´-de-<u>om</u>-e-ter	a device to test hearing
audiometrist	aw´-de-<u>om</u>-e-trist	person who performs hearing tests
computed tomography/ CT scan	com-<u>put</u>-ed <u>to</u>-mog-ra-phy	CT scanner uses X-rays and a computer to create images of the ears and surrounding structures
decibel	<u>des</u>-i-bel	a unit of measure of the intensity of sound
magnetic resonance imaging (MRI)	mag-<u>net</u>-ic <u>res</u>-o-nance <u>im</u>-ag-ing	use of radio waves in a magnetic field; a scanner creates high-resolution images of the ears and surrounding structures
otoscope	<u>o</u>-to-skōp	an instrument used for visual inspection of the eardrum and auditory canal, typically having a light and a set of lenses
otoscopy	o-<u>tos</u>-ko-pe	examination of the ear by means of the otoscope
tuning fork	<u>too</u>-ning	a small metal instrument consisting of a stem and two prongs used to test hearing

Treatment Including Surgery

audiologist	au-di-<u>ol</u>-o-gist	healthcare professional who specializes in the evaluation and rehabilitation of patients with communication disorders related to hearing impairment
cochlear implant	<u>kōk</u>-lē-er im-<u>plant</u>	electronic device surgically placed as treatment for severe to profound hearing loss; cochlear implant sends sound signals directly to the hearing nerve
fenestration	fen´-es-<u>tra</u>-shun	the surgical creation of a new opening in the labyrinth of the ear for restoration of hearing in otosclerosis
hearing aid	<u>hēr</u>-ing	a device used to increase the intensity of sound
hearing ear dogs	hear-ing ear dogs	dogs trained to respond to sounds and alert the person with hearing impairment
mastoidectomy	mas´-toi-<u>dek</u>-to-me	excision of the mastoid cells or the mastoid process
myringotomy	mir´-ing-<u>got</u>-o-me	incision of the tympanic membrane; tympanotomy with placement of tubes to maintain drainage
otoplasty	<u>o</u>-to-plas´-te	plastic surgery of the ear (pinna)
sign language	sine <u>lan</u>-gwij	communication with the deaf by means of manual signs and gestures

(continues)

TABLE 18-6 (*continued*)

Term	Pronunciation	Definition
speech language pathologist (SLP)	speech <u>lan</u>-guage pa-<u>thol</u>-o-gist	health professional trained to diagnose and treat patients with voice, speech, and language disorders; provides services after cochlear implant
stapedectomy	sta´-pe-<u>dek</u>-to-me	excision of the stapes
tympanoplasty	tim´-pah-no-<u>plas</u>-te	plastic surgery on the eardrum
tympanotomy	tim´-pah-<u>not</u>-o-me	myringotomy; incision of the tympanic membrane

BOX 18-1 describes cochlear implants and when they are used.

Box 18-1 What are Cochlear Implants and when are they Used?

Imagine hearing sound for the first time! Activation of a cochlear implant after surgical placement is a joyful occasion for the patient, family, and the entire healthcare team.

A cochlear implant is an electronic device that restores partial hearing to those with severe to profound hearing loss. Unlike a hearing aid, the implant does not make sound louder or clearer. Instead, the device bypasses damaged parts of the auditory system and directly stimulates the nerve of hearing, allowing those who are profoundly deaf to receive sound. An implant does not restore normal hearing. Instead, it can give a deaf person a representation of sounds in the environment and the means to understand speech.

Most often, surgery can successfully treat problems with the outer and middle ear, including the eardrum. However, when there is nerve deafness from damaged hair cells, hearing aids are not beneficial and a cochlear implant is appropriate. Candidates for a cochlear implant are children or adults with profound deafness because of damage to the inner ear. For children who were deaf at birth, the goal is to place the cochlear implant by 18 months of age to allow for the development of language skills comparable to the child's peers. An artificial cochlear placed in a child or adult who became deaf after a hearing loss will require less speech therapy after a cochlear implant than a child who has been deaf from birth. An entire team of health professionals—the physician, audiologist, nurse, social worker and speech and language pathologist—supports the patient and family after cochlear implant surgery.

Source: National Institutes of Deafness and Other Communication Disorders. National Institutes of Health. *Cochlear Implants*. https://www.nidcd.nih.gov/health/cochlear-implants

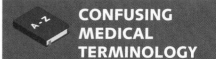

CONFUSING MEDICAL TERMINOLOGY

dysarthria versus **dysarthrosis**

dysarthria (dis-<u>ahr</u>-three-uh) – difficulty with speech, as in stammering or stuttering

dysarthrosis (dis-<u>ahr</u>-thro-sis) – any disorder of a joint

THE ORIGIN OF MEDICAL TERMS

Table 18-7 explains the origin of several terms used in diagnosing and treating diseases of the eye and ear.

TABLE 18-7 The Origin of Medical Terms

Word	Pronunciation	Origin and Definition
amblyopia	am´-ble-o-pe-ah	Greek, *amblyo*, dull or dim + Greek, *opia*, condition of the eye
anisocoria	an´-i-so-ko-re-ah	Greek, *aniso*, unequal + Greek, *kore*, pupil
cochlear	kok-le-er	Greek, *kochlías*, snail (with spiral shell)
diopter	di-op-ter	Greek, *di*, through + Greek, *opter*, visible
emmetropia	em´-e-tro-pe-ah	Greek, *émmetros*, in measure; Greek, *em*, before + Greek, *metr*, to measure + Greek, *opia*, condition of the eye
enucleation	e-nu´-kle-a-shun	Latin, *enucleo*, to remove the kernel French, *e*, out, + Latin, *nucleus*, nut, kernel
labyrinthitis	lab´-i-rin-thi-tis	New Latin, *labyrinthus*, maze, web + Greek, *itis*, inflammation
miotic (myotic)	mi-ot-ik (my-ot-ic)	Greek, *muein*, to shut the eyes + Greek, *osis*, condition
myopia	my-o-pi-a	Greek, *muōps*, shortsighted + Greek, *ōps*, eye
presbycusis	pres´-bĭ-ku-sis	Greek, *presbys*, old man, + Greek, *akousis*, hearing

ABBREVIATIONS

Table 18-8 lists abbreviations frequently used to describe eyes and ears, including clinical disorders, diagnosis, and treatment.

TABLE 18-8 Abbreviations

Abbreviation	Definition	Abbreviation	Definition
AD	auris dextra (right ear)	CT	computed tomography
AMD	age-related macular degeneration	IOL	intraocular lens
AS	auris sinstra (left ear)	IOP	intraocular pressure
AU	auris unitis (both ears) or auris uterque (each ear)	IVFA	intravenous fluorescein angiography
BCVA	best corrected visual acuity	MRI	magnetic resonance imaging
CC	with refractive correction (glasses or lens)	OD	oculus dexter (right eye)
OS	oculus sinister (left eye)	RK	radial keratotomy

(continues)

Abbreviation	Definition	Abbreviation	Definition
OU	oculus unitas (both eyes) or oculus uterque (each eye)	ROP	retinopathy of prematurity
PERRLA/ PERLA	pupils equal, round, react to light, accommodation	SC	without refractive correction (glasses or lens)
PRX	photo refractive keratectomy	SLP	speech and language pathologist
RD	retinal detachment	VA	visual acuity

TABLE 18-8 (continued)

The following box lists two different categories of medications that may be prescribed by a physician treating diseases of the eye or ear.

PHARMACOLOGY AND MEDICAL TERMINOLOGY

Drug Classification	antiviral agent (an-tih-<u>vye</u>-ral)	vitamin (<u>vigh</u>-tah-min)
Function	treats various viral conditions such as serious herpes virus infection, chickenpox, and influenza A	prevents and treats vitamin deficiencies and used as dietary supplement
Word Parts	**anti-** = against; **viral** = pertaining to a virus	pertaining to vital nutrient in the body
Active Ingredients (Examples)	acyclovir (Zovirax); vidarabine (Vira-A)	vitamins A, D, E, etc.; ascorbic acid (vitamin C); cyanocobalamin (vitamin B_{12})

CLINICAL  *Note*

Ophthalmology Initial Office Exam

Ocular History: Twenty-eight-year-old WM with history of mild **hyperopia** with moderate to severe **astigmatism**. Pt. now reports gradually decreasing vision **OS** at distance. Patient works as a truck driver and was unable to pass eye exam for license.

Medical Hx: Neg

Surgical Hx:
1. Tonsillectomy
2. Surgical repair Rt. Ankle

Family Hx: Cataract – Grandmother

Medications: None

Allergies: NKDA

Examination:

Acuity:	**Refraction**:	**BCVA**:
OD: −4.75 + 6.00 × 105	Manifest **Retinoscopy**	OD: 20/20
OS: −4.75 + 9.50 × 080	OD −4.75 + 6.00 × 105	OS: 20/40
	OS −6.25 + 10.00 × 077	

Plan: New Vision Prescription given. Patient to follow up at Work Vision Clinic.

Direction: For the portions of the clinical note shown by a colored font, provide the definition and/or words for abbreviation.

LESSON TWO	Progress Check

MATCHING: EYE STRUCTURES

For the list of terms on the left, select the correct definition on the right:

Eye Structure	Definition
1. Sclera	**a.** Watery liquid in front of the lens
2. Conjunctiva	**b.** Secrete tears
3. Cornea	**c.** Jellylike substance behind the lens
4. Iris	**d.** Innermost layer of the eyeball
5. Pupil	**e.** Refracting mechanism of the eye
6. Lens	**f.** White outer coating of the eye
7. Aqueous humor	**g.** Membrane lining the eyelids
8. Vitreous humor	**h.** Transparent anterior part of the eye
9. Retina	**i.** Pigmented membrane behind the cornea
10. Lacrimal glands	**j.** Opening through which light enters

MATCHING: EYE DISORDERS

For the list of eye disorders on the left, select the correct definition on the right:

Disorder of the Eye	Definition
1. Cataract	**a.** Irregular cornea and lens of the eye
2. Conjunctivitis	**b.** Inflammation of the lacrimal gland
3. Glaucoma	**c.** One eye fails to focus; instead, the eye turns up, down, in, or out
4. Hyperopia	**d.** Dry eye, ulceration of the cornea and possibly blindness; caused by severe vitamin A deficiency
5. Presbyopia	**e.** Pink eye
6. Astigmatism	**f.** Increase in intraocular pressure resulting in blindness
7. Strabismus	**g.** Farsightedness
8. Sty	**h.** Loss of elasticity of the lens; occurs with aging causing farsightedness
9. Xerophthalmia	**i.** Opaque lens resulting in blurred vision; occurs with aging
10. Dacryoadenitis	**j.** Red bump on the eyelid with swelling eyelid; caused by blocking of glands located on the eyelid

MULTIPLE CHOICE: EYE AND EAR

Circle the letter of the correct answer:

1. Deviation from normal color perception is a condition of:
   a. herpes zoster
   b. floaters
   c. cataracts
   d. color blindness

2. Foreign bodies, contusions, lacerations, and burns to the eye are conditions of:
   a. detached retinas
   b. blepharoptosis
   c. injuries
   d. retinopathies

3. The transparent anterior part of the eye is the:
   a. cornea
   b. iris
   c. lens
   d. pupil

4. A tonometer measures:
   a. intraocular pressure
   b. amount of light entering the eye
   c. adjustments for various distances
   d. inequality of size of the pupils

5. Which of the following terms denotes the creation of a new opening in the labyrinth of the ear?

    a.   Fenestration

    b.   Acoustic meatus

    c.   Otoplasty

    d.   Myringotomy

6. Plastic surgery on an eardrum is called:

    a.   tympanotomy

    b.   tympanoplasty

    c.   otoplasty

    d.   stapedectomy

7. The unit of measure of the intensity of sound is called a (an):

    a.   electronystagnometry

    b.   audiometry

    c.   decibel

    d.   tuning fork

8. Which of the following terms describes tinnitus?

    a.   Dizziness

    b.   Nausea

    c.   Intense sound

    d.   Ringing of the ears

9. *Vertigo* is the term used for:

    a.   a sensation of rotation

    b.   ringing of the ears

    c.   intense sound

    d.   sign communication

10. The term for corneal grafting is:

    a.   iridectomy

    b.   radial keratotomy

    c.   vitrectomy

    d.   keratoplasty

ABBREVIATIONS: EYE AND EAR

Write in the definition for the following abbreviations:

1. IOL: _____

2. CC: _____

3. OS: _____

4. OD: _____

5. AMD: _____

6. PERRLA: _____

7. VA: _____

8. AD: _____

9. RK: _____

10. IVFA: _____

MATCHING: STRUCTURES OF THE EAR

For the list of terms on the left, select the correct definition on the right:

Ear Structure	Definition
1. Eustachian tube	**a.** Maintain balance or equilibrium
2. Middle ear	**b.** Convert sound waves to nerve impulses
3. Inner ear	**c.** Eardrum
4. Outer ear	**d.** Contains three small bones: malleus, incus, stapes
5. Hair cells	**e.** Transmits sound wave impulses to the brain
6. Semicircular canals	**f.** Serves as a pressure valve
7. Tympanic membrane	**g.** Contains the vestibule, semicircular canals, and cochlea
8. Auditory nerve	**h.** The auricle (or pinna) and ear canal extending to the tympanic membrane

IDENTIFYING WORD PARTS: EYE AND EAR

For each of the medical terms, list the root word and the prefix and/or suffix:

Word	Root Word	Prefix	Suffix
1. Exotropia			
2. Fenestration			
3. Keratotomy			
4. Labyrinthitis			
5. Myringitis			
6. Neuroma			
7. Otoscope			
8. Subconjunctival			
9. Vertigo			
10. Xerophthalmia			

Endocrine System

OBJECTIVES

After completing this chapter and the exercises, the student should be able to:

1. Locate and name the endocrine glands and list the hormones produced by each gland.
2. Describe the major function(s) of each of the endocrine glands.
3. Build and define medical words related to the endocrine system.
4. Define and explain various pathologic conditions of the endocrine system.
5. Differentiate between diabetes mellitus, diabetes insipidus, and gestational diabetes.
6. Identify laboratory tests and clinical procedures related to endocrinology.
7. Identify and define abbreviations related to endocrinology.

THE ENDOCRINE SYSTEM

The endocrine system interacts with the nervous system to regulate and coordinate body activities (**Figures 19-1** and **19-2**). Integration of nervous and endocrine influences on the body occurs in the *hypothalamus*, a structure of the central nervous system (CNS). The endocrine system is cyclical in nature. Cycles occur over hours or days rather than seconds or minutes.

Endocrine glands have no ducts; instead, they secrete hormones directly into the blood or circulatory system; hormones then travel to cells of the target organ. In contrast, *exocrine* glands, such as salivary glands, secrete saliva into ducts. Endocrine control is regulated by chemical messengers (hormones). The word *hormone* comes from the Greek word *hormon*, which means to excite or stimulate. A *hormone* is a chemical product produced and released by the endocrine glands and transported by the blood to cells and organs of the body on which it has a specific regulatory effect. Hormones produce their effects by binding to receptors that are recognition sites in the various target cells. The target cells are very selective and respond only to specific hormones. Endocrine glands usually secrete more than one hormone. The parathyroid gland is the exception, secreting only parathyroid hormone.

ALLIED HEALTH PROFESSIONS

Emergency Medical Technicians and Paramedics

People's lives often depend on the quick reaction and competent care of emergency medical technicians (EMTs) and paramedics. Incidents as varied as automobile accidents, heart attacks, slips and falls, childbirth, and gunshot wounds all require immediate medical attention. EMTs and paramedics provide this vital service, as they care for and transport the sick or injured to a medical facility.

In an emergency, EMTs and paramedics are typically dispatched by a 911 operator to the scene, where they often work with police and firefighters. Once they arrive, EMTs and paramedics assess the nature of the patient's condition while trying to determine whether the patient has any preexisting medical conditions. Following medical protocols and guidelines, they provide appropriate emergency care and, when necessary, transport the patient. Some paramedics are trained to treat patients with minor injuries on the scene of an accident or they may treat them at their home without transporting them to a medical facility. Emergency treatment is carried out under the medical direction of physicians. EMTs and paramedics may use special equipment, such as backboards, to immobilize patients before placing them on stretchers and securing them in the ambulance for transport to a medical facility.

These healthcare workers generally go out in teams. During the transport of a patient, one EMT or paramedic drives while the other monitors the patient's vital signs and gives additional care as needed. Some paramedics work as part of a helicopter's flight crew to transport critically ill or injured patients to hospital trauma centers.

At the medical facility, EMTs and paramedics help transfer patients to the emergency department, report their observations and actions to emergency department staff, and may provide additional emergency treatment. After each run, EMTs and paramedics replace used supplies and check equipment. If a transported patient had a contagious disease, EMTs and paramedics decontaminate the interior of the ambulance and report cases to the proper authorities.

INQUIRY

National Association of Emergency Medical Technicians: PO Box 1400, Clinton, MS 39060-1400. www.naemt.org
National Highway Traffic Safety Administration, Office of Emergency Medical Services (NDP-400): 1200 New Jersey Ave., SE, Washington, DC 20590. www.ems.gov
National Registry of Emergency Medical Technicians: Rocco V. Morando Bldg., 6610 Busch Blvd., PO Box 29233, Columbus, OH 43229. www.nremt.org

Data from Cross, Nanna and McWay, Dana. *Stanfield's Introduction to the Health Professions*, 7th ed. Burlington, MA: Jones & Bartlett Learning; 2017.

Glands of the endocrine system include:

1. Anterior and posterior pituitary gland
2. Thyroid gland
3. Four parathyroid glands
4. Two adrenal glands
5. Islets of Langerhans in the pancreas
6. Two ovaries
7. Two testes
8. Pineal gland
9. Thymus gland

Three different types of stimuli trigger actions of endocrine glands:

1. *Humoral stimuli*: An example is regulation of blood glucose by the pancreas. High blood glucose levels stimulate the pancreas to secrete *insulin* while low blood glucose levels stimulate the pancreas to secrete *glucagon*. Insulin lowers blood glucose while glucagon raises blood glucose.
2. *Neural stimuli*: An example is the response of the sympathetic nervous system to stress. In response to stress, the adrenal gland secretes *epinephrine* and *norepinephrine*; other names for these hormones are adrenaline and noradrenaline. In times of short-term stress, for example, narrowly escaping a bicycle accident, these hormones increase heart rate and blood glucose to prepare the body for a quick response.

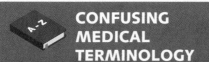

CONFUSING MEDICAL TERMINOLOGY

anter/o versus antr/o

anter/o – front, e.g., anterior (an-<u>teer</u>-eeer) refers to situated before or at the front of the body (as opposed to posterior)

antr/o – a cavity, e.g., nasoantritis (nazo-an-<u>try</u>-tis) refers to inflammation of the nose antrum (cavity)

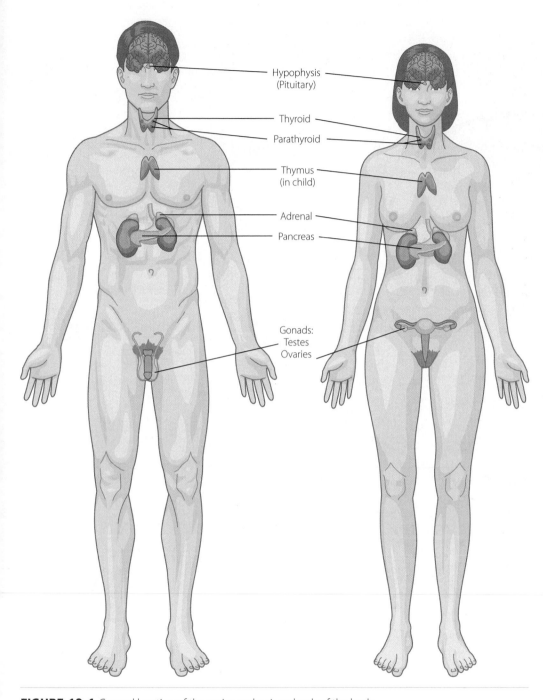

FIGURE 19-1 General location of the major endocrine glands of the body.

3. *Hormonal stimuli*: An example is when the hypothalamus regulates the secretion of the anterior pituitary hormones, *releasing hormones* and *inhibiting hormones* (see Figures 19-3). The cascade of events begins with environmental stress, such as cold environmental temperatures which stimulate the secretion of thyroid-stimulating hormone-releasing hormone (TSH-RH) from the hypothalamus. TSH-RH then stimulates the release of thyroid-stimulating hormone (TSH) from the anterior pituitary gland. TSH travels in the blood stream to the thyroid gland. Direct action of TSH on the thyroid gland is the secretion of thyroid hormone. The thyroid hormone increases heat production to warm the body.

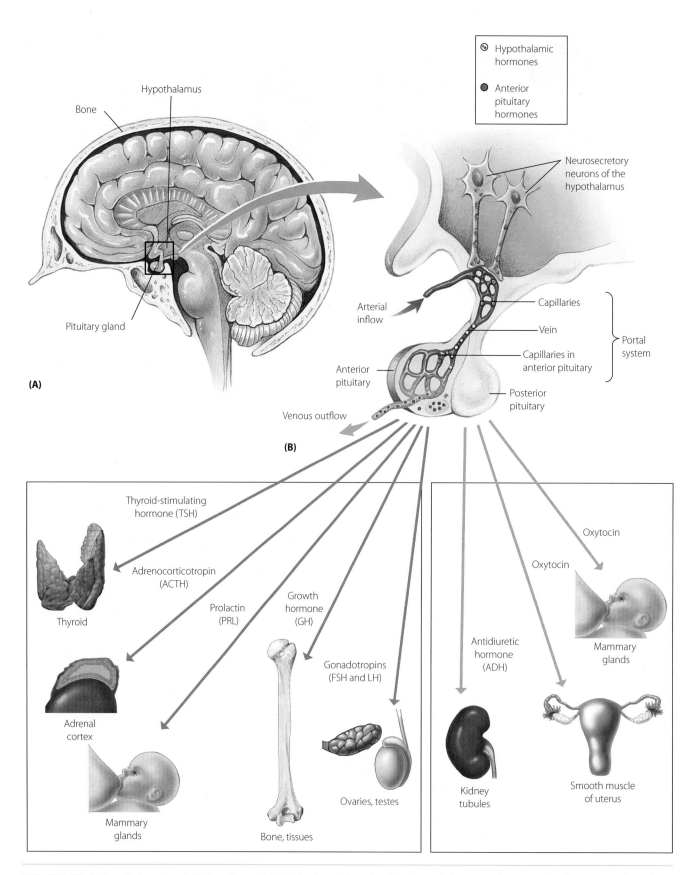

FIGURE 19-2 The pituitary gland: **(A)** Location within the brain and **(B)** role of the hypothalamus on the secretion of hormones from the anterior pituitary and the posterior pituitary.

Negative feedback is the mechanism that controls hormone secretion and maintains stable blood levels of hormones. The feedback loop is the response to changing blood levels of a hormone. As hormone levels rise, negative feedback inhibits the system and hormone secretion decreases. As hormone levels fall, positive feedback stimulates hormone secretion (**Figure 19-3**). Several steps are involved in the control of hormone secretion.

Many activities are regulated or influenced by the endocrine glands, including:

1. Reproduction and lactation
2. Immune system

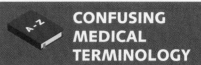

CONFUSING MEDICAL TERMINOLOGY

humor/o versus horm/o

humor/o – moisture, fluid, e.g., humoral (hu-mor-al), related to body fluids, especially blood or serum (liquid part of blood after red blood cells have been removed)

horm/o – to excite or stimulate, e.g., hormonal (hor-mon-al), having a stimulatory effect on the activity of cells in hormonal glands, usually remote from its point of origin

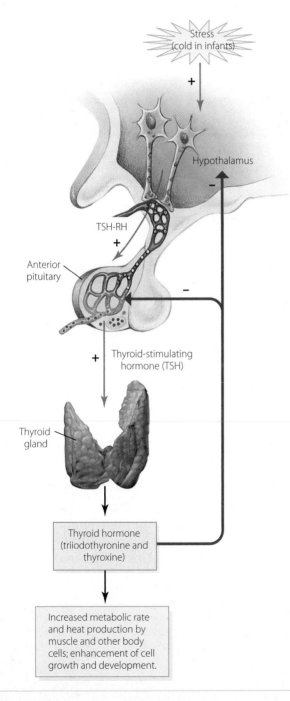

FIGURE 19-3 Negative feedback control of TSH secretion.

3. Acid–base balance
4. Fluid intake and fluid balance
5. Carbohydrate, protein, and lipid metabolism
6. Digestion, absorption, and nutrient distribution
7. Blood pressure
8. Stress resistance
9. Adaptation to environmental change, for example, changes in temperature

More specific details about the function of each of the endocrine glands can be found in anatomy and physiology texts (space limits that discussion in this chapter). The glands are defined and classified in Lesson One (also see Figures 19-1 through 19-3).

Endocrinology is the study of the endocrine system and the disorders and diseases that affect the system. An *endocrinologist* is a physician who specializes in the medical practice of endocrinology.

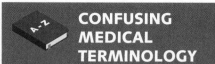

CONFUSING MEDICAL TERMINOLOGY

thym/o versus thyr/o

thym/o – thymus, thymus gland, e.g., thymectomy (thi-<u>mek</u>-to-me) refers to excision of the thymus gland

thyr/o – thyroid, thyroid gland, shield, e.g., thyrotoxicosis (thi-ro-tok-sih-<u>ko</u>-sis) refers to a toxic condition of the thyroid gland or thyroid crisis

LESSON ONE	Materials to Be Learned

CLASSIFICATION AND FUNCTIONS OF THE ENDOCRINE SYSTEM

The endocrine system is a unique body system that uses hormones to help regulate practically all facets of body activity. Glands are body structures (organs) and are divided into two types. A gland may or may not have a duct. Ducted glands secrete by way of a duct into the bloodstream. In this case, the gland is an *exocrine gland.* The exocrine system is made up of all such glands. A ductless gland has no duct and secretes its materials directly into the bloodstream. Thus, the gland is an *endocrine gland*, and the endocrine system is made up of all such glands. The exception is the pancreas, a gland that contains both an endocrine function *and* an exocrine function. The pancreas secretes enzymes into the duodenum through the pancreatic duct (*exocrine function*). Also, the pancreas functions as an *endocrine* gland when insulin and glucagon are secreted into the blood stream. Refer to **Table 19-1** and Figures 19-1 through 19-3 when you study the classification of the endocrine system.

TABLE **19-1** Classification and Functions of the Endocrine System

Gland	Pronunciation	Definition
adrenal	ah'-<u>dre</u>-nal	two adrenal glands sit atop each kidney; each consists of two portions: the central region or *adrenal medulla* and the outer region or *adrenal cortex*. The adrenal cortex is the largest portion of the gland, and it secretes three types of *steroid* hormones called *corticosteroids*. Each has different functions: 1. *Glucocorticoids* affect glucose metabolism and maintain blood glucose levels 2. *Mineralocorticoids* are involved in balance of electrolytes, sodium, and potassium. The most important of these hormones is *aldosterone*, which acts on the kidney to regulate blood levels of sodium and potassium ions 3. *Gonadocorticoids* are sex hormones released from the adrenal cortex instead of the gonads (testes and ovaries), but the small amounts secreted by the adrenal cortex contribute to the secondary sex characteristics, such as breast and beard development, and are necessary for reproduction The adrenal medulla, the inner portion of the adrenal gland, secretes two nonsteroidal hormones called *catecholamines*. The two hormones, adrenaline (*epinephrine*) and noradrenaline (*norepinephrine*), are the stress hormones that exert physiologic changes during times of stress (the fight-or-flight response)

Gland	Pronunciation	Definition
ovaries	<u>oh</u>-vah-reez	female gonads; two small glands located in the upper pelvic cavity, on either side of the uterine wall, near the fallopian tubes; each is almond shaped and held in place by ligaments. Ovaries produce mature ova as well as two hormones (*estrogen* and *progesterone*) responsible for female sex characteristics and regulation of the menstrual cycle. Estrogen promotes maturation of the ova in the ovary and prepares the uterine lining for implantation of a fertilized egg. It is also responsible for the development and maintenance of secondary female characteristics that occur in puberty, such as breast development, growth of pubic and axillary hair, widened pelvis, general growth spurt, and onset of menstruation. Progesterone is responsible for preparation and maintenance of the uterus in pregnancy, and for the development of the placenta after implantation of a fertilized ovum
pancreas	<u>pan</u>-kree-as	an elongated structure located behind the stomach in the left upper quadrant. The specialized cells that produce hormones are called the *islets of Langerhans*; these cells produce two hormones, *insulin* and *glucagon*, and both play a role in maintaining normal glucose levels. The islets of Langerhans carry on the endocrine functions of the pancreas; other cells within the organ carry on its exocrine functions, e.g., the secretion of digestive enzymes. Insulin, produced in the beta cells of the pancreas, is necessary for glucose to pass from the blood into the cells and be used for energy. Insulin also promotes the conversion of glucose into glycogen for storage (*glycogenesis*) in the liver. When blood sugar is high (*hyperglycemia*), the pancreas is stimulated to release insulin and convert the excess glucose into glycogen. Glucagon, produced in the alpha cells, increases blood levels of glucose by stimulating the breakdown of glycogen stored in the liver cells; glycogen is the storage form of carbohydrate in the body. This process, called *glycogenolysis*, helps maintain blood glucose levels between meals; glucagon also helps synthesize glucose from amino acids and glycerol derived from protein and triglycerides, respectively (*gluconeogenesis*), to elevate blood glucose levels
parathyroid	par'-ah-<u>thi</u>-royd	consists of four small nodules of tissue embedded in the back side of the thyroid glands. When blood calcium levels are low, the parathyroid glands secrete parathyroid hormone or *parathormone* (PTH), which increases blood calcium levels in three ways: (1) calcium is released from the bones; (2) less calcium is excreted by the kidneys; and (3) the kidney activates Vitamin D which increases calcium absorption in the gastrointestinal tract
pineal	<u>pin</u>-e-al	the pineal gland is a cone-shaped structure attached by a stalk to the posterior wall of the cerebrum. This gland secretes *melatonin*, the hormone that responds to darkness in the external environment. Darkness stimulates nerve impulses in the eyes to decrease and the secretion of melatonin to increase. The pineal gland functions as a "biological clock" to regulate patterns of sleeping, eating, and reproduction
pituitary gland	pe-<u>tu</u>-i-tar-ee	also known as the *hypophysis*, the pituitary gland is about the size of a pea and is located on the underside of the brain in a depression at the base of the skull, protected by the brain above it and the nasal cavities below it. The pituitary gland is connected by a thin stalk-like projection to the hypothalamus and contains two major parts: the *anterior* pituitary and the *posterior* pituitary lobes. The pituitary is a very complex gland that is often referred to as the "master gland," because it produces many hormones that affect body functions and because it travels throughout the body to stimulate other endocrine glands to secrete hormones. The pituitary gland secretes growth hormone (GH), prolactin (PRL), thyroid-stimulating hormone (TSH), adenocorticotropin (ACTH), gonadotropins (FSH, LH), antidiuretic hormone (ADH), and oxytocin (see Figure 19-2)
testes	<u>tes</u>-teez	male gonads, also known as testicles, are two small egg shaped glands suspended from the inguinal region of the male by the spermatic cord and surrounded by the scrotal sac. After descending from high in the abdominal cavity during fetal growth, testes descend shortly before birth into the scrotum. Testes are the primary organs of the male reproductive system. The testes produce male sperm cells and secrete *testosterone*, the male hormone necessary for secondary sex characteristics that appear in the male during puberty, such as growth of the beard and pubic hair, growth of skeletal muscles, deepening of the voice, and enlargement of the testicles, penis, and scrotum

(continues)

Gland	Pronunciation	Definition
thymus	<u>thi</u>-mus	a single gland located behind the sternum in the mediastinum; it resembles a lymph gland in structure because it not only is a part of the lymphatic system, but it also is a hormone-secreting endocrine gland. The thymus is large in children, but shrinks with age until there is only a trace of active tissue in older adults. The gland secretes *thymosin* and *thymopoietin* which stimulates the production of T cells, the specialized lymphocytes involved in the immune response
thyroid	<u>thi</u>-royd	consisting of a right and left lobe, the thyroid gland is a U- or H-shaped gland located in front of the neck just below the larynx; the lobes are connected by a narrow piece of thyroid cartilage that produces the prominence on the neck known as Adam's apple. Thyroid hormones affect metabolism, brain development, breathing, heart and nervous system functions, body temperature, muscle strength, skin dryness, menstrual cycles, weight, and cholesterol levels. The thyroid gland produces three hormones: 1. *Thyroxin* (T4) helps maintain normal body metabolism 2. *Triiodthyronine* (T3), a chemically similar compound, helps regulate growth and development and control metabolism and body temperature 3. *Calcitonin/thyrocalcitonin* regulates the level of calcium in the blood. It lowers the blood calcium by inhibiting the release of calcium from the bones by a negative feedback loop when blood calcium levels are high

TABLE 19-1 (*continued*)

CLINICAL DISORDERS OF THE ENDOCRINE SYSTEM

Clinical disorders of the endocrine system affect the secretion of hormones from the endocrine gland. *Autoimmune* diseases and tumors (either benign or cancerous) of the endocrine glands are the two main causes of disorders of the endocrine system. These diseases can cause either hypersecretion or hyposecretion of hormones. The most common diseases of the endocrine system are diabetes mellitus and diseases of the thyroid. Once a diagnosis is made, treatment may involve replacement of missing hormones or surgery. Refer to **Table 19-2**, which describes common clinical disorders of the endocrine system, and **Figures 19-4** through **19-8** when reviewing various clinical disorders.

TABLE 19-2 Clinical Disorders of the Endocrine System

Clinical Condition	Pronunciation	Definition
Clinical Disorders of the Pituitary Gland		
acromegaly	ak'-ro-<u>meg</u>-ah-le	hypersecretion of the pituitary growth hormone (GH) after maturity; causes abnormal enlargement of the extremities of the skeleton, nose, jaws, fingers, and toes. Most common cause is a noncancerous tumor of the pituitary gland (see Figure 19-4)
congenital growth hormone deficiency	con-<u>gen</u>-i-tal groth <u>hor</u>-mone de-<u>fi</u>-cien-cy	abnormalities in the development of the pituitary gland and surrounding structures, resulting in short stature in children unless treated with growth hormone (GH); puberty may be delayed or may not occur
Cushing's disease	<u>koosh</u>-ingz di-<u>zez</u>	excessive growth of the pituitary gland caused by a tumor of the pituitary gland; results in the release of too much ACTH, which then leads to overproduction of cortisol. Symptoms of excess cortisol are obesity, weakness, moon face, edema, and high blood pressure

Clinical Condition	Pronunciation	Definition
diabetes insipidus	dye-ah-<u>bee</u>-tez in-<u>sip</u>-ih-dus	insufficient excretion of antidiuretic hormone (ADH; vasopressin) by the posterior pituitary gland; most common cause is damage to the pituitary gland (or hypothalamus) from head injury, surgery, or tumors. Lack of ADH causes the kidney tubules to fail to reabsorb needed water and salts. Clinical symptoms include *polyuria* (increased urination) and *polydipsia* (increased thirst); excessive thirst results in drinking large volumes of water and a very dilute urine
hypopituitarism	hahy-poh-pi-<u>too</u>-i-tuh-riz-uh-m	pituitary insufficiency may be caused by a tumor or injury to the pituitary gland. Usually affects the anterior pituitary and releasing hormones necessary for normal functioning of other endocrine glands (thyroid, adrenal cortex, ovaries and testes)
hyperprolactinemia	hy-per-pro-<u>lac</u>-ti-ne-mi-a	higher than normal amounts of prolactin in the blood and production of breast milk in women when not pregnant or nursing; caused by tumor of the pituitary gland, certain medications, and chronic liver or kidney disease
Simmonds' disease (panhypopituitarism)	<u>sim</u>-ondz di-<u>zez</u> (pan-hi'-po-pi-<u>tu</u>-i-tar-izm)	generalized hypopituitarism owing to absence of or damage to the pituitary gland; results in loss of function of thyroid and adrenal glands as well as gonads, testes, and ovaries; symptoms are exhaustion, emaciation, cachexia, and lack of secondary sex characteristics

Clinical Disorders of the Thyroid Gland

Clinical Condition	Pronunciation	Definition
congenital hypothyroidism (cretinism)	con-<u>gen</u>-i-tal hy-po-<u>thy</u>-roid-ism (<u>kre</u>-ti-nizm)	lack of thyroid secretion that affects infants from birth (congenital). The thyroid gland may be absent or severely reduced in size (*hypoplastic*) or abnormally located. If untreated, congenital hypothyroidism can lead to intellectual disability and slow physical growth. In the United States, infants are tested at birth and treated to allow for normal growth and development (see Figure 19-5)
Graves' disease	Graves di-<u>zez</u>	toxic diffuse goiter; autoimmune disease and most common cause of hyperthyroidism in the United States. Symptoms are nervousness, difficulty sleeping, fatigue, weight loss, goiter, and a protrusion of the eyeballs (see Figure 19-8)
Hashimoto's disease	hash'-i-<u>mo</u>-toz di-<u>zez</u>	chronic lymphocytic thyroiditis; most common cause of hypothyroidism in the United States. An autoimmune disease of the thyroid gland, with replacement of normal tissue with lymphoid tissue. The end result is a lack of production and secretion of thyroid hormone
thyroid nodule	<u>thy</u>-roid <u>nod</u>-ule	solid or fluid-filled lumps within the thyroid gland; most are benign (noncancerous), although in some cases, the nodules produce excessive amounts of thyroxine (see Figure 19-6)
myxedema	mik'-se-<u>de</u>-mah	advanced form of hypothyroidism in adults; a dry, waxy type of swelling with deposits of mucin in the skin, swollen lips, and thickened nose (see Figure 19-7)

Clinical Disorders of the Parathyroid Gland

Clinical Condition	Pronunciation	Definition
primary hyperparathyroidism (PHPT)	<u>pri</u>-ma-ry hy-per-par-a-<u>thy</u>-roid-ism	overactive parathyroid gland with excessive secretion of parathyroid hormone (PTH); most common cause is a benign tumor of the parathyroid gland. PTH increases serum calcium by releasing calcium from bone, reabsorption of calcium by the kidney, and increasing phosphorous excretion by the kidney
Secondary hyperparathyroidism	<u>sec</u>-ond-ar-y hy-per-par-a-<u>thy</u>-roid-ism	overactive parathyroid gland secondary to chronic kidney failure, the most common disease causing secondary hyperparathyroidism

(continues)

TABLE **19-2** (*continued*)		
Clinical Condition	**Pronunciation**	**Definition**
Clinical Disorders of the Adrenal Gland		
Addison's disease (adrenal insufficiency)	ad-i-sonz di-zez (a-dre-nal in-suf-fi-cien-cy)	hypofunction of the adrenal gland; autoimmune disorder with inadequate amounts of hormones secreted by the adrenal gland (cortisol, aldosterone, and androgens); secondary cause is damage to the pituitary gland. Symptoms include a bronze-like pigmentation of the skin, dizziness, low blood pressure, low blood sugar, vomiting, and diarrhea
congenital adrenal hyperplasia (CAH)	con-gen-i-tal a-dre-nal hy-per-pla-si-a	lack of enzymes involved in the biosynthesis of cortisol and aldosterone. In many cases, CAH results in lack of cortisol and overproduction of androgen. causing development of male characteristics in girls and early sexual development in boys
Cushing's syndrome	koosh-ingz syn-drome	adrenal glands produce too much *cortisol*; often caused by high doses of corticosteroid medication treatment for autoimmune diseases, e.g., rheumatoid arthritis or asthma. Untreated Cushing syndrome can lead to diabetes, high blood pressure, and osteoporosis
pheochromocytoma (hyperaldosteronism)	fe'-o-kro'-mo-si-to-mah (hy-per-la-dos-ter-on-izm)	"pheochromo" means dusky color; tumor of the adrenal medulla and excessive production of *aldosterone*. Excessive aldosterone acts on the kidneys to retain sodium and water and to excrete too much potassium resulting in hypertension; symptoms include headache, rapid heart rate, and tremors
Clinical Disorders of the Ovaries		
polycystic ovary syndrome (PCOS)	pol-y-cys-tic o-va-ry syn-drome	hyperandrogenism (abnormally elevated androgen levels); condition in women characterized by the absence of ovulation and menstrual periods, infertility, acne, excess body hair, and metabolic syndrome (obesity, prediabetes, hyperlipidemia)
Clinical Disorders of the Testes		
primary hypogonadism	pri-ma-ry hy-po-go-nad-ism	abnormality in the testicles resulting in lack of testosterone production; can begin during fetal development, before puberty, or during adulthood. Lack of testosterone during fetal development may cause impaired growth of the external sex organs. During puberty, hypogonadism may delay puberty or cause incomplete development
secondary hypogonadism	sec-ond-ar-y hy-po-go-nad-ism	failure of pituitary gland to send chemical messages to the testicles to produce testosterone. Certain diseases and aging can also lower production of testosterone
Clinical Disorders of the Pancreas		
diabetes mellitus, Type 1	dye-ah-bee-tez mel-li-tus	autoimmune disease with destruction of insulin-producing cells in the pancreas. Most commonly diagnosed in children and young adults. Symptoms are high blood sugar, excessive urination (*polyuria*), thirst (*polydipsia*), hunger (*polyphagia*), emaciation, and weakness. Treatment requires daily insulin injections
diabetes mellitus, type 2	dye-ah-bee-tez mel-li-tus	insulin resistance--insulin is produced, but the insulin doesn't function properly--or lack of insulin secretion. Most common form of diabetes; usually diagnosed in those over 40 years of age and in those who are obese
gestational diabetes	jes-tay-shun-al dye-ah-bee-tez	develops during pregnancy, most often in women with a family history of diabetes. Typically, it disappears after delivery, although the condition is associated with an increased risk of developing type 2 diabetes later in life

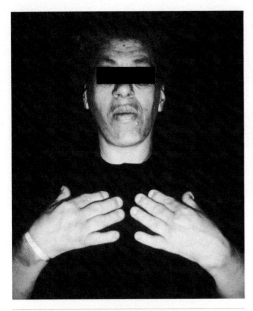

FIGURE 19-4 The appearance of a subject with advanced acromegaly.

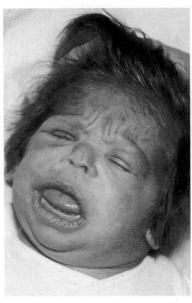

FIGURE 19-5 The characteristic appearance of neonatal hypothyroidism (cretinism) as a result of a congenital absence of thyroid gland; treatment with thyroid hormone reversed manifestations of hypothyroidism.

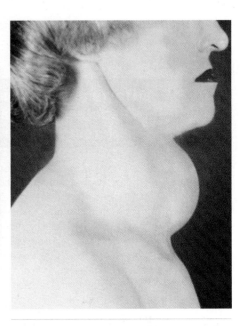

FIGURE 19-6 Large nodular goiter.

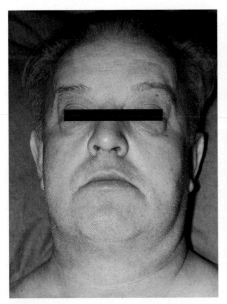

FIGURE 19-7 The appearance of a patient with myxedema.

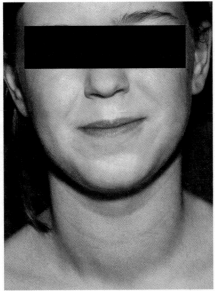

FIGURE 19-8 Small diffuse toxic goiter in a young woman.

BOX 19-1 is a discussion of the similarities and differences of conditions that include the word diabetes.

Box 19-1 How are Diabetes Mellitus, Gestational Diabetes, and Diabetes Insipidus Different and the Same?

Diabetes is derived from the Greek word *dia* (going through) and *bainein* (to pass), for example, body fluid passing through the kidneys instead of being reabsorbed and returned to the blood. The word mellitus originated from the Latin word *mellitus* ("sweet") or sugar in the urine. Diabetes mellitus and gestational diabetes are both diseases in which the insulin hormone, secreted by the pancreas, is either insufficient or does not function properly. As a result, glucose accumulates in the blood (*hyperglycemia*) and urine (*glycosuria*). Diabetes insipidus, however, is a disorder of the pituitary gland in which there is insufficient secretion of the antidiuretic hormone, vasopressin. The characteristic symptom of each of these disorders—diabetes mellitus, gestational diabetes, and diabetes insipidus—is excessive urination (*polyuria*). In diabetes mellitus and gestational diabetes, excessive urination is a method for the kidneys to remove excessive glucose from the blood. However, in diabetes insipidus, excessive urination occurs because of the lack of the antidiuretic hormone that acts on the kidney to promote reabsorption of body fluid. Medications are used for treating all three of these diseases. Diabetes mellitus and gestational diabetes are treated with either insulin or oral hypoglycemic agents while diabetes insipidus is treated with vasopressin.

Diabetes mellitus and gestational diabetes are common disorders while diabetes insipidus is a rare condition.

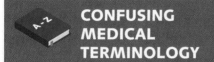

CONFUSING MEDICAL TERMINOLOGY

aden/o versus adren/o

aden/o – gland, e.g., adenohypophysis (ad-en-o-hi-pof-ih-sis) refers to lack of growth in the glands

adren/o – adrenal gland, e.g., adrenocortical hyperplasia (a-dre-no-kor-ti-kal hi-per-pla-se-ah) refers to excessive development of the adrenal cortex

TERMS USED IN THE DIAGNOSIS AND TREATMENT OF DISEASES OF THE ENDOCRINE SYSTEM

Terms in **Table 19-3** are organized into three groups: (1) those documented in the history and physical exam; (2) those used to make a diagnosis; and (3) surgery and other treatments of endocrine disease.

TABLE 19-3 Terms Used in the Diagnosis and Treatment of Diseases of the Endocrine System

Clinical Disorder	Pronunciation	Definition
History and Physical Exam		
acidosis	as'-i-do-sis	a pathologic condition caused by accumulation of acid in or loss of base from the body; symptom of uncontrolled diabetes mellitus
adrenomegaly	ah-dre-no-meg-ah-le	enlargement of the adrenal gland
amenorrhea	a-men-or-rhe-a	absence of menstrual periods in women during reproductive age
anorexia	an'-o-rek-se-ah	lack or loss of appetite for food; found in certain diseases of the pituitary gland

Clinical Disorder	Pronunciation	Definition
cachexia	kah-<u>kek</u>-se-ah	malnutrition, wasting, and emaciation; found in certain diseases of the pituitary gland
congenital	con-<u>gen</u>-i-tal	existing at birth, usually abnormal; nonhereditary
convulsions	kon-<u>vul</u>-shunz	involuntary muscular contractions; characteristic sign of disorders of calcium metabolism
diaphoresis	di'-ah-fo-<u>re</u>-sis	profuse perspiration; often found in conditions of hypoglycemia in diabetes mellitus
emaciation	e-ma'-se-<u>a</u>-shun	excessive leanness, a wasted condition; sign of uncontrolled diabetes mellitus, hyperthyroidism, or diseases of the pituitary gland
exophthalmic goiter	ek'-sof-<u>thal</u>-mic <u>goi</u>-ter	protrusion of the eyeballs; characteristic sign in Graves' disease
glycosuria	gly-cos-u-<u>ri</u>-a	high amounts of glucose in the urine; symptom of uncontrolled diabetes mellitus
goiter (simple)	<u>goi</u>-ter	enlargement of the thyroid gland causing swelling in front of the neck; caused by dietary deficiency of iodine, except in the United States where iodine is added to table salt. Can also be caused by over or under secretion of thyroid hormone (see Figure 19-8)
hypercalcemia	hy-per-cal-<u>ce</u>-mia	blood calcium above normal values
hyperglycemia	hi-per-gli-<u>se</u>-me-ah	blood sugar (glucose) level above normal; sign of uncontrolled diabetes mellitus
hyperthyroidism	hi-per-<u>thi</u>-roi-dizm	excessive secretion of thyroid hormone causing body functions to speed up, e.g., a rapid heartbeat and more frequent bowel movements or diarrhea. Most common cause is Graves' disease
hypocalcemia	hy-po-cal-<u>ce</u>-mia	blood calcium below normal values
hypoglycemia	hi'-po-gli-<u>se</u>-me-ah	blood sugar (glucose) level below normal
hypothyroidism	hi-po-<u>thi</u>-roid-izm	lack of secretion of thyroid hormone causing body functions to slow down, e.g., a slower heart rate and constipation. Most common cause is Hashimoto's disease
ketoacidosis	ke-to-as-i-<u>do</u>-sis	accumulation of ketone bodies in the blood that results in metabolic acidosis; consequences of uncontrolled diabetes mellitus
polydipsia	pol-y-<u>dip</u>-si-a	excessive thirst; sign of uncontrolled diabetes mellitus or diabetes insipidus
polyphagia	pol-y-<u>pha</u>-gi-a	excessive hunger; sign of uncontrolled diabetes mellitus
polyuria	pol-y-<u>u</u>-ri-a	excessive urination; sign of uncontrolled diabetes mellitus or diabetes insipidus
tetany	<u>tet</u>-ah-ne	sharp flexion of the wrist and ankle joints on physical exam; muscle twitching, cramps, and convulsion; caused by abnormal calcium metabolism
thyroiditis	thy-roi-<u>di</u>-tis	inflammation of the thyroid gland
virilization	vir-il-i-<u>za</u>-tion	development of male physical characteristics (muscle bulk, body hair, deep voice) in girls or precociously in a boy; caused by excess androgen production from either the adrenal glands or the gonads (testes in males and ovaries in females)

(continues)

TABLE **19-3** (continued)		
Clinical Disorder	**Pronunciation**	**Definition**
Laboratory Tests		
A1c/HbA1c (glycated hemoglobin)	a-1-c (gly-<u>cat</u>-ed <u>he</u>-mo-glo-bin)	measurement of the level of hemoglobin A1c determines average blood sugar concentrations for the preceding 2–3 months; normal levels below 5.7 percent indicate diabetes mellitus is well controlled
ACTH (adrenocorticotropic hormone)	a-c-t-h (a-<u>dre</u>-no-cor-ti-co-<u>tro</u>-pic <u>hor</u>-mone)	measured in the blood to evaluate for disorders of the pituitary and adrenal glands
cortisol	<u>cor</u>-ti-sol	measured in the blood or saliva to evaluate for diseases of the adrenal gland
estradiol	es-tra-<u>di</u>-ol	measured in the blood to evaluate for normal functioning of the ovaries (in females)
prolactin	pro-<u>lac</u>-tin	measured in the blood when women (who are not pregnant or breastfeeding) secrete breast milk
serum calcium	<u>ser</u>-um <u>cal</u>-ci-um	measured to evaluate for diseases of the parathyroid glands
serum potassium	<u>ser</u>-um po-<u>tas</u>-si-um	measured to evaluate for tumors of the adrenal gland that cause excessive urinary excretion of potassium
testosterone	tes-<u>tos</u>-ter-one	measured in the blood to evaluate for diseases of the adrenal gland or testes (in males)
thyroxine (T4)	thy-<u>rox</u>-ine	measured in the blood to evaluate for diseases of the thyroid
triiodothyronine (T3)	tri-i-o-do-<u>thy</u>-ro-nine	measured in the blood to evaluate for diseases of the thyroid
urine calcium	<u>u</u>-rine <u>cal</u>-ci-um	measured to evaluate for diseases of the parathyroid glands
Radiological Exams and Treatments		
MRI (magnetic resonance imaging)	m-r-i (mag-<u>net</u>-ic <u>res</u>-o-nance <u>im</u>-ag-ing)	use of radio waves and a computer to create pictures of areas inside the body; precise accuracy in detecting structural abnormalities of the body, including tumors
radioactive iodine uptake (RAIU)	ra-di-o-<u>ac</u>-tive <u>i</u>-o-dine <u>up</u>-take	test that measures the amount of radioactive iodine taken up by the thyroid gland; used to evaluate functioning of the thyroid gland
thyroid scan	<u>thy</u>-roid scan	use of radioactive iodine tracer to examine the structure and function of the thyroid gland; used to evaluate for thyroid nodules or goiter or an overactive thyroid gland
Surgery and Other Treatments of Endocrine Diseases		
hypoglycemic agent	hi'-po-gli-<u>se</u>-mik	drug for treating diabetes mellitus to normalize blood glucose
hypophysectomy	hi-pof'-i-<u>sek</u>-to-me	excision of the pituitary gland (hypophysis)
insulin	<u>in</u>-su-lin	genetically engineered preparation used in the treatment of diabetes to restore the normal ability of the body to utilize glucose
thyroidectomy	thi-roi-<u>dek</u>-to-me	surgical excision of the thyroid gland

Clinical Disorder	Pronunciation	Definition
parathyroidectomy	par-a-thi-roi-<u>dek</u>-to-me	surgical excision of the parathyroid glands
thyrotomy	thi-<u>rot</u>-o-me	surgical division of thyroid cartilage
thyrotherapy	thi-ro-<u>ther</u>-ah-pe	treatment with thyroid preparations

THE ORIGIN OF MEDICAL TERMS

Table 19-4 explains the origin of several terms used in this chapter.

TABLE **19-4** The Origin of Medical Terms

Word	Pronunciation	Origin and Definition
acromegaly	ak-ro-<u>meg</u>-ah-le	Greek, *akros*, highest + Greek, *megas*, large+ Greek, *megal*, great, large
androgen	<u>an</u>-dro-gen	Greek, *aner*, man + Greek, *genein*, to produce+ Greek, *genes*, born of, produced by,
calcitonin	cal-ci-<u>tō</u>-nin	Latin, *calx*, lime or chalk + Greek, *tónos*, stretch+ Greek, *tonos*, tone
congenital	con-<u>gen</u>-i-tal	Latin, *com (con)*, together with + Latin, *geni*, to give birth + Latin, *genitus*, born
convulsions	kon-<u>vul</u>-shunz	Latin, *convulse*, spasmodic contractions of the muscles + Latin, *ion*, process
cretinism	<u>kre</u>-tin-izm	French, *cretin*, mentally defective + Greek, *ism*, state or condition
endocrine	<u>en</u>-do-crine	Greek, *endon*, within + Greek, *krinein*, to separate
hormone	<u>hor</u>-mone	Greek, *harmon*, to excite, stimulate
ovary	<u>o</u>-va-ry	Latin, *ovum*, egg
thyroid	<u>thi</u>-royd	Greek, *thyre*, oblong shield + Greek, *oid*, resembles

ABBREVIATIONS

These abbreviations in **Table 19-5** are frequently used to describe the endocrine system including clinical disorders and diagnostic tools.

TABLE **19-5** Abbreviations

Abbreviation	Definition	Abbreviation	Definition
CAH	congenital adrenal hyperplasia	PRL	prolactin
EMT	emergency medical technicians	RAIU	radioactive iodine uptake
GH	growth hormone	RH	releasing hormone
PCOS	polycystic ovary syndrome	T3	triiodo thyronine
PTH	parathyroid hormone	T4	thyroxin
PHPT	primary hyperparathyroidism	TSH	thyroid stimulating hormone

The following box lists two different categories of medications that may be prescribed by a physician treating diseases of the endocrine system.

PHARMACOLOGY AND MEDICAL TERMINOLOGY

Drug Classification	antidiabetic (an-tih-dye-ah-<u>bet</u>-ik)	hormone (<u>hor</u>-mohn)
Function	helps control the blood sugar level in type 2 diabetes	treats deficiency states where a specific hormone level is abnormally low or absent
Word Parts	**anti-** = against, **diabetic** = pertaining to diabetes	pertaining to a natural chemical substance in the body
Active Ingredients (Examples)	chlorpropamide (Diabenese); metformin (Glucophage)	levothyroxine (Levothroid, Synthroid); vasopressin (Vasostrict, Pitressin); insulin (Humalog, Lantus)

CLINICAL

Note

Doctor's Office Progress Note

Sixty-year-old mildly obese white female here for routine follow-up for type 2 diabetes onset at age 53

PMHx - **Type 2 diabetes** onset at age 53

SHx   Divorced, 2 kids

Fx   father **HTN**, Mother with HTN, **DM**, psoriasis

Patient appears to be well nourished with no complaints of **polyphagia** or **polydipsia**. Weight loss of 30 lbs. since last visit. Patient following dietician recommendations. Goal weight loss is an additional 30 lbs. Patient encouraged to continue current diet plan with dietician.

Current **HgA1c** is 7.8 with a gl of <7.0. Lipid panel within normal limits.

Current sliding scale insulin regimen is adequate with 3–5 **hypoglycemic** episodes over 30 days. Glucose is monitored with good overall control. No glucose over 220 noted this quarter.

Patient reports current exercise as x3 weekly cardio workout—walking 1/2 miles daily.

ROS

HEENT: Normal with visual exception noted above.

Ht: 5'6"

Wt: 180 lbs.

BP/Pulse: 80/120, resting pulse rate 75

Fundoscopic examination WNL; Thyroid palpated with no abnormalities or nodules noted. Skin is clear and healthy appearing with no breakdown or inflammation at injection sites.

Neuro Exam: WNL

Foot Exam: WNL

HgA1c ordered prior to next visit in 3 months (fasting not needed)

Direction: For the portions of the clinical note shown by a colored font, provide the definition and/or words for abbreviation.

LESSON TWO	Progress Check

LIST: ENDOCRINE GLANDS

List the nine glands of the endocrine system:

1. _____
2. _____
3. _____
4. _____
5. _____
6. _____
7. _____
8. _____
9. _____

LIST: ACTIVITIES REGULATED BY THE ENDOCRINE SYSTEM

List nine activities regulated by the endocrine system:

1. _____
2. _____
3. _____
4. _____
5. _____
6. _____
7. _____
8. _____
9. _____

MULTIPLE CHOICE: ENDOCRINE GLANDS AND HORMONES

Circle the letter of the correct answer:

1. A gland that secretes its fluids into a duct and then into the bloodstream is a(n) _____ gland.
   a. endogenous
   b. exogenous
   c. endocrine
   d. exocrine

2. The endocrine gland at the base of the brain is the:
   a. pituitary
   b. parathyroid
   c. pineal
   d. pancreas

3. The endocrine gland with a lobe on each side of the trachea is the:
   a. pituitary
   b. pancreas
   c. thyroid
   d. adrenal

4. The two small glands atop the kidneys are the:
   a. pituitary
   b. adrenal
   c. thyroid
   d. thymus

5. The large gland situated transversely behind the stomach is the:
   a. adrenal
   b. thymus
   c. testis
   d. pancreas

6. The gland situated in the pleural cavity that is believed to be part of the body's immune system is the:
   a. pancreas
   b. pituitary
   c. thymus
   d. thyroid

7. The *islets (islands) of Langerhans* refers to:
   a. small bodies in the pituitary gland
   b. the endocrine part of the pancreas
   c. the testes and ovaries
   d. the exocrine part of the adrenals

8. The pineal gland regulates:
   a. digestion and absorption of nutrients
   b. fluid and electrolyte balance
   c. heart rate and body temperature
   d. sleeping and eating

9. Glands responsible for sex characteristics are:
   a. ovaries, testes, and adrenal
   b. testes and thyroid
   c. ovaries and testes
   d. thyroid and parathyroid

10. Hormone that determines the final adult height is:
    a. thyroxine
    b. epinephrine
    c. growth hormone
    d. insulin

WORD POOL: DISORDERS OF THE ENDOCRINE SYSTEM

Select appropriate terms from the word pool below to complete these sentences:

1. Inability to metabolize sugar because of absence of insulin or insulin resistance during pregnancy is

   _____.

2. Arrested mental and physical growth is a sign of _____ caused by congenital lack of thyroxine.

3. Swollen neck, weight loss, nervousness, difficulty sleeping, and fatigue are symptoms of _____.

4. _____ is characterized by headache, hypertension, rapid heart rate, and tremors.

5. _____ is characterized by muscle twitching, cramps, and convulsions.

6. A dry, waxy swelling with swollen lips and thickened nose in adults is diagnosed as _____.

7. Obesity, weakness, moon face, edema, and high blood pressure are symptoms of _____.

8. _____ is production and secretion of breast milk in women who are neither pregnant nor breastfeeding.

9. Iodine deficiency that causes an enlargement of the thyroid gland and swelling of the neck would be diagnosed as

   _____.

10. _____ results in a lack of testosterone production and secretion by the testes.

Word Pool: cretinism, Cushing's disease, gestational diabetes, Graves' disease, hyperprolactinemia, hypogonadism, myxedema, pheochromocytoma, simple goiter, tetany

MATCHING: ENDOCRINE GLANDS AND HORMONES

Match the hormone on the right with the endocrine gland that secretes the hormone on the left:

Endocrine Gland
1. Thyroid
2. Parathyroid
3. Adrenal
4. Pancreas
5. Ovaries
6. Testes
7. Pineal
8. Thymus
9. Pituitary

Hormone
a. Parathormone
b. Testosterone
c. Thymosin
d. Estrogen
e. Thyroxine
f. Prolactin
g. Insulin
h. Corticosteroids
i. Melatonin

MATCHING: DISORDERS OF THE ENDOCRINE SYSTEM

Match the disease with the malfunctioning gland that causes it (answers may be used more than once):

Disease
1. Acromegaly
2. Addison's disease
3. Cretinism
4. Cushing's disease
5. Goiter (simple)
6. Graves' disease
7. Diabetes mellitus
8. Simmond's disease
9. Diabetes insipidus
10. Hishimoto's disease
11. Polycystic ovary syndrome
12. Primary hypogonadism
13. Pheochromocytoma
14. Tetany
15. Hyperprolactinemia
16. Myxedema

Malfunctioning Endocrine Gland
a. Parathyroid
b. Pituitary
c. Adrenal
d. Thyroid
e. Pancreas
f. Testes
g. Ovary

DEFINITIONS: SYMPTOMS OF DISEASES OF THE ENDOCRINE SYSTEM

Define the following terms:

1. Amenorrhea: _____
2. Diaphoresis: _____
3. Emaciation: _____
4. Exophthalmic goiter: _____
5. Ketoacidosis: _____
6. Polyuria: _____
7. Virilization: _____
8. Goiter: _____
9. Convulsions: _____
10. Anorexia: _____

IDENTIFYING WORD PARTS

For each of the medical terms, list the root word and the prefix and/or suffix:

Word	Root Word	Prefix	Suffix
1. Acromegaly	_____	_____	_____
2. Diaphoresis	_____	_____	_____
3. Exophthalmic	_____	_____	_____
4. Glycogenolysis	_____	_____	_____
5. Corticoids	_____	_____	_____
6. Ketosis	_____	_____	_____
7. Panhypopituitarism	_____	_____	_____
8. Polydipsia	_____	_____	_____
9. Progesterone	_____	_____	_____
10. Triiodothyronine	_____	_____	_____

© teekid/iStock/Getty Images

Cancer Medicine

OBJECTIVES

After completing this chapter and the exercises, the student should be able to:

1. Define cancer.
2. Classify cancer.
3. Identify rules and exceptions in naming cancer.
4. Describe the types of cancer normally affecting men and women.
5. Explain the two major clinical phases in cancer medicine: diagnosis and treatment.
6. Describe the details of screening, detection, and diagnosis of cancer.
7. Present the methods of treating cancer.

CANCER MEDICINE

Cancer is the leading cause of death from disease worldwide, and both heart disease and cancer are the leading causes of death in the United States. Lung cancer is the leading cause of death from cancer in both men and women, while the most common new cancer diagnosis is prostate cancer for men and breast cancer for women. Brain cancer and leukemia are the most common cancers in children and young adults.

Normal life processes are characterized by continuous growth and maturation of cells that are subject to control mechanisms that regulate growth. Normally, cells divide to produce more cells only when the body needs them. This ongoing growth process serves the purpose of replacing cells that have been injured or have undergone degenerative changes. If cells keep dividing when new cells are not needed, a *tumor* or *neoplasm* is formed. A neoplasm (neo- = new + plasm = growth) is an overgrowth of cells that serves no useful purpose. Neoplasms lack control mechanisms that normally regulate cell growth and differentiation. The terms neoplasm and tumor have essentially the same meaning and may be used interchangeably.

ALLIED HEALTH PROFESSIONS

Veterinary Technologists and Technicians and Animal Care and Service Workers

Veterinary technologists and technicians typically conduct clinical work in a private practice under the supervision of a licensed veterinarian. They often perform various medical tests as well as treat and diagnose medical conditions and diseases in animals. Besides working in private clinics and animal hospitals, veterinary technologists and technicians may work in research facilities.

Many people like animals, but as pet owners can attest, taking care of them is hard work. Animal care and service workers—who include animal caretakers and animal trainers—train, feed, water, groom, bathe, and exercise animals. They also clean, disinfect, and repair their cages. They play with the animals, provide companionship, and observe behavioral changes that could indicate illness or injury. Boarding kennels, pet stores, animal shelters, veterinary hospitals and clinics, stables, laboratories, aquariums, natural aquatic habitats, and zoological parks all house animals and employ animal care and service workers. Job titles and duties vary by employment setting.

INQUIRY

American Association for Laboratory Animal Science: www.aalas.org

Data from Cross, Nanna, and McWay, Dana. *Stanfield's Introduction to the Health Professions*, 7th ed. Burlington, MA: Jones & Bartlett Learning; 2017.

A *malignant* neoplasm is composed of less well-differentiated cells that grow rapidly and infiltrate and invade the surrounding tissues. The process by which a tumor spreads (meta = change) and the secondary deposits (+ stasis = standing) are called *metastatic* tumors (**Figures 20-1** and **20-2**). Metastatic cancer occurs when cancerous cells break away from where they began (the primary tumor) and travel through the lymph system or blood to form a tumor in another part of the body.

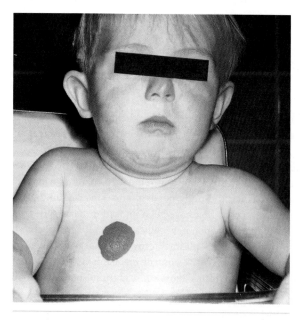

FIGURE 20-1 Clinical appearance of benign blood vessel tumor (angioma) of skin.

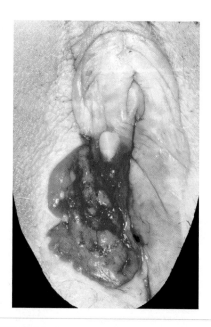

FIGURE 20-2 Large carcinoma of the vulva, the white appearance of the skin adjacent to the carcinoma is caused by preexisting vulva dystrophy.

The *medical oncologist* is a physician who specializes in the diagnosis and treatment of cancer. A *pathologist* is a physician who examines biopsy tissue needed for a cancer diagnosis and staging, the degree to which the cancer has spread. The pathologist's report is used to determine appropriate cancer treatment. The medical oncologist coordinates care as needed, including chemotherapy, surgery, radiation therapy, supportive care, and palliative care.

LESSON ONE | Materials to Be Learned

MEDICAL TERMS IN CANCER MEDICINE

The medical terms associated with cancer medicine are grouped as:

1. Those associated with the word *cancer*
2. Those associated with the cancer site (organ or tissue)
3. Those associated with the diagnosis
4. Those associated with the treatment

General Principles of Naming Tumors

There are many types of malignant tumors, and all can be classified into four groups according to the cancer site and tissue type: (1) carcinomas, (2) sarcomas, (3) leukemias, and (4) lymphomas. The term cancer is a word used to indicate any type of malignant tumor. *Carcinomas*, the most common type of cancer, are formed by epithelial cells, the cells that cover the inside and outside surfaces of the body. A carcinoma is classified further by designating the type of epithelium from which it arose. *Adenocarcinomas* form in epithelial cells that produce fluids or mucus; tissues with this type of epithelial cell are sometimes called glandular tissues. Most cancers of the breast, colon, and prostate are adenocarcinomas. For example, a carcinoma arising from the glandular epithelium of the pancreas is termed an *adenocarcinoma of the pancreas* (aden = gland).

Comparison of Benign and Malignant Tumors

There are two large classes of neoplasms—benign and malignant—with characteristics of each described in **Table 20-1**.

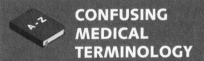

CONFUSING MEDICAL TERMINOLOGY

hematoma versus hematoma

hematoma (hee-ma-<u>toh</u>-muh) – blood tumor if interpreted according to word parts or word origin; this meaning is incorrect under standard clinical circumstances

hematoma (hee-ma-<u>toh</u>-muh) – a mass of blood that has leaked out of a vessel and pooled; this is the accepted meaning in clinical medicine

TABLE **20-1** Comparison of Benign and Malignant Tumors		
Characteristic	**Benign Tumor**	**Malignant Tumor**
cell differentiation	well differentiated	poorly differentiated (cells appear very similar)
character of growth	expansion	infiltration (to nearby tissues)
growth rate	slow	rapid
tumor spread	remains localized	metastasis via the bloodstream and lymph system

Using Root Words to Name Tumors

Most benign tumors are named by adding the suffix "-oma" to the root word that designates the cell of origin (**Table 20-2**). For example, a benign tumor arising from glandular epithelium is called an *adenoma*. A benign tumor of blood vessels is an *angioma* and one arising from cartilage is designated as *chondroma*.

TABLE **20-2** Using Root Words to Name Tumors

Combining Form	Meaning
aden/o	gland
angi/o	vessels (type not specified)
chondr/o	cartilage
fibr/o	fibrous tissue
hemangi/o	blood vessels
lip/o	fat
lymphangi/o	lymph vessels
my/o	muscle
neur/o	nerve
oste/o	bone

Basal cell carcinoma is a cancer that begins in the lower or basal (base) layer of the epidermis, the outer layer of the skin. This cancer is the most common form of skin cancer and is usually found in areas of the body exposed to the sun. It may appear as a small bump that grows slowly and may bleed, but rarely spreads to other parts of the body.

Squamous cell carcinoma is a cancer that forms in squamous cells, epithelial cells that lie just beneath the outer surface of the skin. Squamous cells also line many other organs, including the lining of the respiratory and digestive tracts. Most cancers of the anus, cervix, head and neck, and vagina are squamous cell carcinomas, for example, *cervical squamous cell carcinoma*. *Sarcomas* are cancers that form in bone and soft tissues, including muscle, fat, blood vessels, lymph vessels, and fibrous tissue such as tendons and ligaments. The exact type of sarcoma is specified by using the root word that designates the cell of origin. For example, a malignant tumor of bone is designated as an *osteosarcoma* (oste = bone), the most common cancer of the bone.

The term *leukemia* is applied to cancers of blood-forming tissues. In leukemia, immature blood cells develop into cancerous cells. The abnormal cells proliferate within the bone marrow where they overgrow and crowd out the normal blood-forming cells. The abnormal cells also "spill over" into the bloodstream, and large numbers of abnormal cells circulate in the blood. The low level of normal blood cells can make it harder for the body to get oxygen to tissues, control bleeding, or fight infections. There are four common types of leukemia, grouped based on how quickly the disease progresses (*acute or chronic*) and on the type of blood cell the cancer starts in (*lymphoblastic or myeloid*). A lymphoid stem cell becomes a white blood cell while a myeloid stem cell can become a red blood cell, platelets, or a specific type of white blood cell (lymphocyte).

Lymphoma is a cancer that begins in lymphocytes (T cells or B cells), which are produced in the bone marrow and travel to lymph vessels and nodes throughout the lymph system. Because a lymph tissue is found throughout the body, lymphoma can begin almost anywhere and can spread to the liver and lungs. The two main types of lymphoma are Hodgkin's lymphoma and non-Hodgkin's lymphoma.

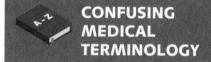

CONFUSING MEDICAL TERMINOLOGY

my/o versus myel/o

my/o – muscle tissue, e.g., myocardial (my-o-<u>car</u>-di-al) refers to cardiac muscle

myel/o – refers to bone marrow, e.g., myelogenous (my-e-lo-<u>gen</u>-ous) relating to or produced by the bone marrow

Tumors are named and classified according to the cells and tissues from which they originate. However, when cancer spreads, the new tumor has the same kind of abnormal cells and the same name as the primary tumor. For example, if lung cancer spreads to the liver, the cancer cells in the liver are lung cancer cells. The disease is called metastatic lung cancer (not liver cancer).

MEDICAL TERMS RELATED TO TYPES OF CANCER

Table 20-3 describes medical terms related to types of cancer.

TABLE **20-3** Medical Terms Related to Types of Cancer

General Term	Pronunciation	Meaning
adenocarcinoma	ad-e-no-car-ci-<u>no</u>-ma	forms in epithelial cells that produce fluid or mucus, e.g., breast, colon, pancreas, and prostate; also called glandular tissues
basal cell carcinoma	<u>ba</u>-sal cell car-ci-<u>no</u>-ma	begins in the lower or basal lower of epidermis, the outer layer of skin; most common form of skin cancer
benign	beh-<u>nine</u>	not cancerous; does not invade nearby tissue or spread to other parts of the body
blastoma	blas-<u>toh</u>-muh	tumor that originates in embryonic tissue and is composed of immature undifferentiated cells
cancer	<u>can</u>-cer	disease in which abnormal cells divide without control; cancer cells can invade nearby tissues and spread through the bloodstream and lymphatic system to other parts of the body
carcinoma	car-ci-<u>no</u>-ma	malignant tumor that begins in the epithelial tissue of the skin or in tissues that line or cover internal organs
cyst	sist	a sac or capsule filled with fluid; noncancerous
ductal carcinoma in situ	<u>duc</u>-tal car-ci-<u>no</u>-ma in <u>si</u>-tu	abnormal cells that involve only the lining of a duct; the cells have not spread outside the duct to other tissues
familial polyposis	fa-<u>mil</u>-ial pah-li-<u>po</u>-sis	inherited condition in which numerous polyps develop on the inside wall of the colon and rectum; increases the risk for colon cancer
hyperplasia	hahy-per-<u>pley</u>-zhuh	increase in number of cells that appear normal; however, cells may become cancerous
large cell carcinomas	large cell car-ci-<u>no</u>-ma	a group of lung cancers that includes squamous cell carcinoma, adenocarcinoma, and large cell carcinoma; also non-small cell carcinoma
leiomyoma	ly-oh-my-<u>oh</u>-muh	benign tumor of smooth muscle of the heart and uterus; leiomyoma of the uterus is commonly called a *fibroid*
leukemia	loo-<u>kee</u>-mee-uh	neoplasm of blood cells; the cancer starts in the bone marrow where the formation of blood cells begins, and large numbers of abnormal blood cells are produced and enter the bloodstream
lymphoma	lim-<u>foh</u>-muh	cancer of the immune system, including lymphocytes and lymph nodes (**Figure 20-3**)

(continues)

TABLE 20-3 (*continued*)

General Term	Pronunciation	Meaning
malignant	ma-<u>lig</u>-nant	cancerous; a growth with a tendency to invade and destroy nearby tissue and spread to other parts of the body
polyp	<u>pah</u>-lip	any benign tumor projecting from surface epithelium; most commonly of the colon and rectum
sarcoma	sar-<u>koh</u>-muh	malignant tumor of connective and supportive tissues, including cartilage, fat, muscle, blood vessels, and fibrous tissue
small cell lung cancer/oat cell cancer	small sel lung <u>can</u>-cer/ot sel <u>can</u>-cer	lung cancer in which the cells are small and round and look like oats when viewed under a microscope
squamous cell carcinoma/ epidermoid carcinoma	<u>skway</u>-mus sel kar-sih-<u>noh</u>-muh/ eh-pih-<u>der</u>-moyd kar-sih-<u>noh</u>-muh	forms in squamous cells, epithelial cells just beneath the outer surface of the skin and cells that line the respiratory and digestive tracts
tumor/neoplasm	<u>too</u>-mer/<u>ne</u>-o-plasm	abnormal mass of tissue as a result of excessive cell division; may be either benign or malignant
Wilms' tumor	wilmz <u>too</u>-mer	malignant tumor of the kidney occurring predominately in children

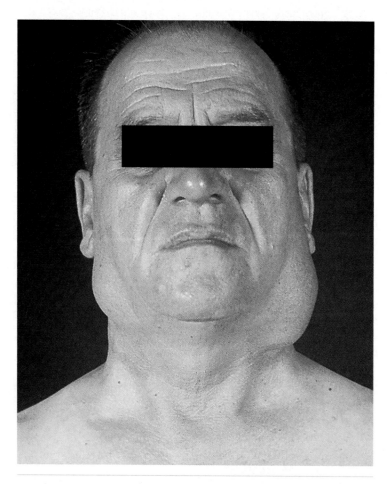

FIGURE 20-3 Marked enlargement of cervical lymph nodes as a result of malignant lymphoma.

CANCER WITH SPECIFIC NAMES

This section explores some tumors with specific names. They do not follow the "rules" discussed earlier (see **Table 20-4**).

TABLE 20-4 Cancer with Specific Names

Tumor	Explanation for Nomenclature
embryonic tumors	derived from persisting groups of embryonic cells of the brain, retina, adrenal gland, kidney, liver, or genital tract. Named from the site of origin with the suffix "-blastoma" added (blast = a primitive cell + oma = tumor); *medulloblastoma*: medulla of the brain; *retinoblastoma*: retina of the eye; *hepatoblastoma*: liver; Wilms' tumor: kidney, exception in naming (*nephroblastoma* not used)
in situ carcinoma (noninfiltrating)	cancer that has not invaded the surrounding tissue or traveled to other parts of the body through the blood or lymph system; common in many locations, including the breast, cervix, colon, skin, and urinary tract; in situ carcinoma can be completely cured by surgical excision of the tumor
lymphoid tumors	all neoplasms of lymphoid tissue are called lymphomas and are malignant: Hodgkin's disease and non-Hodgkin's lymphomas
precancerous conditions	refers to conditions that have a high likelihood of developing into cancer: **1.** Skin cancer: *actinic keratoses* ("actinic" refers to sun rays) or *lentigo maligna* (a latin term meaning "malignant freckle") **2.** Oral cancer: *leukoplakis* (leuko- = white + plakia = patch) may develop in the mucous membranes of the mouth as a result of exposure to tobacco tars from smoking or use of smokeless tobacco **3.** Colon polyps
skin tumors	**1.** Pigment-producing cells of the epidermis benign: *nervus*, a Latin word that means "birthmark" malignant: *melanoma* or *malignant melanoma* **2.** Keratinocytes benign: *basal cell carcinoma* malignant: *squamous cell carcinoma* (sometimes metastasizes)
teratoma tumors	derived from cells that have the potential to differentiate into different types of tissue (bone, muscle, glands, epithelium, brain tissue, hair) and may be either benign or malignant; teratomas occur in ovaries, testicles, central nervous system, chest, or abdomen

SCREENING AND EARLY DETECTION

The early detection of cancers relies on two conditions: the existence of a premalignant or detectable preclinical phase and the availability of appropriate tests that can detect the tumor during the preclinical phase. On an individual basis, the standard history and physical examination provide a comprehensive format for early detection of cancer. Emphasis is placed on:

1. History and physical examination, including family history of cancer, personal habits—smoking, alcohol use, and sexual history—and occupational exposure to chemicals or radiation.
2. Signs and symptoms related to specific organ systems:
   a. Bladder: Hematuria
   b. Breast: Nipple discharge, lump, or mass
   c. Brain: Seizures, loss of balance, problems with vision, hearing, or speech
   d. Gastrointestinal: Change in bowel habits, bleeding

   e. Gynecological: Abnormal vaginal bleeding or discharge, dyspareunia
   f. Lymph system: Abnormal size or number of lymph nodes
   g. Oropharynx: Hoarseness for more than one week, abnormal bleeding, pain, dysphagia
   h. Prostrate: Dysuria
   i. Respiratory system: Cough, pain, dyspnea, hemoptysis
   j. Skin: Slow-healing sore, changing mole

CANCER TREATMENT

Cancer is treated with surgery, radiation therapy, chemotherapy, hormone therapy, immunotherapy, or a combination of these treatments. Treatment may be prophylactic for precancerous lesions, palliative to reduce the size of a tumor when the tumor has metastasized, or reconstructive after a mastectomy for breast cancer. Patients with cancer are often treated by a team of specialists, which may include a medical oncologist (specialist in cancer treatment), a surgeon, a radiation oncologist (specialist in radiation therapy), and others. The choice of treatment depends on the type and location of the cancer, the stage of the disease, the patient's age and general health, and other factors.

TERMS USED IN THE DIAGNOSIS AND TREATMENT OF CANCER

The most common detection and diagnostic tools and treatments or tests are described in **Table 20-5**.

TABLE **20-5** Terms Used in the Diagnosis and Treatment of Cancer		
Term	**Pronunciation**	**Definition**
History and Physical Exam		
anemia	uh-<u>nee</u>-mee-uh	number of red blood cells is below normal; can be a sign of abnormal bleeding from cancer of the gastrointestinal tract or vagina
anorexia	a-nuh-<u>rek</u>-see-uh	abnormal loss of appetite; can be a sign of cancer or some cancer treatments, especially chemotherapy or radiation therapy
dyspareunia	dys-pa-<u>reu</u>-ni-a	painful sexual intercourse in women; can be a symptom of cancer of the cervix or uterus
dyspnea	disp-<u>nee</u>-uh	difficulty breathing, shortness of breath; can be a symptom of lung cancer
dysuria	dys-<u>u</u>-ri-a	discomfort or burning on urination; symptom of cancer in the urinary tract
hematuria	hee-muh-<u>toor</u>-ee-uh	blood in the urine; sign of cancer of the bladder or prostrate
hemoptysis	hee-<u>mop</u>-tih-sis	coughing or spitting up blood from the respiratory tract; sign of lung cancer
lymphadenopathy	lim-fad-n-<u>op</u>-uh-thee	disease or swelling of lymph nodes; sign of lymphoma or metastatic cancer

Term	Pronunciation	Definition
night sweats	night sweats	excessive sweating while sleeping; sign of leukemia or lymphoma
peripheral neuropathy	pe-<u>riph</u>-er-al neu-<u>rop</u>-a-thy	pain, numbness, tingling, swelling, or muscle weakness of the hands and feet; may be a sign of cancer or a complication of cancer treatment such as chemotherapy
thrombocytopenia	throm-boh-sy-toh-<u>pee</u>-nee-uh	lower than normal number of platelets in the blood; symptoms are easy bruising and excessive bleeding from wounds; side effect of some chemotherapy treatments

Laboratory Tests

BRCA1/BRCA2	be-ar-se-a	tissue sample taken to identify inherited mutations that increase the risk of female breast and ovarian cancers
complete blood count (CBC)	<u>kum</u>-pleet blud kownt	blood sample taken for determination of the number and shape of red blood cells, white blood cells, and platelets; especially important for diagnosing and treating leukemia
estrogen/progesterone receptors (ER/PR)	<u>es</u>-truh-jin/proh-<u>jes</u>-teh-rone reh-sep-ter	after diagnosis of breast cancer, cells are taken from breast tissue; used to determine if tumors grow in response to estrogen or progesterone
fecal occult blood test (FOBT)/ guaiac FOBT (gFOBT)	<u>fe</u>-cal oc-<u>cult</u> blood test/ <u>guai</u>-ac	screening for rectal or colon cancer; detects heme, a component of the blood protein hemoglobin (*fecal* refers to stool, *occult* means hidden)
prostate-specific antigen (PSA)	<u>pros</u>-tate spe-<u>cif</u>-ic <u>an</u>-ti-gen	blood test of a substance produced by the prostate; increased levels may be a sign of prostate cancer
sputum cytology	<u>spu</u>-tum cy-<u>tol</u>-o-gy	cells found in sputum (mucus and other matter brought up from the lungs by coughing); checks for abnormal cells for diagnosing lung cancer
urine cytology	<u>u</u>-rine cy-<u>tol</u>-o-gy	sample of urine is checked under a microscope for abnormal cells for diagnosing cancer of the bladder or kidneys

Radiological Exams

barium enema	<u>bah</u>-ree-um <u>en</u>-e-ma	series of X-rays of the colon taken after the person is given an enema that contains barium; used to evaluate for colon cancer
computed axial tomography (CAT, CT)	com-<u>put</u>-ed <u>ax</u>-i-al to-mog-ra-phy	X-ray ± contrast dye with the creation of pictures by a computer linked to an X-ray machine; high specificity, especially for brain tumors
intravenous pyelogram or intravenous pyelography (IVP)	in-truh-<u>vee</u>-nus <u>py</u>-elo-gram py-e-<u>log</u>-ra-hy	dye is injected into a blood vessel and concentrated in the urine to visualize the kidneys, ureters, and bladder
lymphangiography/lymph node mapping	lym-phan-gi-<u>og</u>-ra-phy	blue dye, injected into the lymphatic channel, visualizes lymph nodes; used to evaluate for lymphoma or to evaluate for metastatic cancer
radionuclide scanning/ scintigraphy	ray-dee-oh-<u>noo</u>-klide <u>skan</u>-ing/sin-<u>tig</u>-ruh-fee	radioactive material is injected or swallowed and radioactivity measured with a scanner; used for cancer diagnosis and staging of organs because of specificity

(continues)

TABLE 20-5 *(continued)*

Term	Pronunciation	Definition
sentinel lymph node biopsy (SLNB)	<u>sen</u>-tih-nul limf node <u>by</u>-op-see	biopsy done to determine if cancer has spread beyond the primary tumor; dye or a radioactive substance injected near a tumor flows into the sentinel lymph node(s)—the first lymph node(s) to which cancer is likely to spread from the primary tumor
transrectal ultrasound	tranz-<u>rek</u>-tul <u>ul</u>-truh-sownd	ultrasound probe is inserted into the rectum to check for abnormalities of the rectum and prostate; probe bounces sound waves off body tissues to make echoes that form a sonogram
upper GI series (barium swallow)	<u>uh</u>-per GI <u>seer</u>-eez	X-rays of the esophagus and stomach after the patient has drunk a liquid that contains barium; the liquid coats the esophagus and stomach and shows abnormalities
Surgery for Diagnosis		
biopsy	<u>by</u>-ahp-see	removal of cells or tissues for examination under a microscope to evaluate for cancer
bone marrow aspiration and biopsy	bone <u>mayr</u>-oh as-pih-<u>ray</u>-shun <u>by</u>-op-see	removal of bone marrow, blood, and a small piece of bone by inserting a hollow needle into the hipbone or breastbone; cells are evaluated for leukemia and lymphoma
endometrial biopsy	en-doh-<u>mee</u>-tree-ul <u>by</u>-op-see	removal of tissue from the endometrium by inserting a thin, flexible tube through the cervix and into the uterus to evaluate for uterine cancer
fine-needle aspiration (FNA)	fine <u>nee</u>-dul as-pih-<u>ray</u>-shun	biopsy of the lung using a thin needle to remove tissue or fluid to evaluate cells for cancer; procedure is done during a CT scan, ultrasound, or other imaging procedure
lymph node dissection	limf node dy-<u>sek</u>-shun	*regional lymph node dissection*: some of the lymph nodes in the tumor area are removed *radical lymph node dissection*: most or all of the lymph nodes in the tumor area are removed; cells are examined for cancer
pap smear	pap smear	cells obtained by swab of vagina, endocervical canal, and exocervix
scope	scope	procedure in which a thin, lighted tube is inserted into the body part being examined and a tissue sample (biopsy) is taken to examine under a microscope to determine whether cancer cells are present
bronchoscopy	bron-<u>kos</u>-ko-pee	scope inserted through the nose or mouth to examine the inside of the trachea, bronchi, and lung
colonoscopy	ko-lun-<u>ahs</u>-ko-pee	scope inserted into the rectum to examine the colon
cystoscopy	sis-<u>tos</u>-koh-pee	scope inserted through the urethra into the bladder
endoscopy	en-<u>dos</u>-koh-pee	procedure to look at the throat, trachea, esophagus, stomach, and small intestine
esophagoscopy	ee-<u>sah</u>-fuh-gos-<u>koh</u>-pee	examination of the esophagus using an esophagoscope
hysteroscopy	hys-ter-<u>os</u>-co-py	procedure to look inside the uterus

Term	Pronunciation	Definition
laryngoscopy	lair-in-gos-ko-pee	examination of the larynx (voice box) with a mirror (indirect laryngoscopy) or with a laryngoscope (direct laryngoscopy)
sigmoidoscopy	sig-moid-oss-ko-pee	scope inserted into the sigmoid part of the colon; also called proctosigmoidoscopy
thoracoscopy	thor-uh-kos-koh-pee	surgery to examine organs inside the chest for abnormal areas; an incision is made between two ribs and a thoracoscope is inserted into the chest
thoracotomy	tho-ra-cot-o-my	a larger incision is made between the ribs and the chest is opened to examine internal organs

Treatment

Term	Pronunciation	Definition
Biological/Immunotherapy	bi-o-log-i-cal/im-mu-no-ther-a-py	treatment to stimulate or restore the ability of the immune system to fight infection and disease
Bacille Calmette-Guérin (BCG) vaccine	ba-cille cal-mette gué-rin	an anticancer drug, bacille Calmette-Guérin (BCG) that activates the immune system
colony-stimulating factors (CSF)	col-o-ny-stim-u-lat-ing factor	substances that stimulate the production of blood cells; granulocyte colony-stimulating factors (G-CSF); granulocyte-macrophage colony-stimulating factors (GM-CSF); used to restore blood cells after chemotherapy or radiation therapy
Chemotherapy	kee-mo-ther-a-pee	treatment with anticancer drugs to destroy cancer cells by stopping them from growing or multiplying; the type of chemotherapy varies with the type and stage of cancer
Hormone/Endocrine Therapy	hor-mone/en-do-crine ther-a-py	slows or stops the growth of hormone-sensitive tumors by blocking the body's ability to produce hormones or by interfering with effects of hormones
antiandrogens	an-tee-an-dro-jens	used to block the production or interfere with the action of male sex hormones
antiestrogen	an-ti-es-tro-gen	used to block the production or interfere with effects of estrogen in breast cancer that is estrogen positive
luteinizing hormone-releasing hormone (LH-RH) agonist	loo-tin-eye-zing ag-o-nist	a substance that closely resembles luteinizing hormone-releasing hormone (LH-RH), which controls the secretion of sex hormones; given to decrease secretion of sex hormones in individuals with cancer of the reproduction system
Radiation Therapy	ray-dee-ay-shun ther-a-py	radiotherapy uses high-energy radiation from X-rays, neutrons, and other sources to kill cancer cells or slow their growth
external	ex-ter-nal	uses a machine to aim high-energy rays at the specific part of the body where the cancer is located
internal (brachytherapy)	in-ter-nal brach-y-ther-a-py	given internally by placing radioactive material that is sealed in needles, seeds, wires, or catheters directly into or near the tumor

(continues)

TABLE 20-5 (*continued*)

Term	Pronunciation	Definition
systemic	sys-<u>tem</u>-ic	liquid radioactive substance given by mouth, a vein, or IV line that circulates throughout the body; the treatment travels in the blood to tissues throughout the body, seeking out and killing cancer cells
Stem Cell Transplant	stem sel trans-<u>plant</u>	used to restore stem cells that have been destroyed by high doses of chemotherapy and/or radiation therapy; most often used to treat leukemia and lymphoma
bone marrow transplantation (BMT)	Bone <u>mar</u>-row trans-plan-<u>ta</u>-tion	blood-forming stem cells that are used in transplants can come from the bone marrow bloodstream or umbilical cord
peripheral blood stem cell transplantation (PBSCT)	per-<u>if</u>-er-al cell trans-plan-<u>ta</u>-tion	blood-forming stem cells used in transplants can come from the bloodstream
Surgery	<u>sur</u>-gery	works best to remove solid tumors that are contained in one area; not used for leukemia or metastatic cancer
cryosurgery	cry-o-<u>sur</u>-ger-y	treatment performed with an instrument that freezes and destroys abnormal tissues; used to treat early-stage skin cancer, retinoblastoma, and precancerous growths on the skin and cervix
cystectomy	sis-<u>tek</u>-toe-mee	surgical removal of the bladder
hysterectomy	hiss-ter-<u>ek</u>-toe-mee	surgical removal of the uterus
laryngectomy	lair-in-<u>jek</u>-toe-mee	an operation to remove all or part of the larynx (voice box)
laser	<u>lay</u>-zer	beams of light cut through tissue; used for tumors on the surface of the body or on the inside lining of internal organs, e.g., basal cell carcinoma, cervical, vaginal, esophageal, and non-small cell lung cancer
lumpectomy	lump-<u>ek</u>-toe-mee	surgery to remove the tumor and a small amount of normal tissue around it
mastectomy	mas-<u>tek</u>-toe-mee	surgery to remove the breast (or as much of the breast tissue as possible); may or may not include removal of lymph nodes
modified radical mastectomy	<u>mod</u>-i-fied <u>rad</u>-i-cal mas-<u>tek</u>-toe-mee	surgical procedure in which the breast, some of the lymph nodes in the armpit, and the lining over the chest muscles are removed
orchiectomy	or-kee-<u>ek</u>-toe-mee	surgical removal of one or both testicles
pneumonectomy	noo-mo-<u>nek</u>-toe-mee	surgical removal of an entire lung
prostatectomy	pros-ta-<u>tek</u>-toe-mee	surgical removal of part or all of the prostate
salpingo-oophorectomy	sal-<u>pin</u>-go-o-o-for-<u>ek</u>-toe-mee	surgical removal of the fallopian tubes and ovaries

TERMS USED TO DESCRIBE TREATMENT APPROACHES FOR CANCER

In addition to cancer treatment described in Table 20-5, general approaches used after a cancer diagnosis include those listed in **Table 20-6**.

Approach	Example
palliative	cytoreduction; oncologic emergencies; neurosurgical procedures/pain control; nutritional support
primary/definitive	local excision; en bloc dissection
prophylactic	excision of premalignant lesions
rehabilitative	cosmetic and functional restoration; reconstructive surgery, e.g., after a mastectomy
resection (of metastases)	lung; liver
supportive	insertion of access devices such as a porta catheter for infusion of drugs for chemotherapy; radiation implants

TABLE 20-6 Terms Used to Describe Treatment Approaches for Cancer

BOX 20-1 compares cancer in companion animals and humans.

Box 20-1 Cats and Dogs can have Cancer too

Just like humans, companion animals are living longer because of better diagnosis and treatment of chronic diseases, for example, diabetes and heart disease. Living a long life increases the risk of cancer in both humans and pets, and the leading cause of death in dogs and cats is cancer. Many pet owners consider their pet a part of the family and choose to treat pets with a cancer diagnosis. Companion animal oncology is a specialty within the field of veterinary medicine that requires additional training. The signs and symptoms of cancer in animals are similar to those in humans, and veterinarians use the same methods of diagnosing and treating cancer as physicians. Research findings from companion animal studies can be used to improve cancer treatment for humans and their pets.

Source: American Veterinary Medical Association. *Taking on Cancer*. https://www.avma.org/News/JAVMANews/Pages/140115a.aspx

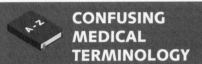

CONFUSING MEDICAL TERMINOLOGY

-ectomy versus -stomy versus -tomy

-ectomy – removal, cutting out, excision, e.g., blepharectomy (blef-ah-<u>rek</u>-to-me) refers to excision of a lesion of the eyelid

-stomy – furnish with a mouth or outlet, new opening, e.g., salpingostomy (sal-pin-<u>jos</u>-to-me) refers to creation of an artificial opening in the fallopian tube

-tomy – cutting, incision, e.g., prostatolithotomy (pros-tat-o-<u>lith</u>-o-to-me) refers to incision in the prostate gland to remove a stone

BREAST CANCER AND MEDICAL ILLUSTRATIONS

This chapter is unable to discuss medical terms associated with each type of cancer.

Figures 20-4 through **20-8** serve as illustrations for breast cancer.

Figure 20-9 shows lymphedema following a mastectomy complicated by lymphosarcoma, a second cancer diagnosis.

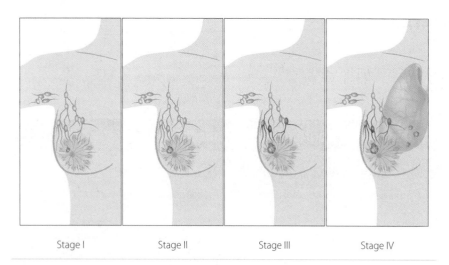

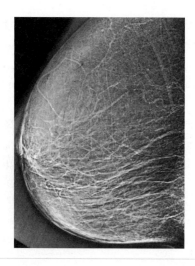

FIGURE 20-4 Stages of breast cancer. Stage I: Localized cancer (*in situ*); Stage II: Invasion of nearby breast tissue; Stage III: Invasion of lymph nodes; and Stage IV: Metastasis to liver.

FIGURE 20-5 A normal mammogram.

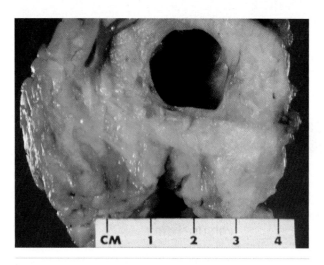

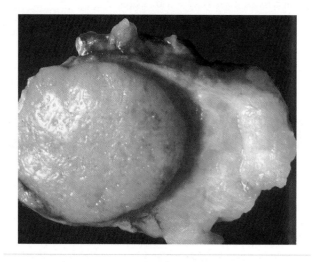

FIGURE 20-6 A benign cyst in the breast viewed in cross section.

FIGURE 20-7 Benign fibroadenoma of the breast.

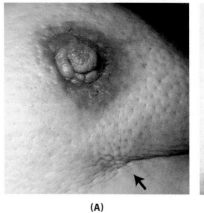
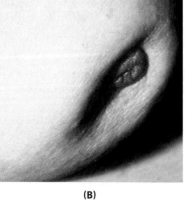

(A)   **(B)**

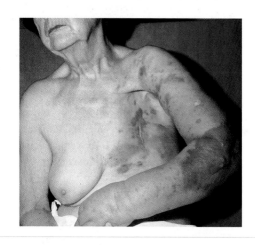

FIGURE 20-8 Changes in the breast caused by advanced carcinoma: **(A)** Skin retraction (arrow) and orange-peel appearance of the skin and **(B)** nipple retraction.

FIGURE 20-9 Severe edema of arm resulting from long-standing lymphatic obstruction. The patient had a radical operation for breast carcinoma many years previously.

Mastectomy

THE ORIGIN OF MEDICAL TERMS

Table 20-7 explains the origin of several terms used in cancer medicine.

TABLE 20-7 The Origin of Medical Terms

Word	Pronunciation	Origin and Definition
astrocytoma	as-tro-cy-to-ma	Greek, *astron*, star + Greek, *kytos*, cell + Greek, *-oma*, tumor
colostomy	co-los-to-my	Greek, *kolon*, large intestine + Greek, *stoma*, mouth
cytology	cy-tol-o-gy	Greek, *kytos*, cell + Greek, *logos*, science
glioblastoma	glio-blas-to-ma	Greek, *glia*, glue + Greek, *blastós*, a bud + Greek, *-oma*, tumor
hemoptysis	hee-mop-tih-sis	Latin, *hemo*, blood + Greek, *ptýsis*, spitting
mastectomy	mas-tek-toe-mee	Greek, *mastos*, breast + Greek, *ektome*, excision, from *ek*, out of
palliative	pal-lia-tive	French, *palliatif*, to relieve or lessen without curing
prophylactic	pro-phy-lac-tic	Greek, *pro*, before + Greek, *phulassein*, to guard
receptor (estrogen)	re-cep-tor	Latin, *receiver*, to receive
teratoma	ter-a-to-ma	Greek, *teras*, monster + Greek, *-oma*, tumor

ABBREVIATIONS

These abbreviations in Table 20-8 are frequently used in cancer medicine, including the naming of cancers and diagnostic tools.

TABLE 20-8 Abbreviations

Abbreviation	Definition	Abbreviation	Definition
ALL	acute lymphocytic leukemia	ER/PR	estrogen receptor/progesterone receptor
AML	acute myeloid leukemia	FNP	fine needle aspiration
BGC	bacille Calmette-Guérin	FOBT	fecal occult blood test
BMT	bone marrow transplantation	gFOBT	guaiac fecal occult blood test
BRCA1/BRCA2	breast cancer 1/breast cancer 2	IVP	intravenous pyelography
CAT/CT	computed axial tomography	LH-RH	leuteinizing hormone-releasing hormone
CBC	complete blood count	PBMCT	peripheral blood stem cell transplantation
CLL	chronic lymphocytic leukemia	PSA	prostate-specific antigen
CSF	Colony-stimulating factors	SNLB	sentinel lymph node biopsy
CML	chronic myeloid leukemia	WBC	white blood cell; white blood (cell) count

The following box lists three different categories of medications that may be prescribed by a physician treating cancer.

PHARMACOLOGY AND MEDICAL TERMINOLOGY

Drug Classification	antiemetic (an-ti-e-<u>met</u>-ic)	antineoplastic (an-tih-nee-oh-<u>plass</u>-tik)	immunosuppressant (im-moo-noh-suh-<u>press</u>-ant)
Function	prevents nausea and vomiting associated with chemotherapy and radiation therapy	prevents the development, growth, or reproduction of cancerous cells	suppresses the body's natural immune response to an antigen, as in treatment for transplant patients
Word Parts	**anti** = against; **emesis** = vomiting; **tic** = pertaining to	**anti-** = against; **ne/o** = new; **plas/o** = formation; **-tic** = pertaining to	**immun/o** = immunity, **suppressant** = pertaining to lower, to control
Active Ingredients (examples)	chlorpromazine (Thorazine); dexamethasone (Baycadron)	fluorouracil (Adrucil); methotrexate (Rheumatrex Dose Pack)	cyclosporine (Sandimmune); azathioprine (Imuran)

CLINICAL *Note*

Discharge Summary

Twenty-eight-year-old, gravida 0, para 0, white female with history of **papillary carcinoma** of the thyroid is admitted for I-131 treatment.

History of Present Illness: Ms. Smith was diagnosed with papillary carcinoma of the thyroid in 12-92 for which she underwent a left **thyroidectomy** on 12-16-92. The pathology revealed evidence of tumor extending through soft tissue with involvement of the lymph nodes. On 1-8-93, she received a dose of I-131, 100 mCi. She was recently seen in follow-up clinic on 4-5-93, at which time she was noted to have a left **anterior cervical lymph node** measuring about 1 × 2 cm in size. The **TSH** was more than 60. The **thyroglobulin** was 370. She denied any other lumps or bumps. The patient was admitted on 4-14-93 for her second **I-131** treatment

Past Medical History: Unremarkable

Past Surgical History: Status post left thyroidectomy in 12-92

Social History: She is single and lives alone

Family History: Unremarkable

Admission Laboratory and X-ray Data: 4-5-93, TSH greater than 60. Thyroglobulin equal 370. CBC unremarkable

Hospital Course: The patient was admitted on 4-14-93 and received a dose of I-131 of 150 **mCi**.

The patient tolerated the treatment well without significant difficulties. She did develop some **bilateral** neck swelling, but denied any soreness or tenderness of the parotid glands. She has noted slight changes in her taste. A final survey was done on 4-17-93 at 1200 hours which showed exposure rate of 4.8 mR/hr.

Disposition: She is scheduled to return on 4-20-93 to undergo whole body I-313 scan

Discharge Medications: Synthroid 0.1 mg one p.o., q. day to start on 4-20-93

Follow-Up: She is scheduled to see Dr. Joseph Simpson in two months.

Direction: For the portions of the clinical note shown by a colored font, provide the definition and/or words for abbreviation.

COMPLETION: CANCER WITH SPECIFIC NAMES

For the type of cancer described, write in the correct term:

1. _____: Benign cancer of the colon
2. _____: Benign skin cancer
3. _____: Cancer of the blood cells
4. _____: Embryonic tumor of the brain
5. _____: Malignant cancer of the lymph system
6. _____: Malignant tumor of cartilage
7. _____: Malignant tumor of the skin
8. _____: Malignant cancer of the bone
9. _____: Benign tumor of the uterus
10. _____: Cancer cells appear the size and shape of oats

MULTIPLE CHOICE: DIAGNOSIS AND TREATMENT OF CANCER

Circle the letter of the correct answer:

1. A biopsy is not used in the diagnosis of this cancer:
   a. Leukemia
   b. Breast
   c. Lung
   d. Bladder

2. Radiation therapy with a radioactive substance given intravenously is:
   a. external
   b. internal
   c. prophylactic
   d. systemic

3. Surgical removal for treatment of bladder cancer is called:
   a. orchiectomy
   b. cystectomy
   c. intravenous pyelogram
   d. cystoscopy

4. A procedure that would not be used to diagnose or treat lung cancer is:
   a. hormone therapy
   b. bronchoscopy
   c. sputum cytology
   d. pneumonectomy

5. Cancer cells in the liver in someone with metastatic cancer of the colon are described as:
   a. liver cancer
   b. colon cancer
   c. colon and liver cancer
   d. lymph cancer

6. Cryosurgery is a method of surgery using:
   a. electricity
   b. light
   c. freezing
   d. radioisotopes

7. Carcinoma of the breast would be treated by any of the following except which method?
   a. Computed axial tomography
   b. Hormone therapy
   c. Radiation therapy
   d. Modified radical mastectomy

8. Surgical excision of basal cell carcinoma of the skin is a type of treatment described as:
   a. definitive
   b. palliative
   c. prophylactic
   d. resection

9. Bone marrow aspiration is a diagnostic tool for:
   a. leukemia
   b. lymphoma
   c. leukemia and lymphoma
   d. neither leukemia nor lymphoma

10. A common symptom of cancer of the bladder or prostrate is:
   a. hemoptysis
   b. dyspnea
   c. lymphadenopathy
   d. hematuria

MATCHING: TOOLS FOR DIAGNOSING CANCER

Match the following diagnostic procedure in the left column to its function in the right:

Diagnostic Procedure
1. Biopsy
2. Barium enema
3. PSA
4. Pap smear
5. Sputum cytology
6. Bone marrow aspiration
7. Estrogen/progesterone receptors
8. Lymphangiography
9. Stool guaiac
10. IVP

Function
a. Used to detect abnormal lung cells
b. Used a dye to visualize kidneys, ureters, and bladder
c. Visualization of lymph nodes
d. Tissue sample taken for microscopic examination
e. Tissue sample taken near a breast tumor
f. Screen for gastrointestinal bleeding
g. Tissue sample taken for diagnosis of uterine cancer
h. Used to detect and monitor treatment of prostate cancer
i. Diagnostic tool for detecting cancer of blood cells
j. Outline of the colon on X-ray

MATCHING: SIGNS AND SYMPTOMS OF CANCER

Match the type of cancer in the left column with the signs and symptoms of cancer in the right:

Cancer
1. Gynecological
2. Skin
3. Brain
4. Gastrointestinal
5. Bladder
6. Respiratory
7. Oropharynx
8. Lymph system
9. Breast
10. Prostrate

Sign or Symptom
a. Hematuria
b. Hemoptysis
c. Nipple discharge
d. Difficulty in swallowing
e. Enlarged lymph nodes
f. Rectal bleeding
g. Change in mole
h. Dysuria
i. Vaginal bleeding after menopause
j. Seizure

IDENTIFYING WORD PARTS

For each of the medical terms, list the root word and the prefix and/or suffix.

Word	Root Word	Prefix	Suffix
1. Antiestrogen			
2. Antineoplastic			
3. Leukemia			
4. Dyspareunia			
5. Hematuria			
6. Hyperplasia			
7. Transrectal			
8. Mastectomy			
9. Pneumonectomy			
10. Precancerous			

Answer Keys

Unit I: Word Parts and Medical Terminology

Answer Key to Chapter 1: Word Pronunciations

⬤ **CLINICAL NOTE**

S = Subjective

A format that is used in the documentation to provide information in a patient's chart. This part of the format is the narration of the patient's current condition in the patient's own words, their complaint, and the reason for the episode of care.

O = Objective

A format that is used in the documentation to provide information in a patient's chart. This part of the format is completed by the health professional and includes facts about the patient's status.

HEENT = Head, Eyes, Ears, Nose, and Throat

Examination of these body parts are part of the overall physical exam given to the patient. It is used to help diagnose the problem.

WNL = Within Normal Limits

Term used by medical professionals to express that the results are normal.

Adenopathy

Term used to describe lymph nodes. Adeno = relating to a gland or glands, and Pathy = disease. When used, it characterizes lymph nodes as large or swollen.

A = Assessment

A format that is used in the documentation to provide information in a patient's chart. This part of the format is completed by the provider and includes the medical diagnoses for the episode of care.

Bell's Palsy

An eponym to describe a condition. The condition is the weakening or paralyses of facial muscles on one side of the face due to damage to the facial nerves.

R/O = Rule Out

Medical abbreviation used by healthcare professional. When used, the term means for the provider to exclude other diagnosis or conditions.

CLINICAL NOTE (*continued*)

TIA = Transient Ischemic Attack
Medical abbreviation used to indicate a mini stroke. A mini stroke is a symptom of a more serious condition, a stroke.

CVA = Cerebrovascular Accident
Medical abbreviation used to indicate a stroke, which is when blood flow to the brain is interrupted and the result is death of brain cells in the affected area.

P = Plan
A format that is used in the documentation to provide information in a patient's chart. This part of the format is completed by the provider and includes the treatment plan for the patient.

CT = Computed Tomography Scan
A procedure that allows a technician to produce multiple images of the body by taking X-rays from different angles. The computer than puts these images together to form a cross-sectional image of the body.

Lesson Two: Progress Check

FILL IN

1. Greek and Latin
2. Synonym
3. Homonym
4. Eponym
5. Diacritical marking
6. Syllable

TRUE OR FALSE

1. True
2. False
3. False
4. False
5. True

Answer Key to Chapter 2: Word Parts and Word Building Rules

CLINICAL NOTE

Gastralgia
Term used to describe pain that is localized to the stomach or abdominal area.

Aphasia
A condition that impairs language, comprehension of speech, and/or the ability to read or write. Aphasia is most commonly associated with stroke or head trauma.

EGD = Esophagogastroduodenoscopy
A procedure to examine the lining of the esophagus, stomach, and duodenum. An instrument with a camera is passed down the throat along the length of the esophagus and into the stomach and upper part of the small intestine.

Cautery
A procedure in which a device is used to destroy tissue by means of heat in order to control bleeding in the upper GI.

Hemostasis
The ability to stop the flow of blood due to bleeding of a blood vessel or organ of the body.

Abdominal quadrants
The abdomen is visually broken into four major regions. Names of the quadrants are based on their location: Right Upper Quadrant, Right Lower Quadrant, Left Upper Quadrant, and Left Lower Quadrant.

Lesson Two: Progress Check Part A

FILL IN

1. sign
2. disorder
3. symptom
4. disease
5. prefix, suffix, and root

MATCHING

1. f
2. d
3. a
4. g
5. b
6. h
7. c
8. e

SPELLING AND DEFINITION

1. (a) oophor/o: ovary
2. (b) proct/o: rectum or anus
3. (c) nephr/o: kidney
4. (b) rhin/o: nose
5. (a) orchi/o: testicle
6. (c) sacr/o: sacrum
7. (b) salping/o: fallopian tube
8. (a) myring/o: eardrum
9. (b) pharyng/o: pharynx
10. (c) spondyl/o: vertebra
11. (c) ureter/o: ureter
12. (a) chondr/o: cartilage
13. (b) cost/o: rib
14. (b) vas/o: vessel
15. (a) ven/o: vein
16. (a) erythr/o: red

DEFINING MEDICAL WORD ELEMENTS

1. andr/o
2. gyne
3. cardi/o
4. cephal/o
5. steth/o
6. dent/o or odont/o
7. encephal/o
8. gastr/o
9. hepat/o or hep/a
10. cholecyst/o
11. stomat/o
12. lingua
13. mast/o or mamm/o
14. my/o or myos
15. neur/o

BUILDING MEDICAL WORDS

1. tendinitis, tendonitis
2. thyroidectomy
3. tracheotomy
4. enteropathy
5. neuralgia
6. cystitis
7. arthritis
8. splenectomy
9. ophthalmologist
10. angiogram
11. cholelithiasis
12. arteriosclerosis
13. pneumonectomy
14. myelogram
15. otoscope
16. phlebotomy
17. prostatectomy
18. cerebrovascular accident
19. esophagitis
20. thoracotomy
21. hyperglycemia

Lesson Two: Progress Check Part B

MATCHING

1. i
2. j
3. g
4. h
5. f
6. e
7. c
8. d
9. a
10. b

SPELLING AND DEFINITION

1. (a) -centesis: surgical puncture
2. (b) -clasis: to break down; refracture
3. (c) -ectasis: to expand, dilate
4. (d) -malacia: softening
5. (a) -plegia: paralysis (stroke)
6. (b) -ptosis: prolapse, falling, drooping
7. (c) -sclerosis: hardening
8. (d) -megaly: enlargement
9. (a) -cele: hernia, swelling
10. (b) -iasis: abnormal condition: presence of, formation of

BUILDING MEDICAL WORDS

1. cephalgia or cephalodynia
2. roentgenography
3. gastritis
4. cholelithiasis
5. polycythemia

6. osteomalacia
7. arthrocentesis
8. phlebotomy
9. rhinoplasty
10. biology
11. hepatomegaly
12. dermatosis
13. appendectomy
14. psychiatry
15. encephalotomy
16. chemotherapy
17. hemostasis
18. carcinogen
19. nephropathy
20. aphasia

DEFINING MEDICAL TERMS

1. surgical fracture or refracture of a bone
2. surgical separation of intestinal adhesions
3. crushing of a stone in the bladder and washing out the fragments
4. death of cells or tissue
5. removal of the foreskin from the penis
6. a gland tumor
7. difficulty in swallowing
8. reduced number of white blood cells
9. paralyzed on one side of the body
10. morbid fear of heights

Unit II: Root Words, Medical Terminology, and Patient Care

Answer Key to Chapter 3: Bacteria, Color, and Some Medical Terms

CLINICAL NOTE

Normocephalic
A term referring to a person's head being of normal shape and size for their age. There is no appearance of significant abnormalities of the head.

Jaundice
Yellow staining of the skin and the whites of the eyes by abnormally high levels of the bile pigment bilirubin in the blood. The yellowing extends to other tissues and body fluids.

Pustules
Small blisters that form on the skin, which contain pus. The pocket of pus forms in either the epidermis or the dermis layer of the skin.

Cirrhosis
A liver disease in which the organ becomes abnormal due to an underlying condition/disease of the liver. The liver structure becomes fibrosis or scarred.

CBC = Complete Blood Count
A test based on a sample of blood drawn from a patient. The test is used to measure and evaluate several components of blood: red blood cells, white blood cells, hemoglobin, hematocrit, and platelets.

SGOT = Serum Glutamic-Oxaloacetic Transaminase
A blood test usually used to detect liver damage or to monitor liver function. This test is typically ordered in addition to other liver tests.

CLINICAL NOTE (*continued*)

SGPT = Serum Glutamic-Pyruvic Transaminase
A blood test used to detect early liver damage by looking at the enzyme ALT. This test is typically ordered in addition to other liver tests.

Rapid strep
A test used to determine whether a person has an infection of the throat caused by bacteria. The test detects antigens and results are available in 10–20 minutes and are read as a positive/negative result.

Lesson Two: Progress Check

FILL IN

1. microbe
2. Genomic medicine
3. Bacteria
4. biotechnology

MULTIPLE CHOICE

1. c
2. c
3. b
4. d
5. b
6. a

MATCHING

1. h
2. e
3. k
4. i
5. f
6. g
7. a
8. h
9. c
10. d
11. h
12. b
13. a
14. j

WRITE IN THE PREFIX

1. acro-
2. aniso-
3. hetero-
4. dys-
5. homo-
6. iso-
7. mal-
8. megaly-
9. pan-
10. post-
11. hemo-

DEFINE THE PREFIX

1. bad, poor
2. bad, painful, difficult
3. enlarged, large
4. excessive, beyond, above normal
5. fast
6. under, below normal
7. slow
8. take away, remove
9. put back
10. water
11. beside
12. around
13. many
14. before
15. before, preceding
16. through
17. together, united
18. night
19. night
20. through
21. around
22. producing pus

Answer Key to Chapter 4: Body Openings and Plural Endings

CLINICAL NOTE

HPI = History of Present Illness
Documentation found in health records. A summary of the symptoms or problems in chronological order from the start of the issue to the time of the episode of care.
Epitaxis
Bleeding from the nose cavity that can vary from mild to severe.
Cavity
A hollow place or space, or a potential space, within the body or one of its organs.
NKDA = No Known Drug Allergies
An acronym used to specify that the patient has no known drug allergies.
Nare
A single nostril.
BP = Blood Pressure
A test performed to measure the blood pressure when the heart beats and when it is between beats.
Supine
A body position where the person is lying down with his face upward.
Otorhinolaryngology Examination
A visual review of the ear, nose, and throat in order to check the function of these organs.
Anterior
Near the front of the object; in this case, near the front of the nose.

Lesson Two: Progress Check

SPELLING AND DEFINITION

1. (c) aperture: opening (orifice)
2. (a) constriction: closed, narrowed
3. (b) foramen: a natural opening or passage

SPELLING AND DEFINITION (*continued*)

4. (d) hiatus: a gap, cleft, or opening
5. (a) orifice: any opening (aperture)
6. (b) introitus: vaginal cavity (opening)
7. (c) ventricle: a small cavity or chamber (especially in the brain or heart)
8. (b) lumen: opening within a hollow tube or organ

WORD CONSTRUCTION

1. ae
2. aces
3. ina
4. es (or) a
5. ices
6. inges
7. ges
8. omata
9. a
10. a
11. i
12. ora
13. ies
14. vertebra
15. thorax
16. lumen
17. crisis
18. ovary
19. artery
20. diverticulum
21. nucleus
22. meninx
23. diagnosis
24. spermatozoon
25. femur
26. appendix
27. ovum
28. thrombus

BUILDING MEDICAL TERMS

1. cavity
2. dilated
3. foramen
4. lumen
5. stoma
6. ventricle
7. patent
8. vaginal canal
9. alimentary canal
10. hiatus (hernia)
11. quadriplegia

DEFINITIONS

1. thigh bone
2. a membrane covering the brain
3. chest
4. small cavity that prevents friction between tissues

5. any bone of the finger or toe

6. blood vessel

7. cavity (orifice) in the body

8. female gonad

9. slender outgrowth from the small intestine

10. male seed (germ) (semen)

11. red blood cell

12. outgrowth (pouch) on large intestine (colon)

13. mouth (oral cavity)

14. general term for the entrance to a cavity or space, e.g., vaginal cavity

15. a small cavity in a chamber

Answer Key to Chapter 5: Numbers, Positions, and Directions

CLINICAL NOTE

Angina

Chest pain caused by a lack of blood flow to the heart muscle. The pain can feel like pressure or squeezing in the chest area. Angina is usually a symptom of a more serious heart disease.

Malaise

A feeling of overall weakness, or lack of well-being. It is usually a symptom of an underlying condition or disease.

Diaphoresis

Sweating or perspiration.

EKG = Continuous Electrocardiogram

A device that records the electrical activity of the heart. Sensors called electrodes are attached to the chest skin. The sensors send the electrical impulses of the heart to the device.

CXR = Chest X-ray

Diagnostic image or radiography of the chest.

AP = anteroposterior

Refers to the position of the patient in relation to the X-ray beam. The patient is positioned such that the beam enters the patient's chest from the front and exits through the upper back.

Lateral

Refers to the position of the patient in relation to the X-ray beam. The patient is positioned such that the beam enters the patient's chest from one side and exits through the other side.

Cardiac Enzymes X 3

Draw a blood sample for the cardiac enzyme test every 8 hours during a 24-hour time period. This procedure is done to note the changes in values and to assess the damage to the myocardium.

Lesson Two: Progress Check

COMPARE AND CONTRAST

1. circum—around/contra—against

2. ecto—outside/endo—inside

3. infra—below/ipsi—same

4. para—near (or beside)/peri—about (around)

5. uni—one/bi—two/tri—three

6. prima—first/multi—many

7. semi—half/hemi—one-sided (half)

8. ambi—both (sides)/quadri—four

9. meso—middle/meta—after (beyond)

10. retro—behind (backward)/trans—across (through)

IDENTIFY THE LOCATION

1. anterior
2. posterior
3. cephalic
4. caudal
5. supine or prone
6. eversion
7. extension
8. oblique
9. medial
10. adjacent

DEFINE THE TERM

1. the system for weighing and measuring drugs and solutions, precious metals, and precious stones
2. the English system of weights and measures for all commodities except drugs, stones, and metals
3. system of measures and weights based on the meter and based on multiples of 10
4. monster
5. small
6. degree of heat or cold based on a specific scale
7. a temperature scale where H_2O boils at 100° and freezes at 0°
8. a temperature scale where H_2O boils at 212° and freezes at 32°
9. change from one scale or system to another
10. conversions that are equal to each other

MATCHING: POSITIONS

1. m
2. o
3. n
4. j
5. a
6. l
7. b
8. c
9. k
10. d
11. i
12. e
13. f
14. h
15. g

MATCHING: METRIC UNITS

1. f
2. g
3. b
4. a
5. d
6. e
7. c

FILL IN

1. 1,000
2. 1,000
3. 100

4. 10
5. 100
6. 1,000
7. 1,000
8. 1
9. 2.2
10. 2.5
11. 1,000; 1,000
12. 9, 5, 32
13. 32, 5, 9
14. 4.18
15. 3
16. 30
17. 240
18. 4.2
19. 0.24

◆ SHORT ANSWER

1. milligram
2. microgram
3. kilogram
4. drops
5. dram
6. fluid dram
7. giga
8. liter
9. joule
10. tera
11. degrees Celsius
12. gram
13. elevated, high
14. take; prescription
15. without
16. with
17. infinity
18. before
19. after
20. female

Answer Key to Chapter 6: Medical and Health Professions

◆ CLINICAL NOTE

Bx = Biopsy
An examination of tissue removed from a patient for diagnostic purposes.
IV = Intravenous
An abbreviation for the term intravenous. A solution administered directly into the venous circulation.
ROS = Review of System
A structured way of gathering the medical history of a patient by reviewing the body functions during a physical examination.
Skin Turgor
The degree of elasticity of the skin. This is a simple assessment to determine the extent of dehydration by pinching up a portion of skin and observing how fast it returns to the normal position.

CLINICAL NOTE (*continued*)

Lesion
An area of the skin tissue that has either changed or suffered damage.
Melanoma in situ
A type of skin cancer that occurrs in the outer layer of the skin.
Rales
Abnormal breath sounds, crackling or rattling, when a patient is taking a breath.

Lesson Two: Progress Check

MULTIPLE CHOICE: SCIENTIFIC STUDIES

1. d
2. b
3. c
4. a
5. c
6. d
7. c

MATCHING

1. h
2. d
3. e
4. i
5. f
6. g
7. l (diseases involving allergic reactions)
8. j
9. k
10. c
11. b
12. a

SHORT ANSWER

1. care and treatment of the teeth and related structures. Dentist (DMD) (DDS)
2. use of diet in promotion of health, and disease prevention and its treatment. Registered Dietitian (RD)
3. care and treatment of the foot. Podiatrist (DMP)
4. care of women throughout pregnancy, delivery, and postpartum. Registered Nurse, Midwife (RN)
5. routine care for persons in acute and chronic institutional facilities or community settings. Licensed Practical Nurse or Licensed Vocational Nurse (LPN or LVN)
6. use of a variety of techniques with persons who have disturbed mental faculties and/or behavior problems. Psychologist (title depends on degree; usually MS or PhD)
7. interpretation and dispensing of drugs. Pharmacist (RPh)
8. direct care of ill persons in a variety of settings under the supervision of a physician. May also function independently. Registered Nurse (RN) or Public Health Nurse (PHN)
9. the practice of medicine and/or surgery as well as research on animals. Veterinarian (DVM)

COMPLETION

1. oral surgeon
2. periodontist
3. dental hygienist
4. dietetic technician
5. podiatrist

6. medical technician
7. physical therapist
8. psychologist
9. pharmacist
10. optometrist
11. environmental scientist
12. exercise physiologist
13. genetic counselor
14. audiologist

MULTIPLE CHOICE: PROFESSIONS

1. a, b, c, d
2. a, b, c, d
3. a, b, c, d
4. a, b, c, d

ABBREVIATIONS

1. OTR
2. RPT
3. PHN
4. RD
5. LPN/LVN
6. RN or PHN
7. RMT
8. RT
9. DDS/DMD
10. DVM
11. OD
12. MD
13. MS/PhD
14. MD
15. RPh
16. ARRT
17. DO
18. MD
19. RHIT

DESCRIBE THE SPECIALTY

1. administration of medications to kill pain sensation
2. study of the endocrine gland functions and illness
3. study of the blood and blood-forming tissue
4. the use of x-ray and radioactive substances to diagnose disease
5. study of body tissues for diagnosis of all diseases, and the nature of disease
6. study of bacteria, especially disease-producing bacteria (pathogens)
7. study of living organisms
8. study of the care of the aging and elderly adults
9. study of the care of children
10. care of the foot
11. promotion of health, and disease prevention and treatment as related to nutrition
12. care of the pregnant woman through delivery
13. practicing medicine and performing surgery on animals
14. assisting families with personal problems resulting from illness

⬤ DESCRIBE THE SPECIALTY
(*continued*)

15. one who designs and implements treatment plans for patients with autism spectrum disorder

16. one who produces still and motion pictures of subjects for the health professions and natural sciences

17. one who designs, measures, fits, and adjusts artificial limbs for amputees and devices for people with musculoskeletal or neurological conditions

18. one trained in the prevention, diagnosis, assessment, treatment, and rehabilitation of muscle injuries, bone injuries, and illnesses

Unit III: Abbreviations

Answer Key to Chapter 7: Medical Abbreviations

⬤ CLINICAL NOTE

D5W = 5% dextrose in water
An abbreviation for a type of intravenous fluid, which contains both sugar and water.
mg = milligram
An abbreviation for a unit of measurement in the metric system.
q = every (quaue)
A Latin abbreviation used in directions to express how often something is to occur.
PO = by mouth (per os)
A Latin abbreviation used in directions to express the route of administration.
GERD = Gastroesophageal Reflux Disease
A disease where the acid from the stomach backs up into the esophagus due to the esophagus muscle between the stomach and esophagus not closing properly.
gtt = drops (guttae)
A Latin abbreviation used in directions to express the quantity of drug to be administered.
OS = left eye (oculus sinister)
A Latin abbreviation used as short hand to denote the left eye.
OD = right eye (oculus dexter)
A Latin abbreviation used as short hand to denote the right eye.
D/C = discharge
An abbreviation to signal a patient's arrangement or event ending their encounter in the reporting facility.
LTC = long-term care (facility)
An abbreviation for a type of facility that offers continuous inpatient health care to patients who have chronic illness or disabilities and are unable to care for themselves.

Lesson Two: Progress Check

⬤ IDENTIFY THE DEPARTMENT

1. admitting and discharge
2. central service
3. operating room
4. physical medicine and rehabilitation
5. radiology
6. laboratory
7. obstetrics
8. pediatrics
9. outpatient department
10. emergency room
11. social service
12. intensive care unit
13. food service

IDENTIFY THE PRESCRIPTION

1. 2 grams by mouth three times a day
2. 60 milliequivalents by rectal suppository at bedtime
3. 6 drops under the tongue every 4 hours
4. 2 liters intravenously every day
5. 30 units intramuscularly before meals
6. 10 milliliters under the skin as needed
7. 2 grains in 10 cubic centimeters of normal saline by needle under the skin once a day
8. one-half of a 5-milligram tablet by mouth after meals

IDENTIFY THE DIET ORDER

1. nothing by mouth
2. diet as tolerated
3. carbohydrate or consistent carbohydrate diet
4. 2 g sodium medical soft
5. mechanical soft
6. clear liquid
7. regular high fiber, force fluids
8. full liquid with interval nourishment at 10 AM to 2 PM and at bedtime; intake and output recorded
9. after meals
10. as required

MATCHING

1. f
2. d
3. g
4. h
5. c
6. e
7. b
8. a
9. i
10. j

SPELL OUT THE ABBREVIATION

1. prepare preoperatively
2. dead on arrival
3. with; without; temperature, pulse, respiration
4. cardiopulmonary resuscitation
5. blood pressure; millimeters; mercury
6. tender loving care
7. discontinue; intravenous (line); as soon as possible
8. carbon dioxide and water
9. treatment; symptoms
10. sodium; potassium
11. diagnosis; iron
12. no known drug allergies
13. past medical history
14. chief complaint

Answer Key to Chapter 8: Diagnostic and Laboratory Abbreviations

🔹 CLINICAL NOTE

Fx = Fracture
A generic term used to describe a broken bone due to an injury or disease.

Bone Scan (scintigraphy)
Nuclear medicine procedure where a tracer agent is injected and taken up into the bone. The nuclear camera is able to take images of the skeleton by visualizing the metabolic process of the bone through the tracer agent. The images locate increased uptake areas.

Hx = history
Abbreviation used to mean relative history of a patient as it pertains to the current encounter.

Lower T-spine = Lower Thoracic spine
Thoracic spine is comprised of 12 vertebral bodies (T1–T12) attached to the ribs and is the mid-region of the spine. The lower T-spine includes the vertebrae that are located in the abdomen region.

Lower L-vertebrae = Lower Lumbar spine
Lower Lumbar Spine is comprised of 5 vertebral bodies (L1–L5) in the lower region of the spine. Lower L-vertebrae refers to the lower back region where the vertebral bodies are located.

Bony Focus
A concentration of compact bone particles within the cancellous bone that is usually benign in nature.

Superior
Refers to the upper portion of the anatomical structure.

Inferior
Refers to the lower portion of the anatomical structure.

Lesson Two: Progress Check

🔹 IDENTIFY THE DISEASE

1. arteriosclerotic heart disease
2. coronary heart disease
3. congestive heart failure
4. cardiovascular disease
5. cerebrovascular accident
6. chronic brain syndrome
7. chronic obstructive pulmonary disease
8. myocardial infarction
9. post traumatic stress disorder
10. rheumatoid arthritis
11. transient ischemic attack
12. sexually transmitted diseases

🔹 SHORT ANSWER

1. auscultation and percussion
2. pupils equal, round, react to light, and accommodation
3. percussion and auscultation
4. rule out
5. systems review
6. tonsillectomy and adenoidectomy
7. physical examination
8. prescription
9. head, eyes, ears, nose, throat
10. diagnosis
11. red blood cell (count)

◆ **MATCHING**

1. c
2. h
3. f
4. b
5. a
6. e
7. g
8. d
9. m
10. p
11. q
12. o
13. n
14. j
15. r
16. l
17. i
18. k

◆ **DEFINE THE ABBREVIATION**

1. chief complaint
2. complains of
3. family history
4. fever of undetermined origin
5. history
6. short of breath
7. upper respiratory infection
8. urinary tract infection
9. murmur
10. present illness
11. symptoms
12. past history

Unit IV: Review

Answer Key to Chapter 9: Review of Word Parts from Units I, II, and III

◆ **CLINICAL NOTE**

Distal Phalanx
Distal means remote; farther from a point of reference. Phalanx means finger. In the context of the note, it would be the final bone at the very tip of the finger.

Aspirated
A medical procedure wherein a thin hollow needle is attached to a syringe and inserted through the skin. The syringe causes body fluid or tissue to be suctioned.

ED = Emergency Department
A department within a hospital where people go to get advanced critical care that is needed in the quickest amount of time.

Erythema
Redness of the skin caused by increased blood flow, which occurs due to a skin injury, infection, or inflammation.

WBC = White Blood Cell
A laboratory test that counts the number of white blood cells (leukocytes) in a sample of blood.

CLINICAL NOTE (continued)

Edema
Medical term for swelling, usually from an injury or inflammation.

C&S = Culture and Sensitivity
A laboratory test that determines the presence of bacteria and determines which antibiotic the bacteria is sensitive to so that the proper medication can be prescribed.

p.o. = by mouth (per os)
A route of administration for medication.

Lesson Two: Progress Check

COMPARE AND CONTRAST

1. lipo: a term for fat; litho: stone
2. para: to bear; pathy: any disease
3. phagia: swallowing; phasia: speech; phonia: voice
4. schizo: split; sclero: hardening
5. thrombo: clot; thermo: heat; trauma: injury
6. abscess: pus; adnexa: accessory structure
7. axilla: armpit; anomaly: defect
8. cervical: neck; coccyx: tailbone
9. edema: excess fluid; embolus: clot in a vessel
10. emesis: vomiting; enema: fluid injected into rectum
11. icterus: jaundice; ischemia: lack of blood to a part
12. palpable: felt by touch; parietal: walls of a cavity
13. prolapse: falling downward; prophylaxis: preventive treatment
14. suture: stitch; sputum: expectorate
15. viscera: interior organ; virus: infectious agent

BUILDING MEDICAL TERMS

1. chondritis
2. colpitis or vaginitis
3. laryngitis
4. paronychia
5. pancreatitis
6. phlebitis
7. salpingitis
8. otitis
9. pleurisy (pleuritis)
10. spondylitis
11. stomatitis
12. ureteritis
13. urethritis
14. esophagitis
15. neuritis
16. aphasia
17. dysphagia
18. carcinoma
19. necrosis
20. lipid
21. scleroderma
22. hemostasis
23. trauma
24. acute
25. anomaly

26. chronic
27. embolus
28. emesis
29. voiding
30. edema
31. coccyx
32. cervical vertebrae
33. excreting
34. exacerbation
35. incontinence
36. inflammation
37. ischemia
38. hemorrhage
39. metastasis
40. obesity
41. palpable
42. prophylaxis
43. sputum
44. virus
45. suture

FILL IN

1. metacarpals
2. laparotomy (celiotomy)
3. oophorectomy (or) ovariectomy
4. podiatry
5. rhinoplasty
6. metatarsals
7. thoracentesis
8. cryptorchidism
9. primigravida
10. multipara
11. salpingitis

MATCHING

1. e
2. d
3. a
4. h
5. j
6. i
7. b
8. c
9. f
10. g

DEFINE THE TERM

1. expulsion of the fetus from the uterus before it is viable
2. listening for sounds within the body
3. strand of collagen from a mammal, used to suture
4. a flexible tube to be passed into body channels
5. stretching; expanding
6. a clot or other plug taken by the blood to a smaller vessel
7. increase in severity of a disease or symptoms

◗ **DEFINE THE TERM (***continued***)**

   8. deep band of fibrous tissue

   9. transfer of disease from one organ or body to another area not connected directly

   10. striking a part with short, sharp blows

   11. existing at the time of birth

◗ **SHORT ANSWER: ROOT WORDS**

   1. carp/o

   2. cervic/o

   3. dent/o, odont

   4. esophag/o

   5. lapar/o, celi/o

   6. onych/o

   7. ophthalm/o

   8. pancreat/o

   9. soma

   10. pod/o

   11. pubis

   12. rhin/o

   13. stomat/o

   14. tars/o

   15. thorac/o

◗ **SHORT ANSWER: BODY PARTS**

   1. vagina

   2. vein

   3. pleura

   4. vertebra

   5. mouth

Unit V: Medical Terminology and Body Systems

Answer Key to Chapter 10: Body Organs and Parts

◗ **CLINICAL NOTE**

Gastroenterologist
Physicians who have training and experience in the management of diseases of the gastrointestinal tract and liver.

Celiac disease
An autoimmune reaction to eating gluten that occurs in the small intestine. Over time, the reaction damages the lining of the intestine and malabsorption of nutrients can occur.

Anemia
Anemia is a condition in which an individual does not have enough healthy red blood cells due to an underlying issue. Anemia can be broken down into categories based on the size, shape, and color of the red blood cells.

Diarrhea
A symptom that includes abnormally frequent bowel movements that is loose and/or watery.

BMI = Body mass index
Body mass index is the measurement of a patient's body fat based on a combination of factors: weight and height. Age and gender play a role in determining and assessing a person's healthy weight.

GFD = Gluten-free diet
A diet that excludes the protein gluten, which is found in certain types of grains. The diet helps patients manage the signs and symptoms of celiac disease.

RDN = Register Dietitian Nutritionist
A professional trained in applying the principles of nutrition to food selection and meal preparation.

Lesson Two: Progress Check

SPELLING AND DEFINITION

1. integumentary; skin, nails, hair, oil and sweat glands
2. cardiovascular; heart and blood vessels
3. musculoskeletal; bones, joints, ligaments, cartilage, and muscles
4. gastrointestinal; mouth, esophagus, stomach, intestines, and accessory organs
5. respiratory; nose, pharynx, larynx, trachea, bronchi, and lungs
6. lymphatic; lymph vessels
7. genitourinary; kidneys, bladder, ureters, urethra, gonads, genitalia, and internal organs
8. endocrine; ductless glands and supporting structures
9. nervous; brain, spinal cord, cranial and spinal nerves

FILL IN

1. cell
2. genetic
3. mitosis
4. multiplying
5. membrane
6. tissues
7. epithelial tissue
8. connective tissue
9. muscle tissue
10. nerve tissue
11. organ
12. systems
13. cavity
14. planes
15. diaphragm
16. chromosomes
17. pancreas, liver, gallbladder, and salivary glands

DEFINITIONS

1. sum of physical and chemical processes that convert food into elements for growth, repair, and energy as well as recycling and excretion
2. when the body systems maintain a balance optimal for survival: a steady state

SHORT ANSWER

1a. epithelial: protects, absorbs, secretes
1b. connective: binds all tissue together
1c. muscle: contracts and relaxes
1d. nerve: controls and coordinates body activity
2. serves as the wall or outer covering; allows some substances to go into the cell but keeps others out
3. contains genes and chromosomes for reproduction
4. it releases the energy required for a body to function
5. allows the body to maintain a stable internal environment despite changes in external conditions

Answer Key to Chapter 11: Integumentary System

◆ CLINICAL NOTE

Eruption
Breaking out in a rash in a localized region.
Erythema
Redness of the skin due to inflammation and underlying condition.
Pruritus
Itching.
AD = Atopic Dermatitis (eczema)
Common skin condition in children during the first year of life; dry, scaly, itchy patches that appear on the scalp, forehead, and face.
OTC = Over-the-counter
Refers to a drug that can be purchased without a prescription and that is considered safe for consumers when directions and warning labels are followed.
b.i.d. = twice a day (bis in die)
A Latin abbreviation used in directions of a prescription to express how frequently a drug should be taken.
Allergy testing
Used to determine an allergy to food items, pollen, or animal dander: a small drop of a suspected allergen is placed on the skin, which is then scratched; a rash or itching indicates an allergic response.

Lesson Two: Progress Check

◆ LIST: SKIN FUNCTIONS

1. a protective barrier from many things
2. enables the body to sense heat, cold, or pain
3. assists in regulating body temperature by insulating
4. eliminates body wastes through perspiration
5. synthesizes vitamin D

◆ SPELLING AND DEFINITIONS: SKIN TERMS

1. (a) epidermis: the outermost nonvascular layer of skin
2. (d) subcutaneous: beneath the skin
3. (b) biopsy: removal of tissue from the body for examination
4. (c) debridement: removal of devitalized tissue
5. (a) escharotomy: removal of burn scar tissue
6. (b) keratosis: any horny growth
7. (c) steatoma: a fatty mass within an oil gland
8. (d) verruca: a wart
9. (b) impetigo: a staphylococcal or streptococcal skin infection marked by vesicles that become pustular
10. (a) pediculosis: infestation with lice
11. (c) eczema: redness in the skin
12. (b) psoriasis: chronic, hereditary, recurrent dermatosis
13. (d) erysipelas: a contagious skin disease
14. (a) varicella: chickenpox
15. (b) actinic: referring to ultraviolet rays reacting on the skin

◆ COMPLETION: SKIN TERMS

1. albinism
2. alopecia
3. dermatology
4. erythema
5. eschar

6. nummular
7. papule
8. urticaria
9. pustule
10. cicatrix
11. keratosis
12. ecchymosis

DEFINITIONS: SKIN TESTS

1. a test for tuberculosis (TB)
2. a test for scarlet fever
3. a test for diphtheria
4. a test to determine an allergy to food items, pollen, or animal dander
5. a test for valley fever
6. a test for systemic fungal disease

MATCHING: SKIN TERMS

1. h
2. j
3. f
4. e
5. i
6. c
7. b
8. a
9. d
10. g

MATCHING: SKIN CONDITIONS

1. d
2. g
3. e
4. c
5. f
6. b
7. j
8. i
9. h
10. a

COMPLETION: SKIN CONDITIONS

1. wart
2. prickly heat, heat rash
3. German measles
4. measles
5. chicken pox
6. Anthony's Fire
7. hives
8. shingles
9. ringworm
10. lice

◆ COMPLETION: SKIN INFECTIONS

1. bacteria
2. fungus
3. virus
4. bacteria
5. parasite
6. bacteria
7. virus
8. parasite

◆ DEFINITIONS: SKIN TESTS

1. a test for tuberculosis (TB)
2. a test for scarlet fever
3. a test for diphtheria
4. a test for valley fever
5. a test to determine an allergy to foods, pollen or animal dander

◆ IDENTIFYING WORD PARTS

Word	Root Word	Prefix	Suffix
1. albinism	albin = white		ism = process
2. debridement	debride = to clean a wound		ment = action
3. epidermis	dermis = skin	epi = above	
4. escharotomy	eschar = scab		otomy = cut into
5. excoriation	corium = skin	ex = out, away from	ation = process
6. hemangioma	oma = tumor	hemangi = blood vessels	
7. neurodermatitis	derma = skin	neuro = nerves, nervous system	itis = inflammation
8. paronychia	onych = nail	para = parallel	ia = abnormal condition
9. pediculosis	pedicul = louse		osis = abnormal condition
10. subcutaneous	cutaneous = pertaining to the skin	sub = under	

Answer Key to Chapter 12: Digestive System

◆ CLINICAL NOTE

Calculus
Formation of solid material composed of salt minerals on teeth due to the hardening of plaque.

Plaque
Bacterial plaque; result of action of bacteria on carbohydrates that initially forms a sticky substance, which hardens to tartar that adheres to the teeth.

Gingivitis
Gum disease. Inflammation of the gums with irritation, redness, and swelling; most common cause is buildup of dental plaque and bacterial growth between the gums and teeth.

Abscess
Tooth infection with pus, pain, and inflammation; common causes are tooth fracture or tooth decay.

Dental caries
Destruction of the tooth enamel due to acids produced by bacterial plaque on dietary carbohydrates; caries can extend to below the enamel.
Molar
Largest and broadest teeth located in the back of the mouth; their function is to crush and grind food.
TID = Three times a day (ter in die)
Latin abbreviation used in directions of a prescription to express the frequency of how often to take a drug.

Lesson Two: Progress Check

LIST: DIGESTIVE PROCESSES

1. ingestion
2. mastication
3. deglutition
4. peristalsis
5. digestion
6. absorption
7. egestion (defecation)

MATCHING: ORAL CAVITY TERMS

1. j
2. e
3. d
4. b
5. a
6. c
7. i
8. f
9. g
10. h

COMPLETION: CLINICAL CONDITIONS OF THE ORAL CAVITY

1. plaque
2. cleft palate
3. abcess
4. gingivitis
5. sialith
6. temporomandibular joint syndrome/disease (TMJ/TMD)
7. peridonitis
8. cavity
9. malocclusion
10. leukoplakia

WORD POOL: ORAL CAVITY

1. extraction
2. root canal
3. cheiloplasty
4. gingivectomy
5. implant
6. gingivoplasty
7. filling
8. crown

MATCHING: DIGESTIVE TRACT TERMS

1. j
2. d
3. e
4. a
5. h
6. f
7. i
8. b
9. g
10. c

COMPLETION: CLINICAL CONDITIONS OF THE GI TRACT

1. achalasia
2. cholelithiasis
3. inflammatory bowel disease (IBD)
4. gastroesophageal reflux disease (GERD)
5. hepatitis
6. pyloric stenosis
7. cirrhosis
8. Celiac disease
9. adhesions
10. hemorrhoids
11. lactose intolerance
12. appendicitis
13. Hirschspring's disease
14. volvulus
15. fistula
16. hernia
17. polyposis
18. irritable bowel syndrome (IBS)
19. peritonitis
20. diverticula

WORD POOL: DIGESTIVE TRACT

1. mouth or oral cavity
2. small intestine
3. cecum
4. gallbladder, liver, pancreas
5. sigmoid colon
6. rectum
7. duodenum, ileum, jejunum
8. large intestine

MATCHING: DIAGNOSTIC AND SURGICAL PROCEDURES FOR TREATING DISEASES OF THE GI TRACT

1. d
2. f
3. a
4. j
5. b
6. c
7. i
8. e
9. g
10. h

IDENTIFYING WORD PARTS

Word	Root Word	Prefix	Suffix
1. achalasia	chala = to loosen	a = not	ia = condition
2. antiemetic	emetic = pertaining to vomiting	anti = against	
3. endodontic	odont = having teeth	end = within	ic = pertaining to
4. epigastric	gastr = stomach	epi = above	ic = pertaining to
5. gingivitis	gingivi = gums		itis = inflammation
6. hypochondrium	chondr = cartilage	hypo = below	ium = structure/tissue
7. hyperalimentation	alimentation = nutrition	hyper = excessive	
8. parenteral	enter = intestines	par = other than	al = pertaining to
9. paracentesis	centesis = puncture (usually to remove fluid)	para = beside	
10. polyposis	polyp = growth hanging from a thin stalk		osis = condition

Answer Key to Chapter 13: Respiratory System

CLINICAL NOTE

Status Asthmaticus
Severe asthma attack considered to be an emergency situation because it does not respond to the initial drug therapy.

H&P = History and Physical
A document created during the episode of care that gives concise information about a patient's history and examination. It is a means of communicating information to all providers who are involved in the care of a particular patient.

Anoxic
Without oxygen; referencing lack of oxygen reaching the lungs.

Dyspnea
Labored or difficult breathing, shortness of breath; can be a symptom of an underlying condition.

Inspiratory
Act of breathing in; oxygen enters the body in this order: nose (mouth), pharynx, larynx, trachea, bronchi, and lungs.

Expiratory
Act of breathing out; oxygen exits the body in this order: lungs, bronchi, trachea, larynx, pharynx, nose (mouth).

Wheezing
The sound of high pitch whistling that occurs in the act of breathing. This occurs usually during an asthma attack.

Pulse Oximeter
Tool used to measure the oxygen saturation of arterial blood. The device is photoelectric and is taped to a finger.

Bronchodilator
An agent, typically a drug therapy, capable of dilating the bronchi.

Lesson Two: Progress Check

◆ LISTS: PARTS OF THE
RESPIRATORY SYSTEM

1. nose
2. pharynx
3. larynx
4. trachea
5. bronchi
6. lungs

◆ MATCHING: SYMPTOMS
RELATED TO DISORDERS OF
THE RESPIRATORY SYSTEM

1. i
2. d
3. e
4. g
5. a
6. h
7. j
8. f
9. c
10. b

◆ MULTIPLE CHOICE: TERMS
THAT DESCRIBE SYMPTOMS,
DIAGNOSTIC TOOLS,
AND DISORDERS OF THE
RESPIRATORY SYSTEM

1. c
2. a
3. b
4. d
5. b
6. b
7. c
8. a
9. d
10. d

◆ MATCHING: DISORDERS
OF THE RESPIRATORY
SYSTEM

1. f
2. g
3. a
4. b
5. j
6. i
7. e
8. d
9. h
10. c

◆ ABBREVIATIONS: TERMS
USED TO DESCRIBE
DISORDERS, DIAGNOSIS
OR TREATMENT OF DISEASES
OF THE RESPIRATORY
SYSTEM

1. upper respiratory infection
2. pulmonary expiration flow rate
3. acute respiratory distress syndrome
4. cystic fibrosis
5. continuous positive airway pressure
6. chronic obstructive pulmonary disease
7. tuberculosis
8. sudden infant death syndrome
9. endotracheal
10. ventilation perfusion

IDENTIFYING WORD PARTS

Word	Root Word	Prefix	Suffix
1. anthracosis	anthrakos = coal		osis = condition
2. asphyxia	sphyxis = to throb	a = without	ia = condition
3. dysphonia	phōnē = voice	dys = abnormal	ia = condition
4. emphysema	physema = a blowing	em = in	
5. epistaxis	staxis = to fall in drops	epi = upon	
6. hypercapnia	capn = carbon dioxide	hyper = excessive	ia = condition
7. pertussis	tussis = cough	per = through, intensely	
8. pneumonia	pneumōn = lung		ia = condition
9. sinusitis	sinus = air-filled space in skull bones		itis = inflammation
10. tuberculosis	tubercle = nodule		osis = condition

Answer Key to Chapter 14: Cardiovascular System

CLINICAL NOTE

ASA = Acetylsalicylic acid (aspirin)
A drug that relieves pain and inflammation. It has the added benefit of decreasing platelet aggregation and is used to prevent myocardial infarction.

SOB = Shortness of Breath
An acronym for the symptom of labored breathing, or not being able to catch breath. It is usually related to a more serious condition such as a lung or heart disease.

Cyanosis
A bluish cast to the skin due to lack of oxygen in the blood, usually occurring in the fingers, lips, or toes. It is a symptom of an underlying condition.

MI = Myocardial Infarction
Gross necrosis of the myocardium, caused by decreased blood supply to the area.

Anterior STEMI = ST-Elevation Myocardial Infarction
A result from an EKG that shows the front wall of the heart tissue damaged due to a blockage of a major artery that supplies blood to that region. This result is the most serious.

Acute thrombotic occlusion
Severe obstruction or closing off of the coronary arteries due to a formation of a blood clot inside the blood vessel. This leads to a heart attack.

Sublingual
Route of administration of a drug, which involves placing the correct drug form under the tongue and allowing it to disintegrate slowly.

CABG = Coronary artery bypass graft
Use of a leg vein or synthetic material to substitute for an occluded artery in the heart.

Lesson Two: Progress Check

LIST: FUNCTIONS OF THE CIRCULATORY AND LYMPHATIC SYSTEMS

1. Transport: Gases, hormones, minerals, enzymes, and other vital substances are carried in the blood to every cell in the body; all waste materials are carried by the blood to the lungs, skin, or kidneys for elimination from the body (*pulmonary circulation*).
2. Body temperature: The blood vessels maintain body temperature by dilating at the skin surface to dissipate heat or by constricting to retain heat.
3. Protection: The blood and lymph systems protect the body against injury and foreign invasion through the immune system; blood clotting mechanisms to protect against blood loss.
4. Buffering: Blood proteins provide an acid-base buffer system to maintain optimum pH of the blood.
5. Returns excess tissue fluid that has leaked from the capillaries. If not removed, this fluid collects in spaces between the cells and results in *edema*.
6. Returns plasma proteins that have leaked out of the capillaries into the circulation. If not returned, these proteins would accumulate, increase the osmotic pressure in the tissue fluid, and upset capillary function.
7. Transports absorbed nutrients. Specialized lymph vessels transport nutrients, especially fats, from the digestive system to the blood.
8. Removes toxic substances and other cellular debris from circulation in tissues after infection or tissue damage.
9. Controls quality of tissue fluid by filtering it through lymph nodes before returning it to the circulation.

COMPLETION: CARDIOVASCULAR SYSTEM

1. ventricles
2. atria
3. vena cava
4. right ventricle
5. aortic
6. pericardium
7. Purkinje
8. arteries, veins
9. diastolic
10. 80/120
11. valves
12. serum
13. universal donor
14. fibrinogen; platelets/thrombocyte

COMPLETION: LYMPHATIC SYSTEM

1. right lymphatic duct
2. tonsils
3. thymus gland
4. capillaries
5. lymph nodes
6. left thoracic duct
7. extracellular
8. spleen
9. phagocytes
10. antibodies

◆ MATCHING: DIAGNOSTIC TOOLS—CARDIOVASCULAR SYSTEM

1. c
2. g
3. j
4. e
5. b
6. a
7. i
8. h
9. f
10. d

◆ MATCHING: CLINICAL DISORDERS

1. c
2. f
3. o
4. l
5. h
6. k
7. n
8. m
9. d
10. e
11. i
12. g
13. j
14. a
15. b

◆ ABBREVIATIONS: CARDIOVASCULAR SYSTEM

1. atrial septal defect
2. blood pressure
3. complete blood count
4. coronary care unit
5. congestive heart failure
6. carbon dioxide
7. cardiopulmonary resuscitation
8. cerebrovascular accident
9. electrocardiogram
10. myocardial infarction
11. oxygen
12. premature ventricular contraction
13. red blood cells
14. transit ischemia attack
15. white blood cells

IDENTIFYING WORD PARTS

Word	Root Word	Prefix	Suffix
1. anticoagulant	coagulant = promotes clotting	anti = against	
2. arrhythmia	rhythm = regular, repeated pattern	ar = without	ia = condition
3. cardiogram	cardi = heart		gram = record
4. cyanosis	cyan = greenish, blue color		osis = abnormal condition
5. dyspnea	pnea = breathing	dys = difficult	
6. endocarditis	cardi = heart	endo = within	itis = inflammation
7. hypertension	tension = stretching	hyper = above	
8. natriuretic	uresis = urination	natr = sodium	tic = pertaining to
9. phagocyte	cyte = cell	phag = eat, swallow	
10. sarcoidosis	sarc = connective tissue	oid = derived from	osis = condition

Answer Key to Chapter 15: Nervous System

CLINICAL NOTE

H/O = History of
An abbreviation used in clinical charting during the episode of care to document any history of a disease or condition in the medical record.

Sz = Seizure
A seizure is a brain disorder where there is a sudden increase in the electrical activity of the brain. The duration, symptoms, and stages of a seizure vary from person to person.

EEG = electroencephalogram
A record/test of electrical activity of the brain that is used to help in the diagnosis of epilepsy.

Dysrhythmia
Abnormal patterns in the function of the electrical activity of the brain.

Paroxysmal
A sudden acute or worsening of a symptom and/or the frequency of a chronic symptom.

CT = Computerized Tomography
Three-dimensional view of brain tissue obtained as X-ray beams pass through layers of the brain. Contrast medium may also be injected by IV to better visualize abnormalities.

Clonic
A symptom of a seizure where the body produces stiff, jerky movements.

O × 3 = Oriented times three
An assessment of a patient's awareness to their surroundings during a mental examination. The patient is aware to all dimensions—person, place, and time/date.

Lesson Two: Progress Check

FILL IN

1. Central or CNS
2. Central or CNS
3. Autonomic
4. Ventricles
5. Plexus

6. Sulcus
7. Limbic
8. Ganglion
9. Hemisphere
10. Encephalon
11. Opening in occipital bone through which the spinal cord passes
12. Cauda equine
13. Peripheral Nervous System or PNS
14. Meninges
15. Somatic Nervous System or SNS

MATCHING: CRANIAL NERVES

1. g
2. e
3. a
4. b
5. c
6. f
7. d

MATCHING: INJURY OR DISEASES OF THE NERVOUS SYSTEM

1. a
2. f
3. e
4. g
5. h
6. d
7. c
8. b

TRUE OR FALSE

1. T
2. F
3. T
4. T
5. T
6. F
7. T
8. T
9. T
10. T

DEFINITIONS: PSYCHIATRIC TERMS AND CONDITIONS

1. Alzheimer's Disease
2. Autism spectrum disorder
3. False personal belief
4. Mental disturbance of short duration; may include illusions or hallucinations
5. Loss of contact with reality
6. Abnormal anxiety about one's health
7. Belief in one's extreme greatness or power
8. Delusions of persecution or self-importance
9. Persistent abnormal dread or fear

DEFINITIONS: PSYCHIATRIC TERMS AND CONDITIONS (*continued*)

10. Chronic, debilitating brain disorder characterized by visual and/or auditory hallucinations, delusions and disordered thoughts
11. Pretending to be ill for personal gain
12. Hearing or seeing things not actually present

SPELLING AND DEFINITION: THE NERVOUS SYSTEM

1. (a) Cerebrum: main portion of the brain; includes right and left hemispheres
2. (c) Meninges: three protective membranes that cover the brain and spinal cord
3. (b) Arachnoid: the middle layer of three protective membranes covering the brain and spinal cord
4. (d) Trochlear: cranial nerve of the peripheral nervous system that controls eye movement
5. (a) Olfactory: cranial nerve of the peripheral nervous system that controls the sense of smell
6. (b) Hypoglossal: cranial nerve of the peripheral nervous system beneath the tongue that is associated with chewing, swallowing and speech
7. (c) Anencephaly: congenital absence of the brain, causing death soon after birth
8. (a) Hydrocephalus: congenital defect of the brain with an accumulation of cerebral spinal fluid within the skull
9. (d) Meningocele: hernial protrusion of the meninges through bone
10. (a) Poliomyelitis: acute viral disease with flu like symptoms that may cause permanent paralysis; rare disease because vaccine is now available

IDENTIFYING WORD PARTS

Word	Root Word	Prefix	Suffix
1. anencephaly	cephal = head	an = without	al = pertaining to
2. aphasia	phasia = speech	a = without	
3. ataxia	tax = coordination	a = without	ia = condition
4. comatose	comat = deep sleep		ose = pertaining to
5. encephalon	cephal = head	en = within	
6. encephalitis	cephal = head	en = within	itis = inflammation
7. hydrocephalus	cephal = head	hydro = water	us = thing, structure
8. megalomania	mania = obsessive	mega = large	
9. meningitis	meninges = membrane covering brain and spinal cord		itis = inflammation
10. meningocele	meninges = membrane covering brain and spinal cord		cele = herniation

Answer Key to Chapter 16: Genitourinary System

CLINICAL NOTE

G1 = Gravida (number of pregnancies)
Number of times a woman has been pregnant. The example in the clinical note is of a woman who has been pregnant once.
P0 = Para (number of births of viable offspring)
A woman who has given birth at least once and the birth resulted in a viable offspring. The example in the clinical note is of a woman who has never given birth.

IUP = Intrauterine pregnancy
A fertilized egg that is implanted in the uterus and the fetus develops to full term.
EDC = Expected date of confinement
An abbreviation used to describe the estimated delivery/due date for a pregnant woman.
Effacement
The thinning of the cervix to enlarge the diameter of its opening during childbirth in the normal processes of labor.
PROM = Premature Rupture of Membranes
Spontaneous rupture of amniotic sac before the onset of labor.
NSVD = Normal spontaneous vaginal delivery
Delivery of a baby through the mother's vagina with the aid of forceps or vacuum.
APGAR = Appearance, Pulse, Grimace Activity, and Respiration
The evaluation of an infant's physical condition, usually performed 1 and 5 minutes after birth, based on a rating of five factors that reflect the infant's ability to adjust to extrauterine life.
EBL = Estimated blood loss
Term used to describe the amount of blood that was lost during a medical/surgical procedure.

Lesson Two: Progress Check

LIST: THE URINARY AND REPRODUCTIVE SYSTEMS

1a. (Two) kidneys
1b. (Two) ureters
1c. (One) bladder
1d. (One) urethra
2a. Removes water and wastes, converts to urine, transports, excretes
2b. Reabsorb substances that the body wants to retain
2c. Maintains body system equilibrium by regulating pH, RBC production, blood pressure, blood glucose
3a. Perpetuation of the species

MULTIPLE CHOICE: ANATOMY OF THE KIDNEY

1. b
2. d
3. c
4. a

COMPARE AND CONTRAST: THE URINARY SYSTEM

1. Albuminuria is the presence of protein (albumin) in the urine; anuria is no (without) urine.
2. Enuresis is bed-wetting while asleep; diuresis is increased excretion of urine.
3. Incontinence is the inability to control bowel or bladder excretion; urinary retention is the inability to excrete urine.
4. Hydronephrosis is distention of the renal pelvis because of the inability to urinate; nephrolithiasis is kidney (renal) stones.
5. Nycturia is excessive night urination; oliguria is diminished urine secretion; and dysuria is painful and difficult urination.
6. Pyelitis is inflammation of the renal pelvis; glomerulonephritis is inflammation of the capillary loops in the glomeruli.

MATCHING: TREATMENT OF THE URINARY SYSTEM

1. d
2. f
3. e
4. a
5. h

MATCHING: TREATMENT OF THE URINARY SYSTEM (*continued*)

6. i
7. j
8. c
9. g
10. b

MATCHING: SURGICAL PROCEDURES OF THE MALE REPRODUCTIVE SYSTEM

1. c
2. d
3. e
4. b
5. a

MATCHING: SURGICAL PROCEDURES OF THE FEMALE REPRODUCTIVE SYSTEM

1. c
2. d
3. e
4. a
5. b

COMPLETION: MALE AND FEMALE REPRODUCTIVE SYSTEMS

1. testis
2. external genitalia
3. vas deferens
4. prostate
5. epididymis
6. seminal duct
7. ovaries
8. fallopian tube
9. uterus
10. vagina

DEFINITIONS: PREGNANCY AND CHILDBIRTH

1. amniocentesis
2. Apgar score
3. cephalopelvic disproportion (CPD)
4. dystocia
5. ectopic or extrauterine
6. gestation
7. gravida
8. neonatal period
9. postpartum
10. placenta

TRUE OR FALSE: SEXUALLY TRANSMITTED INFECTIONS

1. F
2. T
3. F
4. T
5. T
6. T
7. T
8. T
9. T
10. T

IDENTIFYING WORD PARTS

Word	Root Word	Prefix	Suffix
1. azoturia	azot = urea/nitrogen		uria = condition
2. cryptorchidism	orchid = testis	crypt = hidden	ism = condition
3. endometriosis	metri = uterus	endo = in/within	osis = condition (abnormal)
4. episiotomy	episi = vulva		tomy = process of cutting
5. incontinent	continent = able to retain urine or feces	in = not	
6. inseminate	semin = semen/seed	in = within	ate = acted upon
7. laparoscopy	lapar = abdominal wall		scopy = visual inspection
8. neonatal	nat = birth	neo = new	al = pertaining to
9. primapara	para = live births	prima = first	
10. postpartum	partum = birth/labor	post = after	

Answer Key to Chapter 17: Musculoskeletal System

CLINICAL NOTE

CC = Chief complaint
A step in medical history taking. It is the subjective statement given in the patient's own words and describes the main reason for the encounter.

HPI = History of present illness
A step in medical history taking and is an important component in the etiology of the patient's problem. The history of present illness includes the symptoms of the problem from onset to encounter.

Open reduction
A surgery is needed for correction of the fracture by realigning the bone fracture into its normal position.

Internal fixation
The process of making a bone immovable; rods, screws, and wires are placed internally to hold together the bones.

Supracondylar femur fracture
The thigh bone extends from the pelvis to the knee. The supracondylar area is referring to the distal end of the femur where the breaking of the bone occurred.

Osteopenia
Lower than normal bone density; the bones become more porous and this can lead to osteoporosis.

Extension
The movement by which the two ends of any jointed part is drawn away from each other; straightening.

ROM = Range of motion
A term that describes the amount of movement that a joint is able to achieve from extension to flexion.

Flexion
The movement of bending around a joint that decreases the angle between the bones of the limb at the joint.

LIST: FUNCTIONS OF THE MUSCULOSKELETAL SYSTEM

1. Support and protection – vital organs protected
2. Movement – all body movements
3. Red blood cell turnover – bone marrow is the site
4. Storage – minerals and nutrients

MATCHING: LOCATIONS OF BONES

1. f
2. g
3. i
4. h
5. j
6. a
7. b
8. c
9. d
10. e

MULTIPLE CHOICE: BONES

1. b
2. b
3. a
4. c
5. d
6. c
7. b
8. c
9. d
10. a

NAME THE STRUCTURE: JOINTS AND ACCESSORY PARTS

1. bursa
2. fascia
3. lamina
4. ligament
5. aponeurosis
6. hinge joint
7. sutures
8. ball and socket
9. tendon
10. meniscus

MATCHING: MUSCLES

1. c
2. d
3. e
4. b
5. a

MATCHING: MUSCULOSKELETAL INJURY

1. d
2. a
3. b
4. e
5. c

MATCHING: MUSCULOSKELETAL INFLAMMATION

1. g
2. f
3. h
4. e
5. b
6. i
7. a
8. d
9. c

COMPARE AND CONTRAST: MUSCULOSKELETAL DISEASES

1. Kyphosis is humpback (or hunchback); lordosis is curvature of the lumbar spine (swayback).

2. Osteomalacia is softening of the bones, usually in adults with vitamin D deficiency caused by drug-nutrient interaction or a metabolic disorder; rickets is softening of bones in children as a result of vitamin D deficiency.

3. Lyme disease is a bacterial infection transmitted by ticks; rheumatic fever is a complication of strep throat caused by a bacterial infection.

4. Muscular dystrophy is progressive atrophy of the skeletal muscles; myositis is acute inflammation of voluntary muscle.

5. Osteomyelitis is a bacterial infection affecting the bone and bone marrow; osteoporosis is brittle porous bone.

6. Sarcoma is a malignant bone tumor; scoliosis is lateral curvature of the spine.

7. Juvenile rheumatoid arthritis is an inflammatory disease of the joints in children younger than 16 years of age; rheumatoid arthritis is an inflammatory disease of the joints in adults.

8. In a closed fracture, the bone is broken with no open wound; an open fracture involves a broken bone and an external wound, with bone fragments sometimes protruding through the skin.

9. A complicated fracture occurs when a broken bone has injured some internal organ; a comminuted fracture occurs when a bone breaks and splinters into pieces.

10. An impacted fracture occurs when a bone is broken and one edge is wedged into another bone; an incomplete fracture occurs when the fracture does not include the whole bone.

IDENTIFYING WORD PARTS

Word	Root Word	Prefix	Suffix
1. abduction	duct = to lead	ab = away	ion = process
2. acetabulum	acetabul = hip socket		um = structure
3. articulation	articul = joint		ation = process
4. arthroplasty	arthro = joint		plasty = surgical repair
5. bursitis	burs = bursa (sac of fluid near joints)		itis = inflammation
6. fasciitis	fasci = membrane supporting muscles		itis = inflammation
7. intervertebral	vertebr = backbone	inter = between	al = pertaining to

IDENTIFYING WORD PARTS (*continued*)

Word	Root Word	Prefix	Suffix
8. lordosis	lord = sway back		osis = abnormal condition
9. osteomalacia	osteo = bone		malacia = softening
10. subluxation	lux = to slide	sub = below	ation = process

Answer Key to Chapter 18: Eyes and Ears

CLINICAL NOTE

Hyperopia
Farsightedness, a common type of refractive error where distant objects may be seen more clearly than nearby objects.

Astigmatism
Condition characterized by irregular cornea and lens of the eye, which is corrected with lenses.

OS = Oculus sinister
Left eye.

Acuity
Clarity or clearness of vision.

OD = Oculus dexter
Right eye.

Refraction
The determination of the refractive errors of the eye and their correction with glasses or lenses.

Retinoscopy
The procedure used to determine the refraction error of a patient's eyes. The examination/measurement is done with a retinoscope.

BCVA = Best corrected visual acuity
Best vision achieved post correction with glasses or contact lens, as measured on the standard Snellen eye chart.

Lesson Two: Progress Check

MATCHING: EYE STRUCTURE

1. f
2. g
3. h
4. i
5. j
6. e
7. a
8. c
9. d
10. b

MATCHING: EYE DISORDERS

1. i
2. e
3. f
4. g
5. h
6. a

7. c
8. j
9. d
10. b

MULTIPLE CHOICE: EYE AND EAR

1. d
2. c
3. a
4. a
5. a
6. b
7. c
8. d
9. b
10. d

ABBREVIATIONS: EYE AND EAR

1. intraocular lens
2. with correction (glasses or contact lens)
3. oculus sinister (left eye)
4. oculus dexter (right eye)
5. age-related macular degeneration
6. pupils equal, round, react to light, accommodation
7. visual acuity
8. auris dextra
9. radial keratotomy
10. intravenous fluorescein angiography

MATCHING: STRUCTURES OF THE EAR

1. f
2. d
3. g
4. h
5. b
6. a
7. c
8. e

IDENTIFYING WORD PARTS

Word	Root Word	Prefix	Suffix
1. exotropia	tropia = a turning	exo = outside	
2. fenestration	fenestra = small opening		ion = process
3. keratotomy	kerato = cornea		otomy = incision
4. labyrinthitis	labyrinth = maze, web		itis = inflammation
5. myringitis	myringo = tympanic membrane or eardrum		itis = inflammation

IDENTIFYING WORD PARTS (*continued*)

Word	Root Word	Prefix	Suffix
6. neuroma	neur = nerve/nervous tissue		oma = tumor
7. otoscope	oto = ear		scope = instrument for visual examination
8. subconjunctival	conjunctiva = membrane lining the eyelids and covering the eyeball	sub = under	al = pertaining to
9. vertigo	vert = turning around		igo = a condition

Answer Key to Chapter 19: Endocrine System

CLINICAL NOTE

Type 2 diabetes
Insulin resistant condition. Insulin is produced, but the insulin does not function properly.
SHx = Social history
Part of the documentation that is created at an episode of care.
HTN = Hypertension
Elevated blood pressure. A normal blood pressure reading in an adult is less than 120/80 mm Hg.
DM = diabetes mellitus
A lack of insulin, which is secreted by the cells of the pancreas.
Polyphagia
Excessive hunger, often a sign of uncontrolled diabetes mellitus.
Polydipsia
Excessive thirst, often a sign of uncontrolled diabetes mellitus or diabetes insipidus.
HgA1c = Glycated hemoglobin
A lab test to measure the level of hemoglobin A1c determines average blood sugar concentrations for the preceding 2–3 months. Normal levels below 5.7 percent indicate diabetes mellitus is well controlled.
Hypoglycemic
A low level of glucose in the blood, if left untreated, can progress to insulin shock and then coma.
Fundoscopic
An eye examination that looks at the retina. It can help diagnose conditions and identify risk factors for potential vision loss.

Lesson Two: Progress Check

LIST: ENDOCRINE GLANDS

1. Anterior and posterior pituitary gland
2. Thyroid gland
3. Four parathyroid glands
4. Two adrenal glands
5. Islets of Langerhans in the pancreas
6. Two ovaries
7. Two testes
8. Pineal gland
9. Thymus gland

LIST: ACTIVITIES REGULATED BY THE ENDOCRINE SYSTEM

1. Reproduction and lactation
2. Immune system
3. Acid-base balance
4. Fluid intake and fluid balance
5. Carbohydrate, protein and lipid metabolism
6. Digestion, absorption, and nutrient utilization
7. Blood pressure
8. Stress resistance
9. Adaptation to environmental change, for example, changes in temperature

MULTIPLE CHOICE: ENDOCRINE GLANDS AND HORMONES

1. d
2. a
3. c
4. b
5. d
6. c
7. b
8. d
9. a
10. c

WORD POOL: SYMPTOMS OF DISEASES OF THE ENDOCRINE SYSTEM

1. gestational diabetes
2. cretinism
3. Grave's disease
4. pheochromocytoma
5. tetany
6. myxedema
7. Cushing's disease
8. hyperprolactinemia
9. goiter (simple)
10. hypogonadism

MATCHING: ENDOCRINE GLANDS AND HORMONES

1. e
2. a
3. h
4. g
5. d
6. b
7. i
8. c
9. f

MATCHING: DISORDERS OF THE ENDOCRINE SYSTEM

1. b
2. c
3. d
4. c
5. d
6. d

MATCHING: DISORDERS OF THE ENDOCRINE SYSTEM (*continued*)

7. e
8. b
9. b
10. d
11. g
12. f
13. c
14. a
15. b
16. d

DEFINITIONS: SYMPTOMS OF DISEASES OF THE ENDOCRINE SYSTEM

1. Absence of menstrual periods in women during reproductive age
2. Profuse perspiration
3. Excessive leanness, a wasted condition
4. Protrusion of the eyeballs
5. Accumulation of ketone bodies in the blood, causing metabolic acidosis
6. Excessive urination
7. Development of male sex characteristics (in both men and women)
8. Enlargement of the thyroid gland, causing swelling of the neck
9. Involuntary muscle contractions
10. Loss of appetite for food

IDENTIFYING WORD PARTS

Word	Root Word	Prefix	Suffix
1. acromegaly	acro = extremities		megaly = enlargement
2. diaphoresis	diaphor = sweat		esis = condition
3. exophthalmic	ophthalm = eye	ex = out, away from	ic = pertaining to
4. glycogenolysis	glycogen = storage form of glucose (in humans)		lysis = breakdown
5. corticoids	cortic= cortex, outer region		oid = derived from
6. ketosis	ket = ketones		osis = condition
7. panhypopituitarism	pituitary = pituitary gland	pan = all hypo = below, deficient	ism = condition
8. polydipsia	dips = thirst	poly = much	ia = condition
9. progesterone	gester = pregnancy	pro = before	one = hormone
10. triiodthyronine	thyr = thyroid	tri = three iod = iodine	ine = chemical compound

Answer Key to Chapter 20: Cancer Medicine

CLINICAL NOTE

Papillary carcinoma
One of the most common thyroid cancers, where abnormal cancer cells grow in the thyroid gland. As the cancer cells multiply, a bump or nodule can be felt on the thyroid.
Thyroidectomy
Surgical procedure to remove either part or all of the thyroid gland as a treatment for number of thyroid conditions.
Anterior cervical lymph node
A lymph node that is part of a group of lymph nodes—anterior cervical lymph nodes—located down the front of the neck.
TSH = Thyroid stimulating hormone
The hormone produced in the pituitary gland that signals the thyroid to release thyroid hormones into the blood stream. TSH is measured in a TSH test to help diagnose thyroid disorders.
Thyroglobulin
A protein produced in the thyroid gland. It can be used as a tumor marker to evaluate the effectiveness of treatment for thyroid cancer and to monitor for recurrence.
I-131 = Radioactive iodine
Used for treatment of thyroid cancers to eliminate any remaining cancer cells that was not removed during a thyroidectomy.
mCi = millicurie
An abbreviation for the unit of measurement when dealing with radioactive material; one mCi of radioactivity equals one thousandth of a curie (Ci).
Bilateral
Refers to both sides of the body, or two of something.

Lesson Two: Progress Check

COMPLETION: CANCER WITH SPECIFIC NAMES

1. adenoma (polyps)
2. basal cell carcinoma
3. leukemia
4. medulloblastoma
5. lymphoma
6. chondrosarcoma
7. squamous cell carcinoma or melanoma
8. osteosarcoma
9. leiomyoma
10. oat cell lung cancer or small cell lung cancer

MULTIPLE CHOICE: DIAGNOSIS AND TREATMENT OF CANCER

1. a
2. d
3. b
4. a
5. b
6. c
7. a
8. a
9. c
10. d

MATCHING: TOOLS FOR DIAGNOSING CANCER

1. d
2. j
3. h
4. g
5. a
6. i
7. e
8. c
9. f
10. b

MATCHING: SIGNS AND SYMPTOMS OF CANCER

1. i
2. g
3. j
4. f
5. a
6. b
7. d
8. e
9. c
10. h

IDENTIFYING WORD PARTS

Word	Root Word	Prefix	Suffix
1. antiestrogen	estrogen = female sex hormone	anti = against	
2. antineoplastic	neoplastic = uncontrolled growth of abnormal tissue	anti = against	
3. leukemia	emia = blood condition	leuk = white	
4. dyspareunia	pareunia = sexual intercourse	dys = painful or difficult	
5. hematuria	hemat = blood		uria = condition of urine
6. hyperplasia	plasia = formation	hyper = excessive	
7. transrectal	rect = rectal	trans = across	
8. mastectomy	mast = breast		ectomy = excise
9. pneumonectomy	pneumon = lung		ectomy = excise
10. precancerous	cancerous = malignant invasive growth	pre = before	

Bibliography

Barton-Burke, Margaret, and Gail M. Wilkes. *Cancer Therapies*. Sudbury, MA: Jones and Bartlett Publishers, 2006.

Broaddus, V. Courtney, Joel D. Ernst, Talmadge E. King, Robert J. Mason, Stephen C. Lazarus, John F. Murray, Arthur Slutsky, Jay A. Nadel, and Michael Gotway. *Murray and Nadel's Textbook of Respiratory Medicine*, 6th ed. Philadelphia, PA: Elsevier, 2016.

Donnersberger, Anne B, and David R. Donnersberg. *A Laboratory Textbook of Anatomy and Physiology: Cat Version*, 9th ed. Sudbury, MA: Jones and Bartlett Publishers, 2010.

Dorland, W. A. Newman. *Dorland's Illustrated Medical Dictionary*, 32nd ed. Philadelphia, PA: Elsevier, 2011.

Hall, John E., *Guyton and Hall Textbook of Medical Physiology*, 13th ed. Philadelphia, PA: Elsevier, 2016.

Hawkes, Christopher, Jaime Bosch, Guadalupe Garcia-Tsao, and Francis Chan. *Clinical Gastroenterology and Hepatology*, 2nd ed. Malden, MA: Wiley-Blackwell; 2012.

Hay, David W. *Little Black Book of Gastroenterology*, 3rd ed. Burlington, MA: Jones & Bartlett Learning, 2011.

Interprofessional Education Collaborative. *IPEC Core Competencies for Interprofessional Collaborative Practice: 2016 Update*. Washington, DC: Interprofessional Educational Collaborative, 2016.

Mann, Douglas L., Douglas P. Zipes, Peter Libby and Robert O. Bonow. *Braunwald's Heart Disease: A Textbook of Cardiovascular Medicine, Single Volume*, 10th ed. Philadelphia, PA: Elsevier, 2015.

O'Toole, Marie T. ed. *Mosby's Dictionary of Medicine, Nursing & Health Professions*, 10th ed. St. Louis, MO: Elsevier, 2017.

Pagana, Kathleen D., Timothy J. Pagana, and Sandra McDonald. *Mosby's Canadian Manual of Diagnostic and Laboratory Tests*. Philadelphia, PA: Elsevier, 2012.

Patton, Kevin, Gary Thibodeau, and Matthew Douglas. *Anatomy & Physiology Outline for Essentials of Anatomy & Physiology (User Guide and Access Code)*. Philadelphia, PA: Elsevier, 2011.

Ropper, Allan H., and Martin Samuels. *Adams and Victor's Principles of Neurology*, 9th ed. Columbus, OH: McGraw-Hill, 2009.

Stanfield, Peggy S. *Nutrition and Diet Therapy: Self-Instruction Modules*, 5th ed. Sudbury, MA: Jones and Bartlett Publishers, 2010.

Wilkes, Gail M., and Margaret Barton-Burke. *2013 Oncology Nursing Drug Handbook*. Burlington, MA: Jones & Bartlett Learning, 2013.

Wu, Alan. *Tietz Clinical Guide to Laboratory Tests*, 4th ed. Philadelphia, PA: Elsevier, 2006.

Yamada, Tadataka, John M. Inadomi, Renuka Bhattacharya, Jason A. Dominitz and Joo Ha Hwang. *Yamada's Handbook of Gastroenterology*, 3rd ed. Philadelphia, PA: Lippincott Williams & Wilkins, 2013.

Index

Note: Page numbers followed by *f* or *t* indicate material in figures and tables, respectively.